Veterinary Medicine: A Clinical Approach

Veterinary Medicine: A Clinical Approach

Edited by Herbert Dundas

⬜ SYRAWOOD
PUBLISHING HOUSE

New York

Published by Syrawood Publishing House,
750 Third Avenue, 9th Floor,
New York, NY 10017, USA
www.syrawoodpublishinghouse.com

Veterinary Medicine: A Clinical Approach
Edited by Herbert Dundas

International Standard Book Number: 978-1-68286-565-1 (Hardback)

Cataloging-in-Publication Data

Veterinary medicine : a clinical approach / edited by Herbert Dundas.
   p. cm.
Includes bibliographical references and index.
ISBN 978-1-68286-565-1
1. Veterinary medicine. 2. Animals--Diseases. 3. Clinical medicine. I. Dundas, Herbert.
SF745 .V48 2018
636.089--dc23

TABLE OF CONTENTS

Preface...IX

Chapter 1   **Possibilities of Implementing Progesterone EIA Test in the Control
of Reproduction in Dairy Cows**... 1
Barna S. Tomislav, Milovanović M. Aleksandar, Lazarević I. Miodrag
and Gvozdić M. Dragan

Chapter 2   **Effect of Different Extenders and Storage Periods on Motility and
Fertility of RAM Sperm**..10
Rossen Georgiev Stefanov, Georgi Anev and
Desislava Vasileva Abadjieva

Chapter 3   **Screening of Selected Indicators of Dairy Cattle Welfare in
Macedonia**..15
Miroslav Radeski, Aleksandar Janevski and Vlatko Ilieski

Chapter 4   **Pyloric Leiomyoma: Behavioural Aspects in a Shelter Dog**.................... 24
Riccardo Benedetti, Mirko Barabucci, Alessandra Pigliapoco,
Simona Cannas and Clara Palestrini

Chapter 5   **Application of Fluorescence based Molecular Assays for Improved
Detection and Typing of _Brucella_ Strains in Clinical Samples**.....................27
Kiril Krstevski, Ivancho Naletoski, Dine Mitrov, Slavcho Mrenoshki,
Iskra Cvetkovikj, Aleksandar Janevski, Aleksandar Dodovski and
Igor Djadjovski

Chapter 6   **Biliary Clearance of Bromosulfophthalein in Healthy and Ketotic
Holstein Cows**... 37
Kirovski Danijela, Sladojević Željko and Šamanc Horea

Chapter 7   **Detection of Hepatitis E Virus in Faeces and Liver of Pigs Collected
at Two Slovenian Slaughterhouses**..42
Lainšček Raspor Petra, Toplak Ivan and Kirbiš Andrej

Chapter 8   **Influence of the Season on the Metabolic Profile in Chios Sheep**............46
Igor Dzadzovski, Irena Celeska, Igor Ulchar, Aleksandar Janevski and
Danijela Kirovski

Chapter 9   **The Influence of Nutrition (Diet Treatment) in Streptozotocin –
Induced Diabetic Rats**.. 52
Chrcheva-Nikolovska Radmila, Sekulovski Pavle, Jankuloski Dean
and Angelovski Ljupco

Chapter 10   **Fatty Acid Composition of Ostrich (*Struthio Camelus*) Abdominal Adipose Tissue**..59
Daniela Belichovska, Zehra Hajrulai-Musliu, Risto Uzunov,
Katerina Belichovska and Mila Arapcheska

Chapter 11   **Fin Damage of Farmed Rainbow Trout in the Republic of Macedonia**...66
Cvetkovikj Aleksandar, Radeski Miroslav, Blazhekovikj-Dimovska
Dijana, Kostov Vasil and Stevanovski Vangjel

Chapter 12   **Air Quality Measurements in Laying Hens Housing**......................................77
Mirko Prodanov, Miroslav Radeski and Vlatko Ilieski

Chapter 13   **Diagnostic Characteristics of Circovirus Infection in Pigs**.........................82
Ivica Gjurovski, Branko Angelovski, Toni Dovenski, Dine Mitrov and
Trpe Ristoski

Chapter 14   **The Effect of Acute Inflammation on Total Alkaline Phosphatase Activity in Dogs**...88
Zapryanova Dimitrinka

Chapter 15   **Classical and Molecular Characterization of Pigeon Paramyxovirus Type 1 (PPMV-1) Isolated from Backyard Poultry – First Report in Macedonia**...93
Dodovski Aleksandar, Krstevski Kiril and Naletoski Ivancho

Chapter 16   **Effect of Storage on Residue Levels of Enrofloxacin in Muscle of Rainbow Trout (*Oncorhynchus Mykiss*) and Common Carp (*Cyprinus Carpio*)**..100
Ralica Kyuchukova, Anelia Milanova, Aleksandra Daskalova,
Deyan Stratev, Lubomir Lashev and Alexander Pavlov

Chapter 17   **The Paradox of Human Equivalent Dose Formula: A Canonical Case Study of Abrus Precatorius Aqueous Leaf Extract in Monogastric Animals**...106
Saganuwan Alhaji Saganuwan and Patrick Azubuike Onyeyili

Chapter 18   **Immunohistochemical Detection of Estrogen Receptors in Canine Mammary Tumors**...116
Elena Atanaskova Petrov, Ivica Gjurovski, Trpe Ristoski,
Goran Nikolovski, Pandorce Trenkoska, Plamen Trojacanec,
Ksenija Ilievska, Toni Dovenski and Gordana Petrushevska

Chapter 19   **Comparative Clinical and Haematological Investigations in Lactating Cows with Subclinical and Clinical Ketosis**..121
Vania Marutsova, Rumen Binev and Plamen Marutsov

Chapter 20   **Quill Injury – Cause of Death in a Captive Indian Crested Porcupine**
(*Hystrix Indica, Kerr, 1792*)..129
Tanja Švara, Irena Zdovc, Mitja Gombač and Milan Pogačnik

Chapter 21   **Hypodermosis in Northern Serbia (Vojvodina)**...133
Zsolt Becskei, Tamara Ilić, Nataša Pavlićević, Ferenc Kiskároly,
Tamaš Petrović and Sanda Dimitrijević

Chapter 22   **Cardiotoxicity Study of the Aqueous Extract of Corn Silk in Rats**...........138
Adeolu Adedapo, Omotayo Babarinsa, Ademola Oyagbemi,
Aduragbenro Adedapo and Temidayo Omobowale

Chapter 23   **Retrospective Investigation on the Prevalence of Pulmonary
Hypertension in Dogs with Bronchial and Upper Respiratory
Diseases**..145
Chiara Locatelli, Daniela Montrasio, Ilaria Spalla, Giulia Riscazzi,
Matteo Gobbetti, Alice Savarese, Stefano Romussi and
Paola G. Brambilla

Chapter 24   **A Report of a *Hepatozoon Canis* Infection in a Dog with
Transmissible Venereal Tumour**...153
Namakkal Rajamanickam Senthil, Subramanian Subapriya and
Subbaiah Vairamuthu

Chapter 25   **Hematological and Biochemical Parameters in Symptomatic and
Asymptomatic Leishmania-Seropositive Dogs**...158
Igor Ulchar, Irena Celeska, Jovana Stefanovska and Anastasija
Jakimovska

Chapter 26   **Assessment of the Effect of Selected Components of Equine
Seminal Plasma on Semen Freezability**...166
Miroslava Mráčková, Marta Zavadilová and Markéta Sedlinská

Chapter 27   **The Prevalence of *Pasteurella Multocida* from Farm Pigs in Serbia**.......172
Oliver Radanovic, Jadranka Zutic, Dobrila Jakic-Dimic,
Branislav Kureljusic and Bozidar Savic

Chapter 28   **The Art and Science of Consultations in Bovine Medicine: Use
of Modified Calgary – Cambridge Guides**..176
Kiro R. Petrovski and Michelle Mc Arthur

Chapter 29   **PCRAssay with Host Specific Internal Control for *Staphylococcus
Aureus* from Bovine Milk Samples**...187
Zafer Cantekin, Yasar Ergun, Hasan Solmaz,
Gamze Özge Özmen, Melek Demir and Radhwane Saidi

Permissions

List of Contributors

Index

PREFACE

The branch of medicine which studies the health of animals is known as veterinary medicine. It primarily deals with the illnesses and injuries caused to both pets as well as wild animals. Veterinary medicine helps animals as well as humans by controlling the diseases that spread to humans from animals. The various studies that are constantly contributing towards advancing technologies and evolution of this field are examined in detail in this book. Using case studies and examples, constant effort has been made to make the understanding of the difficult concepts of veterinary medicine, as easy and informative as possible, for the readers.

The information shared in this book is based on empirical researches made by veterans in this field of study. The elaborative information provided in this book will help the readers further their scope of knowledge leading to advancements in this field.

Finally, I would like to thank my fellow researchers who gave constructive feedback and my family members who supported me at every step of my research.

Editor

POSSIBILITIES OF IMPLEMENTING PROGESTERONE EIA TEST IN THE CONTROL OF REPRODUCTION IN DAIRY COWS

Barna S. Tomislav[1], Milovanović M. Aleksandar[1],
Lazarević I. Miodrag[2], Gvozdić M. Dragan[2]

[1]Department of Reproduction, Scientific Veterinary Institute „Novi Sad",
Rumenački put 20, 21000 Novi Sad, Republic of Serbia
[2]Faculty of Veterinary Medicine, University of Belgrade,
Bulevar Oslobođenja 18, 11000 Belgrade, Republic of Serbia

ABSTRACT

The aim of this study was to implement the progesterone EIA test, developed in our laboratory by using an anti-progesterone antibody (Yamaguchi University, Japan), in order to determine the optimal moment for artificial insemination (AI) and to detect pregnancy in Holstein-Friesian cows according to the progesterone concentration in the whole milk. Also, the influence of β-carotene, applied at the day of insemination and human chorionic gonadotrophin applied on day 7 after AI on the progesterone level and the pregnancy rate were evaluated.

For the accuracy of oestrus detection, the milk samples from 70 cows were collected on the day of insemination. Milk samples from 148 cows were collected 19-22 days following insemination for pregnancy check.

After detection of naturally occurring oestrus (day 0) and AI, cows were divided into the following groups: group A (n = 19) was treated with 200 mg β-carotene (20 ml Carofertin® i.m. Alvetra u. Werfft Gmbh, Austria), group B (n = 17) was treated with 1500 IU hCG i.m. (Schering-Plough, the Netherlands) and control (non treated) group C (n = 18). The milk samples for EIA progesterone concentration analysis were collected on the day of AI, the 14th and the 20th day of the oestrus cycle.

Oestrus detection errors and inappropriate moments of insemination according to the progesterone concentration were detected in 22.86% animals (16/70). The test accuracy for non-pregnant cows was 90.48% (76/84). The accuracy of the progesterone test in pregnant cows was 75% (48/64). False positive results (high progesterone level, but the cows were not pregnant) was detected in 25% of cows (16/64) as a result of a prolonged oestrus cycles, embrional mortality and endomethritis (10/16 cases). The treatment of cows with 1500 IU of hCG, on the day 7 of the oestrus cycle, resulted in statistically significant increase of progesterone concentration in the dioestrus ($p < 0.01$). The most successful insemination was in the group of cows that was treated with hCG (47.05%; 8/17), then in the control group (38.88%; 7/18) and the least in the Carofertin group - 36.84% (7/19). These differences were only numerical ($p > 0.05$).

The EIA test developed in our laboratory could be used for accurate progesterone determination in the whole milk during implementation of different methods for control of bovine reproduction.

Key words: β-carotene, cows, EIA test, hCG, milk, progesterone

INTRODUCTION

Diagnosis of pregnancy in cattle is of special interest because succesful reproduction is often crucial to cows life time milk production.

Corresponding author: Tomislav Barna, PhD
E-mail address: toma@niv.ns.ac.rs
Present address: Department of Reproduction,
Scientific Veterinary Institute „Novi Sad", Republic of Serbia

Progesterone is a steroid hormone secreted by ovarian *corpus luteum* following ovulation in the luteal phase of the sexual cycle in cattle. Concentration of progesterone in the blood plasma of cows indicates secretory activity of the luteal tissue, since there is no other significant source of progesterone (1).

Progesterone is necessary to preserve the gravidity and luteal deficiency is considered as one of the causes of infertility (2). Progesterone concentration decline in the early period of pregnancy, leads to embryonic death or abortion. As the *corpus luteum* is a main source of progesterone with the task of maintaining pregnancy at the beginning of gestation, stimulating its activity has been the subject of several studies in the last decade. The aim of this research was to find positive effects in the procedures designed to stimulate the *corpus luteum* function in order to increase the conception rate. Numerous authors considered that the application of hCG between 7 to 15 days after oestrus may improve the fertility of the cows (3, 4, 5).

Corpus luteum in cows contains two to five times more β-carotene compared to other tissues (liver, adipose tissue, plasma), even in deficient conditions. In animals with reduced β-carotene in forage, there is only small decrease of progesterone concentration in the *corpus luteum* tissue compared to animals that had enough β-carotene (6). Several studies on the impact of β-carotene in improving reproductive parameters have shown incoherent results (7, 8, 9, 10).

Determining progesterone concentrations in the blood and milk is carried out, not only in terms of diagnosis and exclusion of pregnancy, but also in discovering cyclic dysfunction and disorders of ovarian function. Although the differences in the concentration of progesterone is clearly visible on the 17th day after mating or insemination, the most reliable results in the diagnosis of pregnancy rates are achieved from the 19th to the 24th day of the cycle (11, 12, 13).

Despite significant advances in technology, the measurement of progesterone remains still one of the earliest, indirect ways of detecting nonpregnant cows and an excellent marker for ovarian function.

High reliability progesterone test requires continuous records, which plays a key role in the control of reproduction in dairy farms. The success of reproduction depends on many factors, but oestrus detection and determination of the optimal time of insemination is one of the main problems in management of high-yielding dairy cows.

The aim of this work was to implement the progesterone EIA test developed in our laboratory by using an anti-progesterone antibody (Yamaguchi University, Japan) in order to determine:

1) the accuracy of oestrus detection on the day of insemination;

2) the reliability of the test in detection of pregnant and nonpregnant cows from days 19 to 22 after AI;

3) the effect of application of β-carotene at the moment of insemination on the increase of the progesterone level and the pregnancy rate, and

4) the effect of application of hCG on day 7 after AI on the progesterone level and the pregnancy rate.

MATERIALS AND METHODS

The experiment was conducted on a commercial farm with 450 milking cows. The cows were between 60 and 180 days of lactation and were milked twice a day. The average milk production on the farm was 6,500 l calculated at 305 days of lactation. Oestrus was detected on the basis of external signs of oestrus, rectal examination and vaginal inspection (by speculum).

The pregnancy check was carried out by ultrasound scanner (285 SIUI CTS-V, Shantou, China) using a rectal probe of 7.5 MHz, 27-35th day after insemination. The final confirmation of pregnancy rates was performed by rectal exploration with ≥ 2 months after insemination to detect cases with embryonic mortality.

Approximately 8 ml of milk from clinically healthy quarters (n=232) were sampled in plastic 10 ml tubes (Spectar, Cacak, Serbia). Potassium dichromate tablets of 3.3 mg (Merck, Darmstadt, Germany) were used as a preservative during transportation and storage of milk samples. Samples were stored in a refrigerator at +4 °C until analysed.

Levels of progesterone in whole milk through the use of EIA progesterone tests were determined in the Scientific Veterinary Institute "Novi Sad", Novi Sad. Anti-progesterone antibodies, protocol for assay and protocol of production of HRP-P4 were obtained from the Laboratory of Theriogenology, Department of Veterinary Medicine, Faculty of Agriculture, Yamaguchi University, Japan. Substrates for EIA were produced in INEP, Zemun (Serbia). Optical density (extinction) was recorded by using a plate reader (Rayto Life and Analytical Science Co., Ltd, P. R. China), with filter wavelength of 450 nm.

The "Dairy Quest" (Profit Source, Wi, USA) software program was inplemented on farm for data tracking of production, reproduction, health and results of EIA test. Milk sampling was based on the generated list of cows in the "Dairy Quest" software.

Milk samples from 70 cows were collected on the day of insemination for the accuracy of oestrus detection. One hundred and foury eight milk samples were collected on days 19, 20, 21 or 22 following insemination for indirect early pregnancy check/detecting the resumption of new oestrus. The values of progesterone concentration in whole milk ≥4 ng/ml, obtained in days 19 to 21 of the cycle were used as a possible pregnancy indicator. Values under this levels indicated that the cows were not pregnant.

The influence of β-carotene, applied at the day of insemination and human horionic gonadotrophin (hCG) applied on day 7 after AI, on the progesterone level in milk on day 14 and 20 after insemination on pregnancy rate of Holstein-Friesian cows were also evaluated. After naturally occurring oestrus (day 0) and AI, the cows were randomly divided into the following groups:

- group A ("Carofertin" group, n = 17) was treated with 200 mg β-carotene (20 ml Carofertin® i.m., Alvetra u. Werfft Gmbh, Austria);
- group B ("hCG" group, n = 17) was treated

with 1500 IU hCG i.m. (Schering-Plough, the Netherlands) and
- group C ("control group", non treated, n = 18).

Milk samples for EIA progesterone concentration analysis were collected on the day of AI, at the 14th and at the 20th day of the estral cycle. Cows with high levels of progesterone on the day of insemination were not included in the experiment.

RESULTS

1. Accuracy of oestrus detection at insemination based on the progesterone level

The results for the oestrus detection at insemination based on the progesterone level are showed in Table 1. Out of 70 samples, 16 (22.86%) had a progesterone concentration higher than 2 ng/ml on the day of insemination, which indicates poor oestrus detection technique and insemination at the incorrect time.

Table 1. Progesterone concentration in milk samples collected on the day of insemination

Categories	Number of cows	(%)
low progesterone (0 to 1.9 ng / ml)	54	77,14
suprabasal level (2.0 to 3.9 ng / ml)	12	17,14
high level (≥ 4 ng / ml)	4	5,72
Total:	70	100,00

2. Pregnancy/oestrus detection based on progesterone level at 19th, 20th, 21st or 22nd day after AI

For early detection of pregnancy 148 milk samples between the 19th–22nd day after insemination

were analysed. The results are showed in Table 2. Low levels of progesterone indicated the occurrence of oestrus and high levels of progesterone indirectly pointed to conception (pregnancy).

Table 2. Results of the analysis of milk samples analysed 19-22nd days after AI

Groups according to the level of progesterone	Number of samples	Pregnancy rates			
		Pregnant (No.)	(%)	Non-pregnant (No.)	(%)
High (≥ 4 ng / ml)	64	48	75,00	16	25,00
Low (<4 ng / ml)	84	8	9,52	76	90,48
Total:	148	56	37,83	92	62,17

3. Influence of β-carotene and hCG aplication on the milk progesterone level and the conception rate

3a. Effect at the 14th day of the cycle:

The effect of human chorionic gonadotropin (hCG), applied on the 7th day after AI and β-carotene, applied on the day of insemination (day 0) on the level of progesterone resulted in a statistically significant increase of progesterone concentration in dioestrus-day 14th between hCG and the Control grup ($p < 0.01$). Carofertin treatment resulted in a slight progesterone increase, but this value was only numerical.

Table 3. Descriptive statistics values for the concentration of progesterone on the 14th day of the cycle after AI. The analysis included all cows, regardless of the outcome of insemination (pregnant or nonpregnant)

Groups in the experiment	Concentration of progesterone (ng/ml), 14th day					
	n	$\overline{x}$	SD	S_x	CV%	I.V.
A - Carofertin	19	10,53	9,70	2,23	92,15	0,36-30,5
B – hCG	17	16,97	9,93	2,41	58,52	0,30-34,50
C - Control	18	7,28	5,63	1,33	77,30	0,05-19,50

3b. Results of the determination of progesterone concentration on the 14th day of the cycle between pregnant and nonpregnant cows within Carofertin, hCG and control groups

Mean values of concentrations of progesterone on the 14th day of the cycle, when analyzed on the basis of future outcomes insemination, showed a tendency to increase in the hCG and Carofertin groups of pregnant cows compared to the nonpregnant group. However, a large standard deviation and coefficient of variation could be seen in all groups. A statistically significant increase of progesterone concentration was noted between the hCG pregnant and the Control pregnant group at day 14th ($p < 0.001$).

Table 4. Descriptive statistical parameters for progesterone concentration on the 14th day of the cycle (pregnant and nonpregnant, within the group)

Groups in the experiment	Concentration of progesterone (ng/ml), 14th day					
	n	$\overline{x}$	SD	S_x	CV%	I.V.
Carofertin pregnant	7	14,40	11,43	4,32	79,38	1,50-30,50
Carofertin nonpregnant	12	8,28	8,23	2,38	99,40	0,35-30,00
hCG pregnant	8	21,91	7,03	2,49	32,09	10,75-34,50
hCG nonpregnant	9	12,59	10,39	3,46	82,51	0,30-30,00
Control pregnant	7	5,77	2,99	1,13	51,77	2,15-11,00
Control nonpregnant	11	8,24	6,77	2,04	82,19	0,05-19,50

Table 5. Statistical significance of differences in the concentration of progesterone on the 14th day of the cycle (pregnant and nonpregnant, within groups)

Groups in the experiment	hCG pregnant	Control pregnant	Carofertin nonpregnant	hCG nonpregnant	Control nonpregnant
Carofertin pregnant	p > 0,05 (p=0,281)	p > 0,05 (p=0,2593)	p > 0,05 (p=0,3402)	–	–
hCG pregnant	–	p < 0,001 (p=0,0006)	–	p > 0,05 (p=0,0592)	–
Control pregnant	–	–	–	–	p > 0,05 (p=0,6916)

Mann-Whitney-Wilcoxon rank-sum test

3c. Effect on the 21st day of the cycle

Mean values of concentrations of progesterone on the 20th day after AI were highest in the A-Carofertin and the B-hCG group, but no statistically significant differences were detected between pregnant cows in the groups based on the progesterone values (Mann-Whitney-Wilcoxon rank-sum test). A large standard and coefficient deviation could also be noticed in all the groups.

Table 6. Descriptive statistical parameters for progesterone concentration on the 20th day of the cycle in pregnant cows

Groups in the experiment, 20 days after insemination	Progesterone concentration (ng/ml), 20th day after AI					
	n	$\overline{x}$	SD	S_x	CV%	I.V.
A-Carofertin pregnant	7	22,12	11,78	2,23	53,26	8,00-40,00
B-hCG pregnant	8	19,32	6,62	2,41	34,29	5,53-26,50
C-Control pregnant	7	15,22	10,31	3,90	67,72	3,90-29,67

Pregnancy rates in this experiment were diagnosed by rectal examination in the period of 45 to 60 days after insemination. The results of artificial insemination are shown in Table 7.

Table 7. The results o f artificial insemination of cows in groups according to different treatments

Groups in the experiment	n total	n pregnant	n nonpregnant	% pregnant
A-Carofertin	19	7	12	36,8
B-hCG	17	8	9	47,1
C-Control	18	7	11	38,9

DISCUSSION

In this study we have exeminated the possibilities of implementing progesterone EIA test in the control of reproduction in dairy cows. The absolute incorect time for insemination was determined by the progesterone concentration ≥ 4 ng/ml and the suprabasal progesterone levels were defined as 2-4 ng/ml. The suprabasal level was considered as insemination in proestrus or at the beginning of metoestrus. Out of 70 samples, 16 (22.86%) had a progesterone concentration higher than 2 ng/ml on the day of insemination, which indicates poor oestrus detection technique and insemination at the incorrect time.

The accuracy of oestrus detection in the experiment was 77.14% (54/70). None of the cows that had a high concentration of progesterone on the day of insemination became pregnant (≥ 4 ng/ml). Out of the 12 cows with a suprabasal progesterone concentrations (2.0 to 3.9 ng/ml), two were pregnant, but they were inseminated again after 24 hours. Oestrus detection errors and incorrect moment of insemination according to the progesterone concentration (> 2 ng/ml of progesterone) were detected in 22.86% of the animals (16/70). According to the results reported by other authors (14, 15, 16), 5.1%, 19% and 22.1% of cows, respectively, were inseminated in the luteal phase of the cycle. Comparing with the literature data (15, 21) and based on our clinical experience, it can be concluded that one of the major problems of large farming systems (capacity of 200 or more dairy cows) is poor oestrus detection.

Regarding the oestrus detection based on progesterone level at 19th, 20th, 2nd or 22nd day after AI, we found that out of 64 cows with high progesterone concentrations, pregnancy was confirmed by clinical examination in 48 cows (75%), while 16 cows (25%) were not pregnant. Out of these 16 false positive samples (cows with high-progesterone, but not pregnant), 62.50% (10/16) had embryonic death (finding empty embryonic vesicles with turbid liquor, ondulating membranes and no heart beat at 32-38 post AI - 3 cows) or uterus inflammation process (abnormal vaginal discharge and clinical endometritis, - 5 cows) or hormonal disturbance (luteal cysts - 2 cows). In the 6 remaining cows (6/16; 37.50%) there were no clear indications for the absence of pregnancy, despite high levels of progesterone.

The test accuracy for nonpregnant cows was 90.48% (76/84). All cows with zero progesterone levels from 19-22nd days after AI had characteristic clinical signs on the reproductive organs (estral mucus, postoestrus blood discharge, failed fertilization).

A false negative result (low levels of progesterone, but the cows were pregnant) was detected in 9.52% of the cows (8/84). The average level of progesterone was 1.88 ± 0.68 ng/ml (CV = 36.39%). This is the most critical group for the accuracy of the test and deserves special attention. For more precise control of milk samples with progesterone values close to the "cut off" level, the recommendation is to re-sample milk ater 2-3 days (at the 24th day of cycle) (22).

The effect of human chorionic gonadotropin (hCG), applied on the 7th day after AI and β-carotene, applied on the day of insemination (day 0) on the level of progesterone resulted in a statistically significant increase of progesterone concentration in dioestrus-day 14th between hCG and the Control gruop (p < 0.01). Carofertin treatment resulted in a slight progesterone increase, but this value was only numerical.

On other side, the results of the determination of progesterone concentration on the 14th day of the cycle between pregnant and nonpregnant cows within Carofertin, hCG and control groups showed that the mean values of concentrations of progesterone on the 14th day of the cycle, when analyzed on the basis of future outcomes insemination has a tendency to increase in the hCG and Carofertin groups of pregnant cows compared to the nonpregnant group. However, a large standard deviation and coefficient of variation could be seen in all groups. A statistically significant increase of progesterone concentration was noted between the hCG pregnant and the Control pregnant group at day 14th (p < 0.001).

Additionaly, in this study we have examineted the influence of β-carotene and hCG aplication on the milk progesterone level and the conception rate. The results are in accordance with the results of Mann et al. (17) showing that the concentration of progesterone in early pregnancy has an impact on the outcome of insemination. The concentration of progesterone in dioestrus is lower in open cows than in pregnant cows. Also, Lamming et al. (18) stated that early progesterone increase (from 12 to 17 days after AI) can influence the outcome of insemination, but stressed that there is not strictly a high level of progesterone, which certainly ensures the preservation of embryos.

The concentrations of progesterone on the 20th day after AI were highest in the A-Carofertin and the B-hCG group, but no statistically significant differences were detected between pregnant cows in the groups based on the progesterone values. A large standard and coefficient deviation could also be noticed in all the groups.

Pregnancy rates in this experiment were diagnosed by rectal examination in the period of 45 to 60 days after insemination.

The most successful insemination results were in the group of cows that were treated with hCG (47.05%; 8/17), then in the control group (38.88%; 7/18) and least of all in the Carofertin group (36.84%; 7/19). These differences were only numerical (p>0.05).

The difference in the conception rate between the hCG and the C-control group (+8.17%) and between the hCG and the Carofertin group (+10.21%) may indicate that embryo loss is caused, to a certain extent, by the lack of endocrine communication between mother and embryo.

Delayed embryo development or a poorly developed embryo is not able to produce enough interferone τ, failing to prevent luteolyse and to ensure further development. Fertility reduction of 25-30% occurs because of early embryonal loss and lack of communication between mother and fetus. Further knowledge of the control of embryonal development and production of interferone τ is of great importance in the development of strategies to reduce the high incidence of clinically invisible embryo mortality in dairy cows (19, 20).

In order to have more convincing results of this experiment, a greater number of samples and/or analysis of blood serum, which is expected to have less fluctuations in the progesterone concentration than in whole milk is needed to confirm the hypothesis of Lamming et al. (18) that the amount of progesterone may determine the fate of the embryo from day 7 of the cycle.

The results of our study indicate that treatment of cows with hCG leads to increased levels of progesterone in dioestrus (the middle of the sexual cycle). Application of β-carotene had no effect on milk progesterone concentration and pregnancy rate.

CONCLUSIONS

The accuracy of oestrus detection and determining the optimal time of insemination based on the progesterone concentration in milk was 77.14%. Oestrus detection errors were detected in 22.86% of the animals. The accuracy of the progesterone test in pregnant cows was 75%. False positive results (high progesterone level, but the cows were not pregnant) was detected in 25% of cows and some are recognised as a consequence of a prolonged oestrus cycles, embrional mortality and endometritis.

The treatment of cows with 1500 IU of hCG, on day 7 of the oestrus cycle, resulted in a statistically significant increase of progesterone concentration in dioestrus (p<0.01). The most successful insemination was in the group of cows that were treated with hCG, then in the control group and least of all in the Carofertin group, but these differences were only numerical (p>0.05).

The progesterone EIA test developed in our laboratory by using the anti-progesterone antibody (Yamaguchi University, Japan) could be used for reliable quantitavive detection of progesterone concentration in the whole milk.

ACKNOWLEDGMENTS

Authors are thankful to Professor Dr. Toshihiko Nakao and to his post-doc students from the Laboratory of Theriogenology, Department of Veterinary Medicine, Faculty of Agriculture, Yamaguchi University, Japan for hospitality, support, help and supplying components for establishing a progesterone test in our Lab.

REFERENCES

1. Opsomer, G., Grohn, Y.T., Hertl, J., Leavens, H., Coryn, M., de Kruif, A. (1999). Protein metabolism and resumption of ovarian cyclicity post partum in high yielding dairy cows. Annual ESDAR Conference, 54-57.

2. Parkinson, T.J. (2001). Infertility in the cow. In: Noakes, E.D., T.J. Parkinson, G.C.W. England (Eds.), Arthur's Veterinary Reproduction and

obstetrics. 8th ed. (pp. 383-472). Saunders Company, USA.

3. Sianangama, P.C., Rajamahendran, R. (1992). Effect of human chorionic gonadotropin administered at specific times following breeding on milk progesterone and pregnancy in cows. 38 (1), 85-96.

4. Rajamahendran, R., Sianangama, P.C. (1992). Effect of human chorionic gonadotrophin on dominantfollicles in cows: formation of accessory corpora lutea, progesterone production and pregnancy rates. J Repord Fert, 95, 577-584.

5. De Rensis, F., Valentini, R., Gorrieri, F., Bottarelli. E, Lopez-Gatius, F. (2008). Inducing ovulation with hCG improves the fertility of dairy cows during the warm season. Theriogenology, 69, 1077-82.

6. Ahlswede, L., Lotthammer, K.H. (1978). Untersuchungen über eine spezifische, Vitamin-A-unabhängige Wirkung des ß-Carotins auf die Fertilität des Rindes. 5. Mitteilung, Organuntersuchungen (Ovarien, Corpora lutea, Leber, Fettgewebe, Uterussekret, Nebennieren) - Gewichts- und Gehaltsbestimmungen, Dtsch Tierärztl Wschr, 85, 7-12.

7. Tekpetey, F.R., Palmer, W.M., Ingalls, J.R. (1987). Reproductive performance of prepubertal dairy heifers on low or high ß-carotene diets. Can J Anim Sci, 67, 477-489.

8. Arechiga, C.F., Staples, C.R., McDowell, L.R., Hansen, P.J. (1998). Effects of timed insemination and supplemental beta-carotene on reproduction and milk yield of dairy cows under heat stress. J Dairy Sci, 81, 390-402.

9. Lotthammer, K.H., Ahlswede, L., Meyer, H. (1976). Untersuchungen über eine spezifische Vitamin-A-unabhängige Wirkung des ß-Carotins auf die Fertilität des Rindes. 2. Mitteilung: Weitere klinische Befunde und Befruchtungsergebnisse, Dtsch Tierärztl Wschr, 83, 353-8.

10. Veličković, M., (2005). Uticaj parenteralnog davanja beta karotina na plodnost krava i zdravstveno stanje teledi. (Master thesis on Serbian) Fakultet veterinarske medicine, Beograd.

11. Nakao, T., Sugihashi, A., Saga, N., Tsunoda, N., Kawata, K., (1983). Use of milk progesterone enzyme immunoassay for differential diagnosis of follicular cyst, luteal cyst, and cystic corpus luteum in cows. Am J Vet Res, 44, 888-90.

12. Wimpy, T.H., Chang, C.F., Estergreen, V.L., Hillers, J.K. (1986). Milk Progesterone Enzyme Immunoassay: Modifications and a Field Trial for Pregnancy Detection in Dairy Cows. Journal of Dairy Science, 69, 1115-1121.

13. Shrestha, H.K., Nakao, T., Higaki, T., Suzuki, T., Akita, M. (2004). Resumption of postpartum ovarian cyclicity in high producing Holstein cows. Theriogenology, 61, 637-649.

14. Reimers, T.J., Smith, R.D., Newman, S.K. (1985). Management Factors Affecting Reproductive Performance of Dairy Cows in the Northeastern United States. J. Dairy Sci, 68 (4), 963-972.

15. Sturman, A., Oltenacu, B., Foote, H. (2000). Importance of inseminating only cows in oestrus. Theriogenology, 53, 8, 1657-67.

16. Ranasinghe, R.M.S.B.K., Nakao, T., Kobayashi, T. (2009). Incidence of Error in Oestrus Detection Based on Secondary Oestrus Signs in Tie-Stalled Dairy Herd with Low Fertility. Reprod Dom Anim, 44, 643-6.

17. Mann, G.E., Lamming, G.E. (1999). The Influence of Progesterone During Early Pregnancy in Cattle. Reprod in Dom Anim, 34, 269-74.

18. Lamming, G.E., Darwash, A.O., Back, H.L. (1989). Corpus luteum function in dairy cows and embryo mortality. J Reprod Fertil, 37, 245-252.

19. Mann, G.E., Mann, S.L., Lamming, G.E. (1996). The inter-relationship between the maternal hormone environment and the embryo during the early stages of pregnancy in the cow. J Reprod Fertil, 17, 21.

20. Mann, G.E., Lamming, G.E., Fisher, P.A. (1998). Progesterone control of embryonic interferon-t production during early pregnancy in the cow. J Reprod Fertil., Abst Series 21, abstr 37.

21. Samardžija, D., Barna, T., Milovanović, A., Gvozdić, D. (2013). Monitoring the reproductive status of dairy cows on farms in R. of Serbia, using the software program and progesterone test. XIII Middle European Buiatrics Congress, Belgrade, Serbia, June 5-8, 2013. Congress Proceedings, 592-596, Belgrade, Serbian Buiatrics Association.

22. Pennington, J.A., Schultz, L.H., Hoffman, W.F. (1985). Comparison of Pregnancy Diagnosis by Milk Progesterone on Day 21 and Day 24 Postbreeding: Field Study in Dairy Cattle. Journal of Dairy Science, 68, 10, 2740–45.

EFFECT OF DIFFERENT EXTENDERS AND STORAGE PERIODS ON MOTILITY AND FERTILITY OF RAM SPERM

Rossen Georgiev Stefanov[1], Georgi Anev[2], Desislava Vasileva Abadjieva[1]

[1]*Institute of Biology and Immunology of Reproduction-BAS,*
bul. Tsarigradsko Shose 73, p.c. 1113, Sofia, Bulgaria
[2]*Agricultural Institute, BG – Turgovishte, Bulgaria*

ABSTRACT

The aim of this study was to test the effect of extenders containing different sugar in their composition on ram sperm motility and pregnancy rate of ewe's following artificial insemination. Semen were collected from ten North-east Bulgarian fine-fleece breed and tested for quality. Semen was diluted with different extenders, with di- and trisaccharides. A series of experiments were repeated in triplicate. Total motility was determined by using Sperm Analysis (SCA, Microptic, Spain). A total of 200 North-east Bulgarian fine-fleece breed mature ewes were used for cervical insemination with a sperm dose at the concentration of 100×10^6 spermatozoa. Pregnancies were diagnosed 60 days after AI by - a real-time ultrasonic scan device (Alloka SSD 500). In conclusion, our experiments demonstrated that higher sperm motility after storage at 4°C for 24 hours and 48 hours has a ram spermatozoa diluted with extender 1, with combination of disaccharides (sucrose and lactose) and trisaccharides (rafinosa). This semen extender (number 1) can be used for successful insemination of ewes and to enhance pregnancy rate after artificial insemination.

Key words: ram, sperm extenders, motility, fertility

INTRODUCTION

Artificial insemination with chilled-stored semen has become a technique in sheep breeding (1). Efforts have been made to improve the preservation of ram semen by the modification of extender composition (2), as well as with the addition of various components to maintain motility, fertilizing capacity and preserve sperm membrane integrity (3,4,18). The preservation of functional properties of sperm in the storage medium is dependent on the quantities of non-electrolytes. The spermatozoa require exogenous substrates to obtain energy through mitochondrial oxidative phosphorylation and glycolysis by the consumption of glycolysable sugars, such as glucose, fructose, mannose (5).

Corresponding author: Assoc. Prof. Rossen Stefanov, PhD
E-mail address: stefanovrossen@gmail.com
Present address: Institute of Biology and Immunology of Reproduction-BAS, bul. Tsarigradsko shose 73, p.c. 1113, Sofia, Bulgaria

Fructose is thought to be a major energy source for ejaculated spermatozoa, and together with glucose is found in the seminal plasma in many mammalian species. In many species, glucose and fructose have been investigated for their different effects on gametes in terms of metabolizable energy and fertility potential, but the beneficial effects vary between species (6). The effects of sugars on the metabolism of freshly ejaculated spermatozoa has been studied in rams, but metabolize glucose and fructose use different pathways, resulting in separate systems of energy management as indicated by their different roles in glycogen metabolism and motility patterns (7). Sugars are the most commonly used components for semen extenders; however, the concentration of these sugars in the extenders varies markedly.

To optimize the extender medium for the achievement of best storage semen characteristics which would infer greater fertility, it is important to study the influence of different sugars on rams spermatozoa. The aim of this study was to test the effect of three extenders with different ratios of sugar in their composition on ram sperm motility and pregnancy rate of ewe's following insemination.

MATERIAL AND METHODS

Animals

The experiment was carried out on June and July in the Experimental station of agriculture (Targovishte, Bulgaria). Ten clinically healthy rams from north-east Bulgarian fine-fleece breed, around three years old and 70-98 kg of live weight were used as a semen source. Semen was collected using an artificial vagina two times a week. Fresh semen with ≥ 70% motility was eligible for experimentation.

Extenders

The extenders were used to dilute the samples of semen to be chilled. Semen was diluted with two different extenders (Table 1), which gave the best result after prior experiment with twelve extenders with mono-, di- or three disacharide. The third extender served as a control (8). All series of experiments (I–III) were repeated in triplicate.

Prior to sugar measurement, each egg-yolk was mixed in distilled water to the same final concentration as in the extenders, i.e., 20% (v:v). To make the extenders, fresh egg-yolks were pooled and mixed to reduce the biological variation found in the eggs.

and concentrations by using sperm analyzer SCA (Microptic, Barcelona, Spain). For each sample, at least 200 sperm cells from four randomly selected fields were evaluated.

Pregnancy rate experiment

A total of 200 North-east Bulgarian fine-fleece breed mature ewes (2-3 years old) were used for insemination. The detection of ewes in clinically manifested oestrus was performed in the morning by ram tester. The ewes were cervically inseminated with a sperm dose at the concentration of 100×10^6 spermatozoa. The insemination was reiterated second time after 10 h with the same sperm, which was stored 48 h.

Pregnancy was diagnosed 60 days after AI by ultrasonic scan device (Alloka SSD 500).

Statistical analyses

The statistical analyses were performed by GraphPad software, using the pairwise t-tests for comparison of the least-squares means. The pregnancy rate (number of pregnant ewes to number of inseminated) in all groups was statistically analyzed using a chi-square test. A value of $p < 0.05$ was considered statistically significant.

Table 1. Compositions of semen extenders used in the experiments

Ingredients	I	II	III
Na-citrate (g)	2.8	2.8	2.8
Saccharosa (g)	0.267	0.4	0.4
Lactose (g)	0.267	-	0.4
Rafinosa (g)	0.267	0.4	-
Egg-yolk (mL)	0.25	0.25	0.25
Distilled water (mL)	to 100	to 100	to 100

Experimental design

The pooled semen was divided into three equal aliquots and placed in three screw cap closed sterile plastic tubes. The resulting sperm samples were divided and re-suspended in ratio 1:4 with different extenders to reach a final sperm concentration of 2×10^6 cells/mL. To avoid cooling too rapidly, the extended semen samples were placed in a room temperature cooler, which reached a temperature of 4°C within 45 min. Subsequently, all samples were stored at 4°C in a refrigerator for 24 and 48 hours and after that semen samples were evaluated daily during the first three days, as motility was determined on 15 min; 60 min; 120 min; 180 min; 240 min; 300 min and 360 min, after incubation in the water bath at 39°C. The semen samples were evaluated microscopically which included percentage of motile spermatozoa

RESULTS

Three different extenders were used for the motility of the spermatozoa at different postdilution intervals.

Total motility (%) decreased with storage time in all cases (Table 2). However, the type of extender significantly (P<0.05; P<0.001) affected the percent sperm motility. Combination of sucrose, lactose and rafinosa in extender 1 showed highest values than other extenders (P<0.001) regarding this characteristic after 240 min to 360 min.

Data indicate that the survival of sperm cells on fresh ram semen in extender 1 and 3 had similar values after 6 hours incubated at 39°C (P<0.001). Extender 2 showed significantly lower protective qualities (P<0.001). After 48 hours, only semen diluted with extender 1 showed living and motile

Table 2. Effect of extender with different sugar contents on the sperm motility in rams on 24 h and 48 h at 39°C

Semen extender	Total motility (%)							
	0'	15'	60'	120'	180'	240'	300'	360'
After 24 h								
1 M	77.0±0.90	70.8±1.3	63.33±0.38	53.67±0.62	34.67±0.81	33.60±0.43	25.67±0.33	**19.83±0.16**
S*	n.s.	n.s.	a	D, E	b, F	A_1, B_1	D_1, c	F_1, A_2
2 M	77.8±0.66	72.2±1.7	64.00±0.17	50.00±0.32	9.00±1.40	25.00±0.73	15.00±0.31	**8.00±0.60**
S*	n.s	n.s.	C	D	b	A_1, C_1	D_1, E_1	F_1, B_2
3 M	78.0±0.52	71.0±2.6	62.17±0.28	49.50±0.40	39.83±0.45	30.93±0.20	24.67±0.27	**17.43±0.19**
S*	n.s.	n.s.	a, C	E	F	B_1, C_1	c, E_1	A_2, B_2
After 48 h								
1 M	70.0±0.11	65.33±1.36	62.4±1.54	41.6±1.65	32.1±0.98	22.3±1.32	18.0±1.07	**10.1±0.39**
S*	n.s	A	a	n.s.	d	A, e	B	
2 M	70.0±0.24	68.50±1.28	57.1±1.30	41.8±1.30	28.3±1.50	13.2±0.96	0	**0**
S*	n.s.	A,B	a	n.s.	n.s.	A		
3 M	70.0±0.45	65.83±1.52	58.6±1.71	43.2±1.19	26.3±1.65	15.6±1.85	9.3±1.00	**0**
S*	n.s.	B	n.s.	n.s.	d	e	B	

S*-values with same superscripts are significant a, b, c – P≤0.05; d, e- P≤0.01; A_{n-2}, B_{n-2}, C, D, E, F – P≤0.001

sperm cells (total motility =10.1%). Samples, which were diluted with extenders 2 or 3 showed no protective effect on ram semen, since all spermatozoa were dead.

The beneficial effect of more sugar concentrations in maintaining higher TM% was consistent.

Values for pregnancy rates are presented in Table 3. There were significant differences between the extender 1- sucrose, lactose and rafinosa (80 %) and extender 2 – sucrose and rafinosa (71 %), also between extender 1 and control extender 6A- with sucrose and lactose (71.20 %; Table 3).

different metabolism (7). Sperm motility gives a measure of the integrity of the sperm axoneme and tail structures as well as the metabolic machinery of the mitochondria, and sperm morphology is a surrogate measure of the integrity of DNA packaging and the quality of spermatogenesis (9). The results from the present study clearly demonstrated the major effect of sucrose, lactose and rafinosa in semen extenders on chilled ram sperm motility. Total motility is an important indicator of sugar utilization by spermatozoa as the sugars provide the external energy source essential

Table 3. Ewe´s pregnancy rate after cervical insemination with ram sperm diluted in extenders

Semen extender	No of inseminated ewes (n)	No of pregnant ewes (n)	Pregnancy rate (%)
1	65	52	80.00 % a, b
2	69	49	71.01 % a
3	66	47	71.21 % b

Values with same superscripts are significant a, b – p≤0.05

DISCUSSION

Different sugars were tested and compared to the untreated control because they have been shown to have protective effects on motility patterns and

for maintaining motility. In this study, TM% (>70%) remained high during the first 48 hours and subsequently, as could be expected, decreased with storage time. The decrease in the percentage of total motile spermatozoa in 0'-15'(71-78%) may be due to the fact that there are subpopulations of ram spermatozoa with different sensitivities to changes in the environment, particularly reduced temperature. Decreased sperm motility after 60' has been postulated to be due to temperature sensitivity of the ATPase-linked sodium–potassium pump and subsequently a leakage of ions (10). Preservation with increasing variety of sugars resulted in better maintenance of sperm motility with extender 1. The combination of sucrose, lactose and rafinosa as a part of semen extender for ram semen provided beneficial effect on the survival of sperm more than as sole component. Bohlooli et al. establish that only sucrose and lactose in extenders was less effective at protecting spermatozoa during the storage process, which was indicated clearly by lower osmotic resistance of spermatozoa (11). In addition, the increased concentration of buffer solutions in the extender reduces the deleterious effects of the great amount of hydrogenic ions produced from the metabolic activity of spermatozoa. In addition, egg yolk is known to contain many specific components like lecithin, phospholipids and lipoprotein fractions (12). The significantly higher sperm motility after storage for 24 hours and 48 hours could explain the evolution of fertilizing ability and was probably sufficient to achieve gestation. A dose of $25–50 \times 10^6$ sperm for intrauterine insemination, $75–100 \times 10^6$ sperm for transcervical insemination and $150–300 \times 10^6$ for cervical insemination is recommended in ewes (13). In the present study, concentration of 100×10^6 ram spermatozoa was selected for in vivo use. The change in the motility parameter was less dramatic in samples diluted with extender 1 and significant difference was observed between the groups regarding the fertilization rate or the establishment of pregnancy. It was reported that low motile sperm injection may have a negative effect on fertilization and pregnancy rates (14). On the other hand Vildan Karpuz et al. found no correlation in fertilization and pregnancy rates with either morphology or motility (15).

The possible physiological reasons for the decline in motility might be due to extracellular oxidative stress, effects of seminal plasma volume-constituents and endogenous free radical production. Substances from seminal plasma protect spermatozoa from premature aging during storage (16). The most sugars in content of extender 1. may be one of the reasons for better preservation of functional and motility parameters in our study.

In conclusion, our experiments demonstrated that higher sperm motility after storage at 4°C for 24 hours and 48 hours has the ram spermatozoa diluted with extender 1. with combination of disaccharides (sucrose and lactose) and trisaccharides (rafinosa). This semen extender (number 1) can be used successfully for the insemination of ewes and it might improve the pregnancy rate after artificial insemination.

REFERENCES

1. Ax, R. L., Dally, M. R., Didon, B. A, Lenz, R. W., Love, C. C., Varner, D.D., Hafez, B., Bellin, M. E. (2000). Artificial insemination. In: Hafez, B.Hafez, E.S.E. (Eds.), Reproduction in farm animals. (7th Eds.) (pp. 376-389). Philadelphia, Lea and Febinger ISBN 0-683-30577-8

2. Marti, J. I., Marti, E., Cebrian-Perez, J. E., Muino-Blanco, T. (2003). Survival rate of antioxidant enzyme activity of ram spermatozoa after dilution with different extenders or selection by a dextran swim-up procedure. Theriogenology 60, 1013-1020. http://dx.doi.org/10.1016/S0093-691X(03)00105-5

3. Riha, L., Apolen, D., Pivko, J., Grafenau, P., Kubovica, E. (2006). Influence of implememtors on sheep fertility out of season. Slovak J. Anim. Sci., 4, 180-182. http://www.cvzv.sk/index.php/en/volume-39-2006/number-4

4. Sarlos, P., Molnar, A., Kokai, A., Gabor, G., Ratky, J. (2002). Evaluation of the effect of antioxidants in the conservation of ram semen. Acta Vet. Hung., 50, 2, 235-245. http://dx.doi.org/10.1556/AVet.50.2002.2.13 PMid:12113179

5. Adeoya-Osiguwa S., Fraser, L. R. (1993). A biphasic pattern of 45 Ca^{2+} uptake by mouse spermatozoa in vitro correlates changing functional potential. J. Reprod. Fertil., 99, 187-194. http://dx.doi.org/10.1530/jrf.0.0990187 PMid:8283437

6. Williams, AC, Ford, WCL., (2001). The role of glucose in supporting motility and capacitation in human spermatozoa. J. Androl., 22, 680–695. PMid:11451366

7. Rigau, T., Farrem, M., Ballester, J., Mogas, T., Peňa, A., Rodriguez-Gil, J.E. (2001). Effects of glucose and fructose on motility patterns of dog spermatozoa from fresh ejaculates. Theriogenology 56, 801–815. http://dx.doi.org/10.1016/S0093-691X(01)00609-4

8. Zahariev Z., Georgiev, G., Chelebiyski, S. (1988). Diluent for storage of ram semen for 24 hours at 3-4 ° C. Journal of Livestock Breeding (BG), 6, 65-66.

9. Pacey, A.A. (2006). Is quality assurance in semen analysis still really necessary? A view from the andrology laboratory. Hum Reprod., 21, 1105-1109. http://dx.doi.org/10.1093/humrep/dei460 PMid:16396933

10. Saito, K., Kinoshita, Y., Kanno, H., Iwasaki, A. (1996). The role of potassium ion and extracellular alkalization in reinitiation of human spermatozoa preserbed in electrolyte-free solution at 4°C. Fertil Steril., 56, 1214–1218.

11. Bohlooli, Sh., Cedden, F., Jang, J. P., Razzaghzadeh, S., Bozoğlu, Ş. (2012). The effect of different extenders on post-thaw sperm viability, motility and membrane integrity in cryopreserved semen of Zandi Ram. J. Basic. Appl. Sci. Res., 2 (2): 1120-1123.

12. Demianowicz, W., Strzezek, J. (1996). The effect of lipoprotein fraction from egg yolk on some of the biological properties of boar spermatozoa during storage of the semen in liquid state. Reprod. Dom. Anim., 31: 279–280.
http://dx.doi.org/10.1111/j.1439-0531.1995.tb00051.x

13. Buckrell, B. (1997). Reproductive technologies in commercial use for sheep, goats and framed deer. In: Proceedings for Annual Meeting of the Society for Theriogenology. (pp.185–192). Montreal, Quebec, Canada

14. Lui, J., Nagy, Z., Tournaye, H., et al. (1995). Analysis of 76 total fertilization failure cycles out of 2732 intracytoplasmic sperm injection cycles. Hum Reprod, 10: 2630-36.
http://humrep.oxfordjournals.org/content/10/10/2630

15. Karpuz, V., Gokturk, A., Koyuturk, M. (2007). The effects of sperm morphology and motility on the outcome of intracytoplasmic sperm injection. Marmara Medical Journal 20(2): 92-97.
http://www.marmaramedicaljournal.org/pdf.php3?id=418

16. Kasimanickam, R., Pelzer, K. D., Kasimanickam, V., Swecker, W.S., Thatcher, C.D. (2006). Association of classical semen parameters, sperm DNA fragmentation index, lipid peroxidation and antioxidant enzymatic activity of semen in ram-lambs. Theriogenology 65, 1407–1421.
http://dx.doi.org/10.1016/j.theriogenology.2005.05.056

17. Varisli, O., Uguz, C., Agca C., Agca, Y. (2009). Motility and acrosomal integrity comparisons between electro-ejaculated and epididymal ram sperm after exposure to a range of anisosmotic solutions, cryoprotective agents and low temperatures. Animal Reproduction Science 110, 256-268.
http://dx.doi.org/10.1016/j.anireprosci.2008.01.012
PMid:18294786

18. Nikolovski, M., Mickov, Lj., Dovenska, M., Petkov, V., Atanasov, B., Dovenski, T. (2014). Influence of glutathione on kinetic parameters of frozen-thawed spermatozoa from Ovchepolian Pramenka rams. Mac Vet Rev, 37 (2): 121-128.
http://dx.doi.org/10.14432/j.macvetrev.2014.05.014

3

SCREENING OF SELECTED INDICATORS OF DAIRY CATTLE WELFARE IN MACEDONIA

Miroslav Radeski, Aleksandar Janevski, Vlatko Ilieski

Animal Welfare Center, Faculty of Veterinary Medicine
Lazar Pop Trajkov 5-7, 1000 Skopje, Macedonia

ABSTRACT

The welfare state of cattle in dairy farms in Macedonia has never been assessed previously. The objective of this study was to perform screening analysis of dairy cows welfare and to test the practical implementation of the Welfare Quality® Assessment protocol for cattle in dairy farms in Macedonia. In ten small scale and large scale tie stall farms 23 measures were recorded related to 9 welfare criteria of 4 welfare principles (WP) described in the Welfare Quality® Assessment protocol for dairy cows. The mean percentage of very lean cows was 40.5±9.1%. All assessed farms were not providing access to pasture and an outdoor loafing area. Regarding cleanliness, the presence of dirty udder, upper leg/flank and lower leg was 65.2±9.0%, 85.5±8.0% and 86.5±5.8%, respectively. The overall prevalence of lameness was 5.6±5.0%, and for mild and severe alterations it was 30.8±5.8% and 54.1±4.6%, respectively. The ocular and vulvar discharge, diarrhea, dystocia, percentage of downer cows and mortality rate exceeded the warning and alarm threshold. The avoidance – distance test classified 70.4±6.8% as animals that can be touched or approached closer than 50cm, with overall score of 42.9±3.5. This screening reveals that the most welfare concerns are found in the WP Good Feeding and Good Housing. The on-farm welfare assessment using the full protocol on a representative sample of farms in the country is highly recommended for emphasizing the key points for improving the animal welfare in Macedonian dairy farms.

Key words: welfare assessment, cattle, dairy farms, animal based measures

INTRODUCTION

The maintenance of good animal welfare is an essential part of dairy production systems. Farmer's strong commitment to animal welfare in dairy cattle and appropriate dairy herd management is driven by fulfilling the physiological and behavioral needs of the animal, compliance with the relevant international (1, 2) and national animal welfare regulations (3, 4), and respecting the consumer expectations for animal welfare standards in the food industry (5).

The implementation of welfare standards must be accompanied by proper assessment which

Corresponding author: Prof. Vlatko Ilieski, PhD
E-mail address: vilieski@fvm.ukim.edu.mk
Present address: Faculty of Veterinary Medicine-Skopje
University "Ss. Cyril and Methodius" in Skopje
Lazar Pop-Trajkov 5/7, 1000 Skopje, R. Macedonia

should be based on valid and reliable indicators of animal welfare. The recently adopted EU Strategy for the Protection and Welfare of Animals 2012–2015 highlights that the possibility of using scientifically validated outcome-based indicators complementing prescriptive requirements in EU legislation should be considered when necessary (6). Factors affecting animal welfare include the physical environment, resources available to the animal and management practices on the farm. Depending on its characteristics (breed, sex, age, etc.) the animal will respond to these inputs and the animal's responses are assessed using animal-based measures. Animal-based measures are evaluative, quantitatively and qualitatively, and may be obtained in a reliable way. To have an objective indication of an animal's welfare and to perform a good welfare assessment, a set of measures are needed to be measured. Animal-based measures can be collected on-farm either by observation or inspection of the animal on individual and herd level. Animal-based measures usually have been used to identify animals whose welfare is poor, as an early warning for animals with deteriorating welfare, as well as, for immediate recognizing of improvements in welfare in order to maximize benefits (7). The European Welfare Quality® Project was set out to develop scientifically sound tools to assess animal welfare on-farm. The acquired data provides feedback to animal unit managers about the welfare status of their animals and is translated into accessible and understandable information on the welfare status of food producing animals, including dairy cattle (8). This paper uses selected indicators for assessment of animal welfare designed by this project.

Currently, a total number of 238 000 of cattle are kept in the dairy sector in Macedonia (9) out of which about 50% are milking cows with a total milk production of 350 million liters and an annual average of milk yield of 2,928 L per cow (10). The dairy farms are categorized in three categories: 1) traditional farmers with up to 3 cows; 2) family farms with 5 – 20 milking cows; and 3) specialized farms with more than 20 milking cows. The most dominating farms are in the first two categories

study in order to identify the possible challenges and obstacles in implementing a more comprehensive analysis of dairy cattle welfare in Macedonia.

MATERIAL AND METHODS

The study was conducted on eleven dairy farms in Macedonia, four large-scale tie stall farms with at least 30 milking cows and seven small – scale tie stall farms with less than 15 milking cows. The number of tested animals and categories for each farm is presented in Table 1. At the Farm F only the avoidance distance test was performed and no other measures were taken into account, while at the Farm K the avoidance distance test was not possible to perform due to the conditions and physical obstacles. Hence, the total number of included farms in the assessment for each measure in this study is ten (4-large and 6-small scale farms).

Table 1. Allocation of farms according to category and number of animals assessed

Farm type	Farm	No. of milking cows	No. of dry cows	No. of heifers	Total no. of animals	No. of animals tested
Large scale tie-stall	A	43	0	17	60	37
	G	39	0	5	44	32
	H	120	0	0	120	55
	I	30	0	7	37	28
Small scale tie-stall	B	8	3	0	11	11
	C	5	0	2	10	7
	D	11	1	6	18	18
	E	3	1	1	5	5
	F	5	0	2	7	7
	J	2	0	0	2	2
	K	6	0	1	7	7
Total number:	11	272	5	41	321	209

(up to 20 cows) with 97% of all farms in the country, while only 1% of the dairy farms keep more than 50 milking cows (10). The most prevalent housing system is the tie stall system without grazing periods.

Assessing the welfare state of dairy cows in Macedonia, the neighboring countries and in the Balkan Peninsula has received only little attention so far. Studies concerning the welfare assessment in dairy farms in this region were conducted in Serbia (11), Croatia (12) and Romania (13-16). Until now, on-farm welfare assessment in dairy farms in Macedonia has not been performed. Therefore, the objective of this study was to assess selected indicators of dairy cattle welfare from the Welfare Quality® Assessment protocol (8) and to identify the main welfare concerns and challenges in Macedonian farms. This study also served as a pilot

The welfare assessment and sampling procedure were performed according to the Welfare Quality® Assessment protocol for cattle (8).

For the on-farm assessment, nine out of twelve welfare criteria as proposed by Welfare Quality® were selected, consisting of 23 measures. Welfare principles (WP), criteria and measures applied in this study are summarized in Table 2. The majority of the measures were performed in individual animals and few measures were referring to housing resources and management.

The gathered data was translated into criterion scores expressed on a 0 to 100 value scale, where 0 corresponds to the worst and 100 corresponds to the best level of welfare. The calculation of criterion scores was performed using an on-line Welfare Quality® scoring system (http://www1. clermont.inra.fr/wq).

Table 2. Welfare principles, criteria and measures applied in the screening study

Welfare principle	Welfare Criteria	Measures
1. Good feeding	1.1 Absence of prolonged hunger	1.1.1 Body Condition Score
	1.2 Absence of prolonged thirst	1.2.1 Water provision
		1.2.2 Cleanliness of water points
		1.2.3 Water flow
2. Good housing	2.1 Comfort around resting	2.1.1 Cleanliness of udders
		2.1.2 Cleanliness of flank/upper legs
		2.1.3 Cleanliness of lower legs
	2.2 Ease of movement	2.2.1 Presence of tethering
		2.2.2 Access to outdoor loafing area or pasture
3. Good health	3.1 Absence of injuries	3.1.1 Lameness
		3.1.2 Integument alterations
	3.2 Absence of disease	3.2.1 Nasal discharge
		3.2.2 Ocular discharge
		3.2.3 Hampered respiration
		3.2.3 Diarrhea
		3.2.4 Vulvar discharge
		3.2.5 Mortality
		3.2.6 Dystocia
		3.2.7 Downer cows
	3.3 Absence of pain induced by management procedures	3.3.1 Disbudding/Dehorning
		3.3.2 Tail docking
4. Appropriate behavior	4.1 Expression of other behaviors	4.1.1 Access to pasture
	4.2 Good human - animal relationship	4.2.1 Avoidance distance

All data processing and statistical analyses were performed using MS Excel® 2010, MS Office Professional Plus 2010 (©2010 Microsoft Cooperation) and StatSoft, Inc. (2007), STATISTICA (data analysis software system), version 8.0. The statistical analysis was based on descriptive statistical indicators (mean, standard error of the mean and quartiles) for the measures and criteria used in the study. Tests for statistically significant differences between large-scale and small-scale farms were performed by the Mann-Whitney U Test, except for data from the avoidance distance test, which were analyzed by the Chi-Square test for independence. The significance level was set at $p < 0.05$.

RESULTS

The mean percentage of very lean cows per farm was $40.5 \pm 9.1\%$ ($Q_1 = 14.29$; $Q_3 = 54.72$) with no differences between large and small scale farms ($p = 0.14$).

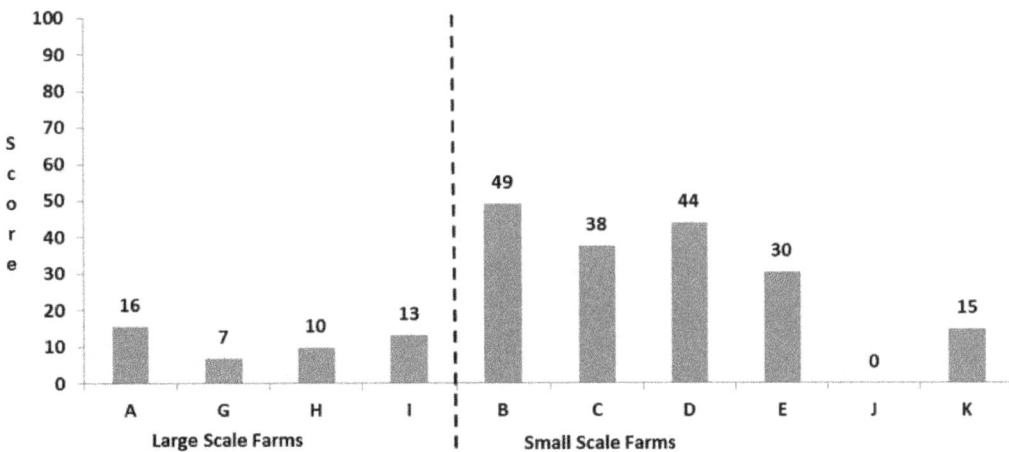

Figure 1. Scores for the criterion Absence of prolonged hunger

Consequently, the criterion scores for Absence of prolonged hunger ranged between 0 (Farm J) and 49 (Farm B), (Fig. 1). The water supply in the farms was one bowl per two animals and the majority of bowls were assessed as clean except in two farms (E and G). Two farms (G and J) did not provide continuous water supply - some animals did not have free access to water and the water flow was lower than 10 l/min. Therefore, the scores for the criterion Absence of prolonged thirst were 3 in two farms, 32 in four farms and 60 in the remaining four farms. Overall, considering the scores for both criteria, Absence of prolonged hunger and thirst, there was no significant difference with regard to the size of the farm (p=0.35).

In all farms, cows were kept in a tie-stall system and were not provided access to pasture or outdoor loafing area throughout the year. This resulted in the lowest possible score (score of 15) for the criterion Ease of movement. In addition, as part of the WP Good Housing, the prevalence of dirty udder, upper leg/flank and lower leg were assessed, with a mean prevalence of 65.2±9.0% (Q_1=50.00; Q_3=84.62), 85.5±8.0% (Q_1=85.71; Q_3=100.00), 86.5±5.8% (Q_1=77.78; Q_3=100.00), respectively. According to the Welfare Quality Assessment protocol (8) all farms, with the exception of Farm E for cleanliness of the udder, were classified as farms with "serious problem" considering the three measures of cleanliness. Although the percentage of cows with dirty udder, upper and lower leg was

numerically lower in the small scale farms, there were no differences between large scale and small scale farms (udder, p=0.14; upper and lower leg p=0.29) (Fig. 2).

Three welfare criteria were assessed concerning the WP Good Health. The criterion Absence of pain induced by management procedures was measured in terms of the percentage of animals submitted to the procedures of disbudding/dehorning and tail docking. At two farms, the small scale farm D - 50% of the animals and the large scale farm H - all animals at the farm were submitted to the disbudding procedure at the age of 4 and 2 weeks, using caustic paste and without any analgesia or anesthesia. Milking cows with docked tail were not found in any of the assessed farms. Regarding the welfare criterion Absence of injuries, lameness prevalence was 5.6±5.0%, and 30.8±5.8% were cows with mild (hairless patch) alterations and 54.1±4.6% of the cows showed severe alterations (lesions and swellings), without any differences considering the size of the farms. The overall mean score for the criterion Absence of injuries was 57.0±7.4. The measurements taken concerning the criterion Absence of disease showed that the prevalence of ocular discharge at farms B and J (9% and 50% of tested animals); diarrhea at farms B, D and I (9 %, 28% and 7% of tested animals); vulvar discharge at farm E (20%); the incidence of dystocia at farms A, C and H (17%, 7% and 5% of all animals in the last twelve months); the incidence of downer cows

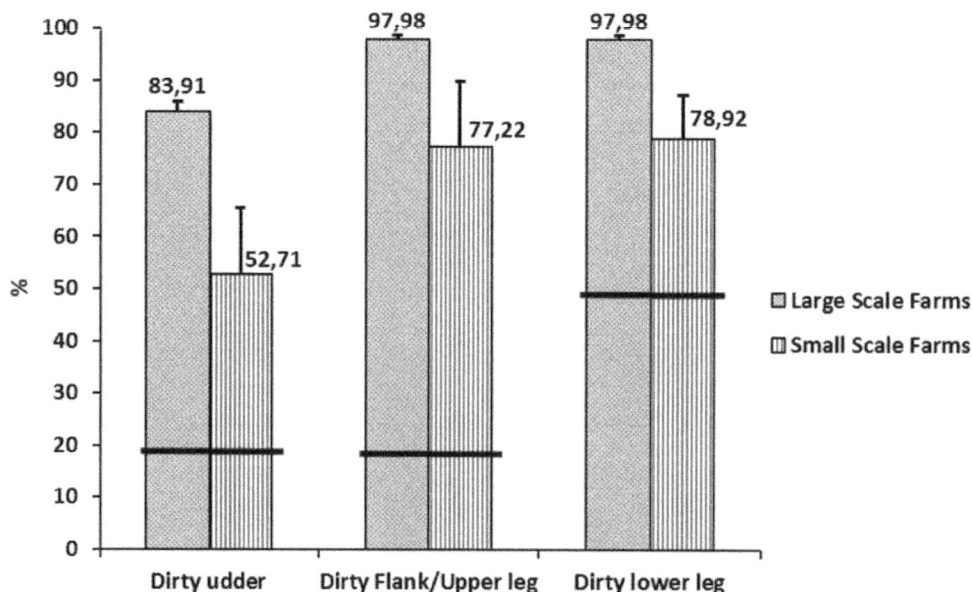

Figure 2. Percentage of animals (mean ± SE) with dirty lower leg, upper leg and udder in large and small scale farms. Black lines are showing the threshold for the level of cleanliness being considered a "serious problem"

Table 3. Prevalence in percentage and comparison between small and large scale farms for measures from the welfare criteria Absence of disease

Measure	Small Scale Farms			Large Scale Farms			p
	Mean±SE	Q_1	Q_3	Mean±SE	Q_1	Q_3	
Nasal Discharge	2.4±1.6	0.0	5.6	4.5±2.7	0.0	9.0	0.61
Ocular Discharge	9.9±8.2[a]	0.0	9.1	1.4±0.9	0.0	2.7	1.00
Hampered respiration	0.0	0.0	0.0	2.6±0.9	1.6	3.6	0.07
Diarrhea	6.1±4.6[w]	0.0	9.1	3.7±1.12[w]	2.3	5.1	0.47
Vulvar discharge	3.3±3.3[w]	0.0	0.0	2.6±0.9[w]	1.6	3.6	0.26
Dystocia	1.2±1.2	0.0	0.0	6.0±3.8[a]	1.0	11.0	0.17
Downer cows	4.0±2.6[w]	0.0	10.0	1.9±1.9	0.0	3.9	0.76
Mortality rate	9.5±8.2[a]	0.0	7.0	3.8±1.8[w]	1.0	6.5	0.61

Measures above the ([a]) Alarm Threshold and ([w]) Warning Threshold, defined in the Welfare Quality® Assessment Protocol for cattle

– farms A, C and I (8%,10% and 14% in the last twelve months) and mortality rate in farms B, H, I and J (7%, 5%, 8% and 50%, respectively) were above the defined alarm or warning thresholds in the protocol (8), (Tab. 3).

The welfare criterion Good Human – Animal Relationship, as part of the WP Appropriate Behaviour, was measured using the Avoidance distance towards an unknown observer and the animals were categorized in four categories: 1) animals that can be touched, 2) animals that can be approached closer than 50cm, 3) between 50 – 100 cm and 4) animals that cannot be approached closer to 100cm. From 200 cows which were assessed in all farms, 70.4±6.4% were classified as animals that can be touched or approached closer than 50cm. The mean overall score for this criterion was 42.9±3.5 (Q_1=36.00; Q_3=53.00). Similar findings were found in small and large scale farms (p=0.18), where 72.5±11.2% and 67.2±5.7% were cows classified in the first two categories of this measure (Fig. 3).

During the welfare assessment process in the assessed farms, the following findings were observed regarding the implementation of the Assessment protocol for Cattle: a) all selected indicators could be measured according to the suggested methodology in the protocol (8), except the Avoidance distance test, where due to the physical obstacles in front of the cows, in one farm failed to be performed; b) there were no reliable records kept by the farmers for presence of diseases, mortality level, milk production and other information requested by the Assessment protocol; and c) no continuous analysis of the somatic cell counts in milk on individual level in all assessed farms.

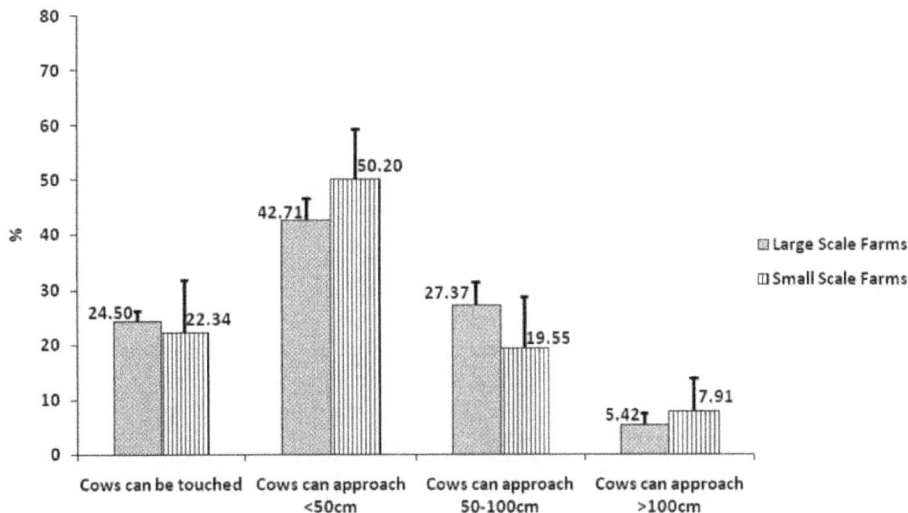

Figure 3. Mean ± SE percentage of cows categorized in four categories in the Avoidance distance test, considering the size of the farms

DISCUSSION

The present screening of cattle welfare in dairy farms in Macedonia has indicated the major welfare concerns in dairy production in the country. Since this is the first screening performed in Macedonia, the results from this study are compared with a number of publications from Serbia, Croatia and Romania. In these studies the number of farms involved in the assessment varies from 2 in Croatia (12) up to 52 in Romania (14). The results of this study are not representing the overall dairy cattle welfare in Macedonia, due to the small sample size (10 farms for each measure), and are preliminary findings. Hence, the discussion focuses on the findings for tie stall housing systems considering the cultural and traditional similarities in dairy production.

Using most of the measures suggested by the Welfare Quality® Assessment protocol for cattle (8), the main overview for dairy cattle welfare was established for the assessed dairy farms. Considering the WP Good Feeding, the percentage of very lean cows per farm was high resulting in low scores for the criterion Absence of prolonged hunger. Although, there were no significant differences considering the size of the farms, still in most of the small scale farms the presence of very lean animals was numerically lower in comparison with the large scale farms. The comparison with results from studies in other countries for tie stall systems shows that the percentage of very lean cows in our study is higher than the findings in Serbia (11) and Romania (13, 16), almost equal to the results in Croatia (12) and lower than North - Eastern Transilvania (14). Although, this pilot study covered only 10 farms in Macedonia, the findings for the absence of prolonged hunger are alarming and it is expected to be one of the most serious disturbances of cattle welfare. Regarding provision of water, all farms are complying with the minimal standards suggested by the Assessment protocol (8); however, the assessed farms are far from fulfilling the recommendations for this criterion by the Assessment protocol and Anderson et al. (1984), which is at least one water bowl for each animal and water flow of 15 l/min (8, 17). For the WP Good Feeding, according to the classification thresholds in the Assessment Protocol (8), seven farms were classified as "acceptable" and three farms as "not classified".

The hygiene level, in terms of cleanliness of the animals was classified as a serious problem in all farms. Lower percentages of soiled animals, using the same assessment methods, were found in the studies performed in UK (18), Romania (13, 16), Switzerland (19), while almost equal percentage

of dirty body regions with our results was found in Serbia (11) and Croatia (12). The main reason for the findings in the present study were inappropriate lying areas, in terms of improper length of the cubicles, insufficient amount of bedding material and too infrequent and irregular cleaning of the stalls. The high percentage of dirty body regions on the animal is highly related to the traditional and cultural way of dairy farming in this region, characterized with hard surfaces and poor bedding resulting in low hygiene. Additionally, keeping the animals tethered during the whole year is quite common in dairy farms in Macedonia. Therefore, all assessed farms have no access to outdoor run and pasture during the whole year which has high impact on the welfare criteria "Ease of movement" and "Expression of other behaviour", resulting in the lowest scores for these criteria.

Most of the low scores in the WP Good Health are likely to be related to poor housing and hygiene conditions. This is supported by the high percentage of animals with integument alterations, where the percentage of animals with at least one swelling or lesion is dominating over the mild skin alterations. The main factors for these findings are poor bedding conditions and inappropriate lying areas (20, 21), confirmed by the location of integument alterations on the body, which were predominantly on the hock and carpal regions. Mild alterations were less prevalent and severe alterations more prevalent in comparison with the findings in tied cattle in Romania (13) and Switzerland (19), but similar to the findings in tie-stalls in Ontario (21) and Serbia (11), especially for the mild alterations. Additionally, some studies suggest that continuously tethered animals tend to have more skin injuries compared with systems with access to loafing areas, pasture and loose housed cattle (13, 19). Although the proposed method for assessing the lameness in tied cows is different from the one for loose animals (8), at least severely lame may be reliably detected (22). The prevalence of lameness had wide range in the assessed farms, but not exceeding 16.2% per farm. Lameness in cattle is highly related to the bed surface, bedding material, cleanliness, hock skin alterations, regular exercise and feeding management (21, 23, 24, 25) – factors observed in poor condition in the assessed farms.

The measures of criterion "Absence of disease", ocular discharge, diarrhea, vulvar discharge, dystocia, percentage of downer cows and mortality rate exceeded the warning and alarm threshold set up by the protocol. The study conducted in Serbia revealed similar findings as regards the percentage of animals with ocular discharge, diarrhea, dystocia and mortality rate (11), while the respective prevalences found in Romania (13, 16) were lower for all parameters than ours. Although there were no significant differences in the above mentioned measures, ocular discharge, mortality rate, diarrhea, downer cows and vulvar discharge were higher in small scale, while dystocia, nasal discharge and hampered respiration were higher in large scale farms. This pilot study found that testing for milk somatic cell count in milk samples per individual animal did not exist in all visited farms. This confirms the categorization of this measure as "parameters which should be included but lack reliability in most countries" (26). Testing for milk somatic cell count is only done for the bunk tank milk – which is not useful for welfare assessment. This should be taken in consideration for complete implementation of the Welfare Quality® Assessment Protocol for cattle (8).

Tail docking is not practiced in Macedonian dairy farms, thus avoiding unnecessary pain of the animal. However, all the disbudding / dehorning procedures are performed without any use of anesthesia and analgesia which contributes to the presence of pain during the management procedures and lowers the welfare score in the farms with dehorned animals.

Human – animal relationship represents the mutual perception of stockman and animals and is essential for good animal welfare (27). Many studies confirmed that negative handling experiences of animals result in higher levels of fear of humans which may have negative effects on production, reproduction, welfare and the risk of injuries for both, animal and man (28, 29, 30). Positive handling might improve the welfare (31), resulting in good animal health, performance and stockman's confidence in the animals. In this study, most of the assessed cows allowed to be touched or approached in a distance of less than 50cm by the assessor. These findings indicate that the animals are not exposed to severe handling experiences by the farmers. Considering the size of the farms in the study, there were no differences between small and large scale farms, while similar findings for the avoidance distance test was found in other studies with tie (13) and loose (18) stalls. The assessed farms were without access to pasture, but according to Matiello et al. (32) farms with access to pasture are expected to have a larger avoidance distance. Additionally, in one farm (Farm K) the Avoidance Distance Test could not be performed due to the placement of the tethered animals in the shed (the cows were facing very closely to the wall). Such cases represent a real obstacle in full implementation of the Assessment Protocol (8). The other criteria and measures of the WP Appropriate Behaviour were not included in this study, therefore, for further detailed analysis of this principle complete assessment measures defined in the protocol (8) must be performed.

Considering the present dairy production in Macedonia, where most of the farms have less than 20 animals (9, 10) with predominantly tie stalls, the acquisition of farms was focused on tie stalls, while the categorization of large and small scale farms was set up only by the number of animals (more than 30 and less than 15 milking cows). Since this study was performed only as initial screening and for the first time the Welfare Assessment Protocol (8) was performed in Macedonian dairy farms, the number of farms was very low for complete representation of the present welfare state of milking cows. Therefore, the absence of any differences between large and small scale farms could be due to the low number of farms included in the study. Since there is considerable variability within small scale farms this could have biased the representation of the current welfare status on state level. In future analyses, proper sampling, in terms of valid geographic distribution and representative number of small and large scale dairy farms, is highly recommended for any detailed analysis on the dairy cattle welfare.

CONCLUSION

This study confirms that the Welfare Quality® Assessment Protocol for cattle could be put in practice and implemented in Macedonian dairy farms with precautions while measuring some of protocol's defined measures. Therefore, implementation of the whole protocol and on-farm welfare assessment on a representative sample of farms with different housing systems in Macedonia is highly necessary. Subsequently, a baseline study for animal welfare of dairy cattle could be created which will point out the key areas for improvement in the welfare of dairy cattle in Macedonian farms.

REFERENCES

1. European Communities (EC) (1976). European Convention for the Protection of Animals kept for Farming Purposes. Strasbourg, 10.3.1976. European Treaty Series No. 87.
www.conventions.coe.int/Treaty/EN/Treaties/Html/087.htm

2. Council Directive 98/58/EC of 1998 concerning the protection of animals kept for farming purposes. OJ L 221/23 8.8.98 (July 20, 1998)

3. Animal welfare and protection law (2007). OJ Republic of Macedonia 113 (September 20, 2007)

4. Regulation for conditions and methods for protection of farm animals (2009). OJ Republic of Macedonia 140 (November 20, 2009)

5. European Commission (2007). Attitudes of EU citizens towards Animal Welfare. Special Eurobarometer 270. Wave 66.1. TNS Opinion and Social http://ec.europa.eu/public_opinion/archives/ebs/ebs_270_en.pdf

6. European Commission (2012). Communication from the commission to the European Parlament, the council and the European economic and social committee on the European Union Strategy for the Protection and Welfare of Animals 2012-2015 (Text with EEA relevance), European Commission, Brussels, Belgium

7. EFSA Panel on Animal Health and Welfare (AHAW) (2012). Statement on the use of animal-based measures to assess the welfare of animals. EFSA Journal 2012; 10(6): 2767, 29.

8. Welfare Quality®, (2009). Welfare Quality® assessment protocol for cattle. Welfare Quality® Consortium, Lelystad, Netherlands, 180.

9. State Statistical Office, Skopje – News release (2014). Number of livestock, poultry and beehives in 2013. Skopje, Macedonia. www.statgov.mk

10. Ministry of Agriculture, Forestry and Water Economy (2013). Annual report for agriculture and rural development, 2012. Skopje, Macedonia

11. Ostojić-Andrić, D., Hristov, S., Novaković, Ž., Pantelić, V., Petrović, M. M., Zlatanović, Z., Nikšić, D. (2011). Dairy cows welfare quality in loose vs tie housing system. Biotechnol Anim Husb. 27 (3): 975-984. http://dx.doi.org/10.2298/BAH1103975O

12. Vučemilo, M., Matković, K., Štoković, I., Kovačević, S., Benić, M. (2012). Welfare assessment of dairy cows housed in a tie-stall system. Mljekarstvo 62 (1): 62-67.

13. Popescu, S., Borda, C., Diugan, E., Niculae, M., Stefan, R., Sandru, C. (2014). The effect of the housing system on the welfare quality of dairy cows. Ital J Anim Sci. 13 (1): 2940. http://dx.doi.org/10.4081/ijas.2014.2940

14. Popescu, S., Borda, C., Sandru, C.D., Stefan, R., Lazar, E. (2010). The welfare assessment of tied dairy cows in 52 small farms in north-eastern Transylvania using animal-based measurements. Slov Vet Res. 47 (3): 77-82.

15. Popescu, S., Borda, C., Lazar, E.A., Hegedus, I.C. (2009). Assessment of dairy cow welfare in farms from Transylvania. Proceedings of the 44th Croatian and 4th International Symposium on Agriculture. Opatija, Croatia. 2009 Feb 16-20; 752-756.

16. Popescu, S., Borda, C., Diugan, E. A., Spinu, M., Groza, I. S., Sandru, C. D. (2013). Dairy cows welfare quality in tie-stall housing system with or without access to exercise. Acta Vet Scand. 55 (1): 43. http://dx.doi.org/10.1186/1751-0147-55-43 PMid:23724804 ; PMCid:PMC3674972

17. Andersson, M., Schaar, J., Wiktorsson, H. (1984). Effects of drinking water flow rates and social rank on performance and drinking behaviour of tied-up dairy cows. Livest Prod Sci. 11, 599-610. http://dx.doi.org/10.1016/0301-6226(84)90074-5

18. Heath, C., Lin, C., Mullan, S., Browne, W.J., Main, D.C.J. (2014). Implementing Welfare Quality® in UK assurance schemes: evaluating the challenges. Anim Welf. 23 (1): 95-107. http://dx.doi.org/10.7120/09627286.23.1.095

19. Regula, G., Danuser, J., Spycher, B., Wechsler, B. (2004). Health and welfare of dairy cows in different husbandry systems in Switzerland. Prev Vet Med. 66 (1–4): 247-264. http://dx.doi.org/10.1016/j.prevetmed.2004.09.004 PMid:15579346

20. Brenninkmeyer, C., Dippel, S., Brinkmann, J., March, S., Winckler, C., Knierim, U. (2013). Hock lesion epidemiology in cubicle housed dairy cows across two breeds, farming systems and countries. Prev Vet Med. 109 (3–4): 236-245. http://dx.doi.org/10.1016/j.prevetmed.2012.10.014 PMid:23174217

21. Zurbrigg, K., Kelton, D., Anderson, N., Millman, S. (2005). Stall dimensions and the prevalence of lameness, injury and cleanliness on 317 tie-stall dairy farms in Ontario. Can Vet J. 46 (10): 902-909. PMid:16454382; PMCid:PMC1255592

22. Leach, K. A., Dippel, S., Huber, J., March, S., Winckler, C., Whay, H.R. (2009). Assessing lameness in cows kept in tie-stalls. J Dairy Sci. 92(4): 1567-1574. http://dx.doi.org/10.3168/jds.2008-1648 PMid:19307637

23. Cook, N. (2003). Prevalence of lameness among dairy cattle in Wisconsin as a function of housing type and stall surface. J Am Vet Med Assoc. 223 (9): 1324–1328. http://dx.doi.org/10.2460/javma.2003.223.1324 PMid:14621222

24. Wells, S., Trent, A., Marsh, W., Williamson, N., Robinson, R. (1995). Some risk factors associated with clinical lameness in dairy herds in Minnesota and Wisconsin. Vet Rec. 136 (21): 537–540. http://dx.doi.org/10.1136/vr.136.21.537 PMid:7660557

25. Dippel, S., Dolezal, M., Brenninkmeyer, C., Brinkmann, J., March, S., Knierim, U., Winckler, C. (2009). Risk factors for lameness in cubicle housed Austrian Simmental dairy cows. Prev Vet Med. 90 (1–2): 102-112. http://dx.doi.org/10.1016/j.prevetmed.2009.03.014 PMid:19409629

26. Winckler, C., Capdeville, J., Gebresenbet, G., Hörning, B., Roiha, U., Tosi, M., Waiblinger, S. (2003). Selection of parameters for on-farm welfare-assessment protocols in cattle and buffalo. Anim Welf. 12 (4): 619-624.

27. Estep, D.Q., Hetts, S., (1992). Interactions, relationships, and bonds: the conceptual basis for scientist–animal relations. In: Davis, H., Balfour, A.D. (Eds.), The Inevitable Bond–Examining Scientist–Animal Interactions (pp. 6–26). CAB International, Cambridge

28. Seabrook, M.F. (1972). A study to determine the influence of the herdsmans personality on milk yield. J Agric Labour Sci. 1, 45–59.

29. Hemsworth, P.H., Coleman, G.J. (1998). Human–Livestock Interactions: The Stockperson and the Productivity of Intensively Farmed Animals. CAB International, Wallingford, Oxon, United Kingdom

30. Waiblinger, S., Menke, C., Coleman, G. (2002). The relationship between attitudes, personal characteristics and behaviour of stock people and subsequent behaviour and production of dairy cows. Appl Anim Behav Sci. 79 (3): 195–219. http://dx.doi.org/10.1016/S0168-1591(02)00155-7

31. Waiblinger, S., Menke, C., Fölsch, D.W. (2003). Influences on the avoidance and approach behaviour of dairy cows towards humans on 35 farms. Appl Anim Behav Sci. 84 (1): 23–39. http://dx.doi.org/10.1016/S0168-1591(03)00148-5

32. Mattiello, S., Klotz, C., Baroli, D., Minero, M., Ferrante, V., Canali, E. (2009). Welfare problems in alpine dairy cattle farms in Alto Adige (Eastern Italian Alps). Ital J Anim Sci. 8 (2s): 628-630.

4

PYLORIC LEIOMYOMA: BEHAVIOURAL ASPECTS IN A SHELTER DOG

Riccardo Benedetti[1], Mirko Barabucci[2], Alessandra Pigliapoco[2],
Simona Cannas[3], Clara Palestrini[3]

*[1]Department of Environmental Science, University of Camerino,
Via Gentile III da Varano 62032 Camerino (MC), Italy*
*[2]Veterinary Clinic "Pigliapoco, Leoni, Barabucci", C.da Valle 6,
62100 Macerata (MC), Italy*
*[3]Department of Veterinary Science and Public Health, University of Milan
Via Celoria 10, 20133, Milan, Italy*

ABSTRACT

The present report describes a case of pyloric wall leiomyoma in a shelter dog with a history of vomiting, pica, licking and chewing the walls of the kennel. The clinical, radiological, ultrasound, hematological and blood chemistry examinations showed no abnormalities. A compulsive oral disorder was diagnosed and treatment with behaviour therapy instigated. The compulsive oral behaviours stopped following behaviour therapy, however, the vomiting persisted, suggesting the need to proceed with further diagnostic exams. The ultrasound examination, repeated after 6 months, had revealed the presence of a hypoechoic mass (3.52 cm) in the pyloric-antrum obstructing the gastric outflow. Following gastric dilatation the mass was surgically excised. Histological examination revealed a pyloric leiomyoma. In clinical practice this case highlights the importance of gastrointestinal diseases in the development of behaviour changes related to pica.

Key words: dog, pica, gastrointestinal disease, compulsive disorders

INTRODUCTION

The term pica indicates the ingestion of non-nutritive and inedible substances, such as tissue, plastic, sticks and stones. Pica is most common in puppies, but can be also found in adult dogs. The behaviour of pica should be carefully evaluated for various reasons. First, because it may indicate the existence of an organic problem such as dental and/or oral disease, central nervous system disorders such as tumours or hydrocephalus, electrolyte imbalances, metabolic diseases, toxins, brain aging, cognitive dysfunction or gastrointestinal disorders and secondly, because it can have dangerous effects on the health of dogs and may cause intestinal obstructions or transmit parasitic diseases (1). Pica can be a disorder linked to learning and/or sometimes be a manifestation of an obsessive compulsive disorder (OCD) (2).

CLINICAL CASE

A female neutered, 12 year old, mixed breed dog had been housed in a shelter for 11 years. The dog presented with behavioural changes of one month duration, consisting of destruction and ingestion of the plastic and metal coating of the kennel, and vomitus consisting of food plastic and metal. The dog shared the kennel with another male neutered dog, 8 years old. The kennel was an area of 20 m^2 which was partially covered. The kennels had an automatic watering bowl and the dogs were fed once a day, in the morning with fish and rice dog kibble. The dogs were exercised in a run area for an hour twice a week. During the clinical examination the dog showed on abdominal palpation, pain in

Corresponding author: Dr. Riccardo Benedetti, PhD
E-mail address: riccardo.benedetti@unicam.it
Present address: Department of Environmental Science,
University of Camerino, Via Gentile III da Varano,
62032 Camerino (MC), Italy

the left hypochondric area. The examination of the oral cavity excluded dental and/or oral disease and the neurological examination was normal. A faecal examination was negative for parasites. A gastric foreign body was suspected due to the history of pica and vomiting. The diagnostic plan was to do a complete blood count, blood biochemistry, urinalysis, Leishmania testing (IFI), radiography and ultrasonography. A lateral and ventro-dorsal abdominal radiograph showed the presence of small radiopaque foreign bodies within the stomach. Symptomatic treatment was initiated consisting of pantoprazole (Nycomed SpA, Milano, Italy) (1 mg/kg PO, SID for 5 days) and metoclopramide (Eurovet Animal Health, Ozzano dell'Emilia, Bologna, Italy) (0.2 mg/kg SC, BID for 5 days), in order to protect the stomach and facilitate gastric emptying. During the treatment, the dog did not vomit and appetite was preserved. However, the dog continued to show pica accompanied with destruction of the kennel. Repeat radiological examination and ultrasonography were carried out, but no abnormalities were found. The dog was referred for a behavioural examination. The behavioural consultation excluded behaviours relating to cognitive dysfunction, typical of aging, and diagnosed an oral Compulsive Disorder (CD). The treatment was aimed to decrease stress, which may develop due to life in kennels (3, 4, 5) and to enrich the environment where the dog lived. First, the dog and its dog kennel companion were moved to another kennel, where the surfaces were perfectly intact. The dog was also given the Kong® (Kong Company, LTD), a game dog food dispenser for mental stimulation at specific times of the day (periods during which there were no visitors and staff in kennels) and chewing bones for dogs were always available. The dog was given a daily routine which included an increase in exercise, which provided a daily output of at least one hour. During the following four months, the patient vomited with a frequency of 1-2 times per month but showed no more destructive behaviours or ingestion of inedible material, making extensive use of bones. The dog was presented to the clinic staff after six months with a decreased appetite and weight loss. A full blood count, biochemistry and urinalysis were performed. No abnormalities were detected in the complete blood count. Serum creatinine levels were increased (2.54 mg/dl; range 0.5-1.25mg/dl) and urea was increased (166 mg/dl; range 15-45 mg/dl).

Urinalysis showed a specific gravity of 1.010 (range 1.025-1.035) and a protein:creatinine ration of 0:23. The patient was placed alone in a kennel, and 1 day later started vomiting and had a mild gastric dilatation. Ultrasound examination showed the presence of a hypo-echoic mass (3:52 cm) at the

antrum of the pylorus blocking the gastric outflow. An ultrasound-guided fine needle aspirate was taken of the mass. Cytological examination was non diagnostic due to significant blood contamination. Two days later the dog showed an evident gastric dilatation and an emergency decompression and gastric lavage was performed. Later the mass was surgically excised and sent for histological examination. The histology report indicated a leiomyoma of the pyloric wall (Fig. 1) with large areas of necrosis and haemorrhage of an ischemic regressive character. The dog was followed up for a period of one year after the surgery. During this period there was no recurrence of the vomiting or pica and no abnormalities were detected in the serum creatinine levels, urea and urine specific gravity in the following biochemistry and urinalysis performed.

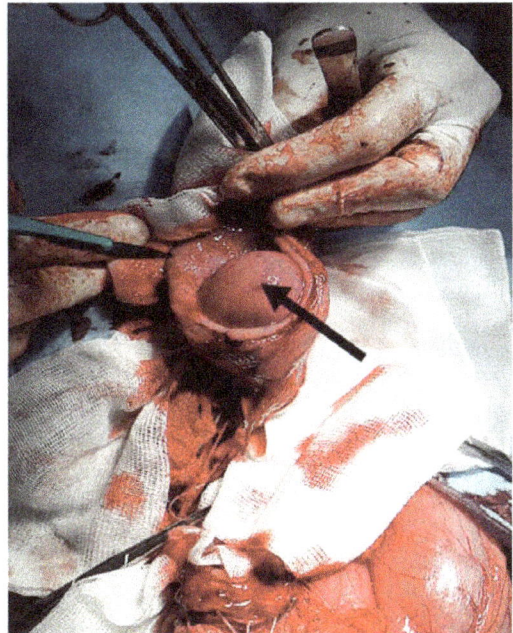

Figure 1. Pyloric leiomyoma: the arrow indicates the mass (3:52 cm) at the antrum of the pylorus

DISCUSSION

Pica and the biting and/or licking of surfaces such as floors, carpets and finishes with a frequency, duration and intensity excessive compared to a normal exploratory behaviour, are often classified as compulsive disorders (6, 7, 8). According to authors these repetitive and exaggerated behaviours can be caused by situations of conflict, stress and anxiety, and can be generalized out of this context and interfere with the daily activities (7, 8). Life in kennels can have significant negative effects on the welfare of dogs causing physiological (9) and behavioural changes (10, 11, 12) contributing to the development of potential CD (13) conditions. Pica should be considered primarily as a nonspecific sign that may be the consequence of several clinical conditions, including behavioural disorders (14).

In the submitted clinical case, though the CD disappeared because the dog was redirected to appropriate targets following the behavioural therapy, the persistence of the vomiting, the time lived in kennels, the sudden evolution and the age of the subject are factors that suggest the possible presence of an organic disease. In presentations of pica, in an adult or geriatric dog population, according with the existing literature, it is therefore necessary first to rule out differential diagnoses that take into account the presence of possible organic diseases (especially gastrointestinal) (15); only after having excluded the latter, will it be possible to direct the suspected diagnosis towards a compulsive behaviour.

CONCLUSION

In conclusion, the case report highlights the difficulty of a correct diagnosis and the importance of gastrointestinal disease in the differential diagnosis of pica in dogs. However, more investigations should still be done around pica in an adult or geriatric dog population, by finding a more significant sample data that can highlights further possible causes.

REFERENCES

1. Manteca Vilanova, X. (2003). Etologia clinica veterinaria del perro y del gatto, 3th ed. (pp. 206–208).

2. Overall, K.L. (2001). Paure, ansie e stereotipie: condizioni specifiche che possono rientrare in una diagnosi di OCD; pica. In Prima Edizione Italiana, C.G. Edizioni Medico Scientifiche s.r.l, La Clinica Comportamentale del Cane e del Gatto (pp. 327). PMid:11605091

3. Coppola, C.L., Enns, R.M., Gradin, T. (2006). Noise in the animal shelter environment: building design and the effects of daily noise exposure. J Appl Anim Welf Sci. 9(1): 1–7.
http://dx.doi.org/10.1207/s15327604jaws0901_1
PMid:16649947

4. Sales, G., Hubrecht, R.C., Peyvandi, A., Milligan, S., Shield, B. (1997). Noise in dog kenneling: Is barking a welfare problem for dogs? Appl Anim Behav Sci. 52, 321–329.
http://dx.doi.org/10.1016/S0168-1591(96)01132-X

5. Gazzano, A., Mariti, C., Cozzi, A. et al. (2005). Modificazioni comportamentali nel cane ospitato in canile sanitario. Atti VI Congresso Nazionale So.Fi. Vet., 2-5 giugno, Stintino (Ss).

6. Landsberg, G, Hunthausen, W, Ackerman, L. (2003). Stereotypic and compulsive disorders. In: Handbook of behaviour problems of the dog and cat. (pp. 195-225). Saunders Ltd, Toronto, ON, Canada.

7. Luescher, A.U. (2003). Diagnosis and management of compulsive disorders in dogs and cats. Vet Clin North Am Small Anim Pract. 33, 253-267.
http://dx.doi.org/10.1016/S0195-5616(02)00100-6

8. Tynes, V.V. (2008). Help! My dogs lick everything. Vet Med. 103, 198-211.

9. Hennessy, M.B, Voith, V.L, Mazzei, S.J. et al. (2001). Behaviour and cortisol levels of dogs in a public animal shelter, and an exploration of the ability of these measures to predict problem behaviour after adoption. Appl Anim Behav Sci. 73, 217-273.
http://dx.doi.org/10.1016/S0168-1591(01)00139-3

10. Beerda, B., Schilder, M.B., Bernadina, W. et al. (1999). Chronic stress in dogs subjected to social and spatial restriction: II. Hormonal and immunological responses. Physiol Behav. 66, 243–254.
http://dx.doi.org/10.1016/S0031-9384(98)00290-X

11. Wells, D.L., Hepper, P.G. (2000). Prevalence of behavior problems reported by owners of dogs purchased from an animal rescue shelter. Appl Anim Behav Sci. 69, 55–65.
http://dx.doi.org/10.1016/S0168-1591(00)00118-0

12. Diesel, G., Pfeiffer, D., Brodbelt, D. (2008). Factors affecting the success of rehoming dogs in the UK during 2005. Prev Vet Med. 84, 228-241.
http://dx.doi.org/10.1016/j.prevetmed.2007.12.004
PMid:18243374

13. Stephen, J.M., Ledger, R.A. (2005). An audit of behavioural indicators of poor welfare in kennelled dog in the United Kingdom. JAAWS 8 (2): 79–95.

14. Becuwe-Bonnet, V., Belanger, M.C., Frank, D. et al. (2012). Gastrointestinal disorders in dogs with excessive licking of surfaces. J Vet Behav. 7, 194-204.
http://dx.doi.org/10.1016/j.jveb.2011.07.003

15. Myers, N.C., Penninck, D.G. (1994). Ultrasonographic diagnosis of gastrointestinal smooth muscle tumours in the dog. Veterinary radiology and ultrasound 35(5): 391-397.

5

APPLICATION OF FLUORESCENCE BASED MOLECULAR ASSAYS FOR IMPROVED DETECTION AND TYPING OF *BRUCELLA* STRAINS IN CLINICAL SAMPLES

Kiril Krstevski[1], Ivancho Naletoski[2], Dine Mitrov[1], Slavcho Mrenoshki[1], Iskra Cvetkovikj[1], Aleksandar Janevski[1], Aleksandar Dodovski[1], Igor Djadjovski[1]

[1]Veterinary Institute, Faculty of Veterinary Medicine, Ss. Cyril and Methodius University in Skopje, Republic of Macedonia
[2]Animal Production and Health Section, Joint FAO/IAEA Division, International Atomic Energy Agency, Vienna, Austria

ABSTRACT

Bacteria from the genus *Brucella* are causative agents of brucellosis – a zoonotic disease which affects many wild and domestic animal species and humans. Taking into account the significant socio-economic and public health impact of brucellosis, its control is of great importance for endemic areas. The chosen control strategy could be successful only if adapted to the current epidemiological situation. This implies that a choice of appropriate diagnostic procedures for detection and typing of *Brucella spp.* strains are of essential importance. Significant advancement of molecular techniques and their advantages compared to classical methods, give strong arguments in promotion of these techniques as a powerful tool for comprehensive diagnostics of brucellosis. Considering this, the major tasks of the study were to select and implement molecular tests for detection and genotyping *Brucella* spp. and evaluate their performances using DNA from cultivated *brucellae* (islolates) and limited number of tissue samples from seropositive animals. The obtained results confirmed that implemented real time PCR for *Brucella* spp. detection, as well as MLVA-16 used for genotyping, have excellent analytical sensitivity (4.2 *fg of Brucella* DNA were successfully detected and genotyped). Furthermore, compared to bacteriological cultivation of *Brucella* spp., real time PCR and MLVA-16 protocols showed superior diagnostic sensitivity and detected *Brucella* DNA in tissues from which *Brucella* could not be cultivated. Based on the summarized study results, we propose a diagnostic algorithm for detection and genotyping of *Brucella* spp. bacteria. Routine use of proposed diagnostic algorithm will improve the effectiveness of infection confirmation and help for accurate evaluation of epidemiological situation.

Key words: brucellosis, clinical samples, DNA, real time PCR, MLVA-16

INTRODUCTION

Bacteria from the genus *Brucella* are causative agents of brucellosis – a zoonotic disease which affects many wild and domestic animal species and humans. Currently, ten *Brucella* species are officially recognized: *B.melitensis, B. abortus, B. suis,*

Corresponding author: Assist. Prof. Kiril Krstevski, DVM, MSc, PhD
E-mail address: krstevski@fvm.ukim.edu.mk
Present address: Veterinary Institute, Faculty of Veterinary Medicine, Ss. Cyril and Methodius University in Skopje, Republic of Macedonia

B. canis, B. ovis, B. neotomae, B. pinnipedialis, B. ceti, B. Microti and *B. inopinata.* This classification of the genus *Brucella* is based on the differences in host preference, pathogenicity, phenotypic traits and genetic structure. However, it is very likely that novel species will be included in the genus soon, mainly as a result of advancement and increased use of molecular diagnostic tools (1).

Infections in animals result in significant economic losses due to induced abortions, infertility, reduced milk and body weight production. Moreover, the presence of brucellosis in animals represents a constant risk for human infections, which are commonly characterized with fever, malaise, sweating and lymphadenopathy (2). In the absence of vaccine for human use, control of human brucellosis remains largely dependent on the control of the disease in animals (3).

Taking into account the significant socio-economic and public health impact of brucellosis, its control is of great importance for endemic areas. Different scientifically approved approaches are available for brucellosis control. However, the chosen control strategy could be successful only if it is adapted to the current epidemiological situation, as well as to the economic and political situation in the country or the region (4, 5). Epidemiology of brucellosis is very complex due to the possible involvement of different mammal (animal) and different *Brucella* species. This fact highlights the importance of the diagnostic procedures for detection and typing of *Brucella*, as powerful epidemiological tools which are indispensable for a successful control program.

The only unequivocal confirmation of *Brucella* spp. infections is laboratory detection and identification of the *brucellae* in the affected organism. Until recently, isolation of *Brucella* has been considered as a gold standard assay for brucellosis diagnosis (6, 7). However, significant advancement of molecular techniques and their increased application in the diagnostic laboratories during the past two decades, has led to the formal recognition of these techniques as valid assays for definite diagnosis of brucellosis (8). Unlike isolation, PCR based molecular tests do not require the presence of vital bacteria in the samples, provide quick and objective results and are safe and relatively easy to perform (7, 9). Moreover, due to the possibility for detection of bacterial DNA even in the samples with small number of *Brucellae*, they have better sensitivity compared to isolation (6, 7, 10). Numerous molecular assays using different targets for *Brucella* spp. identification have been published in the last twenty five years (11-16). Different methods are available for determination of species (17-21), as well as for typing at subspecies level (22-25). Molecular typing based on the analysis of variable number of tandem repeats analysis (VNTRs) in multiple loci (MLVA), provides valuable epidemiological results and is of great value for investigating outbreaks. MLVA testing scheme consisting of 16 genetic loci (MLVA-16) has high discriminatory power at subspecies level and enable differentiation of unrelated *Brucella* spp. strains, which could not be differentiated by classical microbiological methods (26-35). The existence of public database with MLVA-16 allelic profiles (http://mlva.u-psud.fr/brucella/) allows comparison of the typed *Brucella* spp. strains at regional and international level (36). In addition, allelic profiles could be used for species identification or confirmation, if necessary.

The purpose of this study was to establish and evaluate a diagnostic algorithm (flowchart) for *Brucella* spp. detection and typing, which will exploit the advantages of fluorescence-detection based molecular techniques in terms of sensitivity, safety and testing time and hence provide improved brucellosis diagnostics when clinical samples are tested.

MATERIAL AND METHODS

Samples

One isolate of *B. abortus* (field strain MKD-1027), derived from culture collection of the Faculty of Veterinary Medicine-Skopje, and organs from 11 slaughtered seropositive ruminants (Table 3) were used for extraction of genomic DNA. Organs from one animal (spleen, supramammary, iliac and inguinal lymph nodes) were grinded and macerated together in a form of suspension suitable for cultivation, inoculated on selective (*Farrell's*) media and archived at -80°C as "tissue sample". Eleven tissue samples used in the study were randomly selected from the FVMS's collection of tissue samples kept at -80°C.

DNA extraction

Pure bacterial DNA used for implementation and optimization of the test protocols for detection and molecular typing was obtained from the MKD-1027 isolate using *PureLink Genomic DNA kit* (Life Technologies, USA), according to the manufacturer's instructions for Gram negative bacteria. Concentration and purity of extracted bacterial DNA was determined spectrophotometrically (A_{260} and A_{280}) using NanoDrop 2000c (Thermo Scientific, USA). Total genomic DNA was extracted from tissue samples using the same commercial kit, according to the manufacturer's instructions for tissues. The genomic DNA extracted from tissue samples was used to evaluate the performance of implemented testing scheme.

Real time PCR

Genomic DNA from field strain MKD-1027 was used for optimization and performance evaluation of implemented real time PCR for *Brucella* spp. detection. Primers and probe used in the test are targeting *IS711* and are described elsewhere (11). Eight tenfold dilutions corresponding to a DNA concentration range between 1.7 ng/µL and 0.17 fg/µL were prepared from the purified DNA sample and tested in duplicate. Real time PCR reaction was prepared in a final volume of 25 μL using 12.5 μL 2x RT PCR reaction mix for probes (Bio-Rad, USA), 8 μL nuclease-free water, 2 μL primer-probe mix and 2.5 μL of DNA sample. Final concentrations of primers and probe were 0.5 μM and 0.2 μM, respectively. Amplification was performed in IQ5 Thermal Cycler (Bio-Rad, USA) under the following conditions: initial denaturation at 95°C for 5 min and 42 cycles of denaturation at 95°C for 15 s, and combined annealing-extension at 60°C for 30 s. Efficacy of the reaction (E), coefficient of determination (R^2) and slope of the standard curve were calculated using IQ5 software. One of the DNA dilutions with high quantification cycle (*Cq*) value has been defined as a future "positive control sample" and was independently tested ten times. Obtained *Cq* values were used for calculation of coefficient of variation (CV) standing for inter-assay reproducibility and upper and lower limits of the positive control (95% and 99% confidence levels).

MLVA-16 genotyping

For achieving the best analytical sensitivity and repeatability of the capillary electrophoresis system used, all loci from the MLVA-16 panel (22, 24) were amplified in singleplex PCR reactions using 5' - fluorescently (6-FAM) labeled forward primers and *Taq PCR Master mix kit* (Qiagen, USA). Depending on the amount of input DNA, three different protocols for PCR reaction set-up and cycling were used (Table 1).

PCR reactions were set in a total volume of 15 μL (PCR-1 and PCR-2) and 25 μL (PCR-3), containing 1 x Qiagen master mix and 0.5 μM of each primer. All PCR amplifications were performed in a TC412 thermal cycler (Techne, UK).

The size of the PCR products was determined using capillary electrophoresis on ABI 310 system (Applied Biosystems, USA). Briefly, undiluted (PCR-3) or diluted (PCR-1, PCR-2) products have been prepared for electro kinetic injection by adding deionized formamide (Applied Biosystems, USA) and *GS LIZ500* or *GS LIZ1200* (Applied Biosystems, USA) size standards. Amplified loci from referent *B. abortus S19* and *B. melitensis Rev-1* strains were used as a control strains. Fragment sizing was performed by *GeneMapper* software ver. 4.0, according to a generated standard curve. Obtained raw data for the size of each locus was recorded in an excel sheet. Measured fragment size was corrected for the previously determined measuring aberration of the instrument. Corrected values were converted in tandem repeat units using *Table for allele assignment* freely available at MLVA Net for *Brucella* website (http://mlva.u-psud.fr/brucella/spip.php?article93). Aberration in size measuring was determined for each locus by sequencing. Complete sequences of all 16 loci for referent *B. abortus S19* and *B. melitensis Rev-1* strains were obtained using *ABI Prism Big Dye Terminator (v3.1) cycle sequencing ready reaction kit* (Applied Biosystems, USA).

RESULTS

Real time PCR – culture dilutions

Bacterial DNA was detected in seven out of eight tenfold DNA dilutions when tested with the real time PCR assay for detection of *Brucella* spp., corresponding to analytical sensitivity of 4.2 fg bacterial DNA (Fig. 1, Table 2). The implemented test protocol amplified broad range of DNA concentrations (4.2 ng to 4.2 fg) with excellent linearity ($R^2 = 0.997$) and 85.5% reaction efficacy (Fig. 2).

Table 1. Cycling conditions for amplification of VNTR loci for *Brucella* genotyping

STEP	PCR-1	Cycles	PCR-2	Cycles	PCR-3	Cycles
Initial denaturation	94°C, 5 min	1	94°C, 5 min	1	94°C, 5 min	1
Denaturation	94°C,30 s		94°C,30 s		94°C,30 s	
Primer annealing	60°C,30 s	30	60°C, 50 s	35	60°C, 50 s	40
Extension	72°C, 60 s		72°C, 60 s		72°C, 60 s	
Final extension	72°C,5 min	1	72°C, 7min	1	72°C, 10min	1

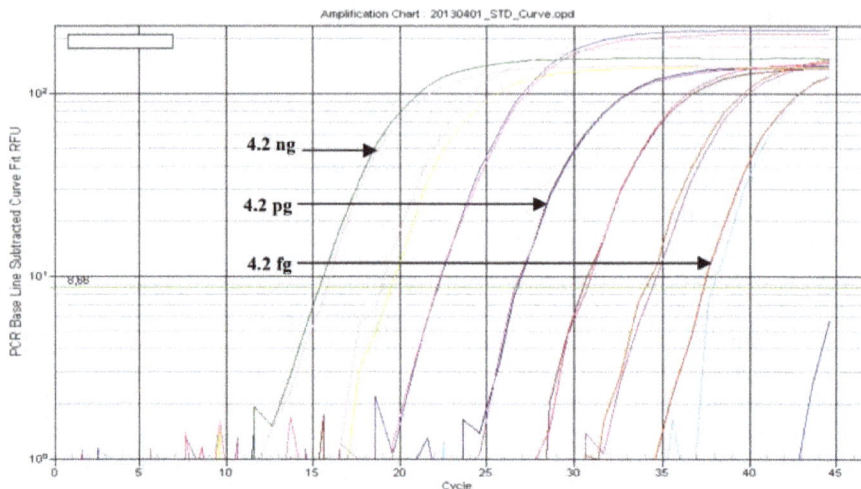

Figure 1. Amplification curves of *B. abortus* (MKD-1027) DNA (log view). Tenfold dilutions (from 4.2 ng to 0.42 fg) were tested with the implemented IS711 real time PCR. Fluorescence data is baseline subtracted

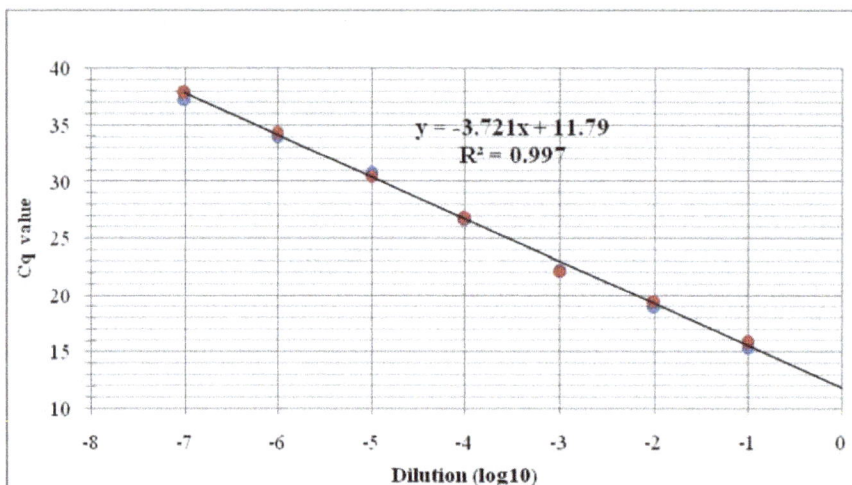

Figure 2. Standard curve obtained after testing tenfold dilutions of *B. abortus* (MKD-1027) DNA with the implemented IS711 real time PCR

Table 2. Tenfold dilutions of *B. abortus* (MKD-1027) DNA with appropriate amounts of DNA in reaction and obtained Cq values (tested in duplicate)

DNA dilution (MKD-1027)	Total amount of DNA in reaction (ng)	*Cq*-1	*Cq*-2	*Cq*-mean
10^{-1}	4.2	15.35	15.78	15.56
10^{-2}	0.42	18.87	19.47	19.17
10^{-3}	0.042	22.07	22.14	22.10
10^{-4}	0.0042	26.63	26.71	26.67
10^{-5}	0.00042	30.71	30.46	30.59
10^{-6}	0.000042	33.97	34.37	34.17
10^{-7}	0.0000042	37.25	37.81	37.53
10^{-8}	0.00000042	/	/	/

Analysis of Cq values obtained in ten independent tests of 10^{-6} *B. abortus* (MKD-1027) DNA dilution, indicated very good reproducibility and inter-assay CV of 1.8%. This DNA dilution has been defined as a positive control for all future runs, with upper and lower Cq limits in the following range: 33 – 34.2 (95% confidence level) and 32.5 – 34.7 (99% confidence level) (data not shown).

MLVA-16 genotyping

The modified PCR protocol (PCR-3) used for amplification, combined with fluorescence based capillary electrophoresis system for detection, enabled detection of all loci from the MLVA-16 scheme, even in the highest real time PCR positive dilution (10^{-7}) of *B. abortus* DNA (Fig. 3). Next dilution (10^{-8}) was negative, meaning that the lower limit of detection of the implemented MLVA-16 typing system was equal to the lower limit of detection observed in the implemented real time PCR for detection of *Brucella* spp. However, PCR-3 protocol should be used only for samples with minor DNA amounts (close to the lower limit of detection), which could not be genotyped using agar-gel electrophoresis. Otherwise, unspecific fragments are likely to appear (Fig. 4), especially if DNA is extracted from clinical samples. The appearance of unspecific fragments could compromise the interpretation of results in situations when their size is very close to the size of existing alleles.

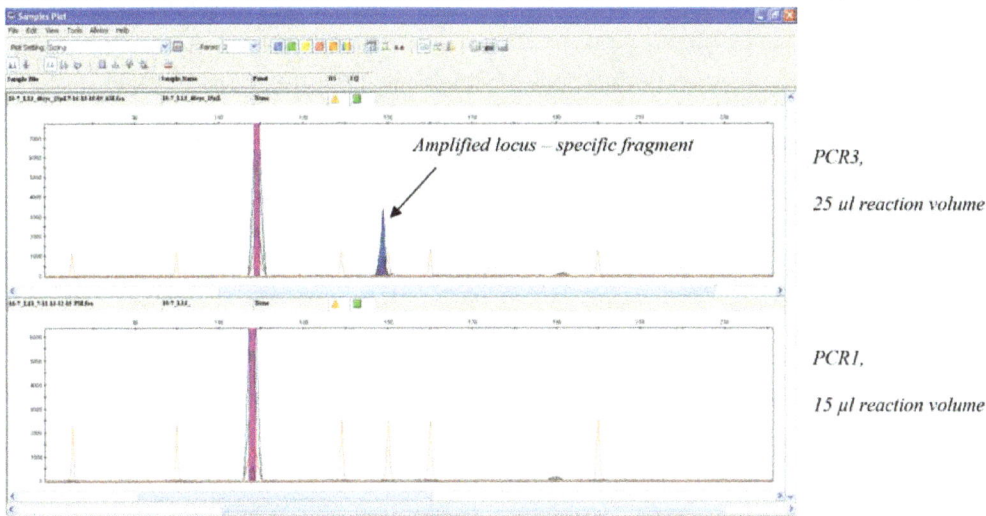

Figure 3. Electropherograms of the products obtained after two different PCR amplifications of bruce30 locus in highest detectable dilution (10^{-7}) of *B. abortus* DNA. Amplified locus was detected only with the modified (PCR-3) protocol (upper electropherogram)

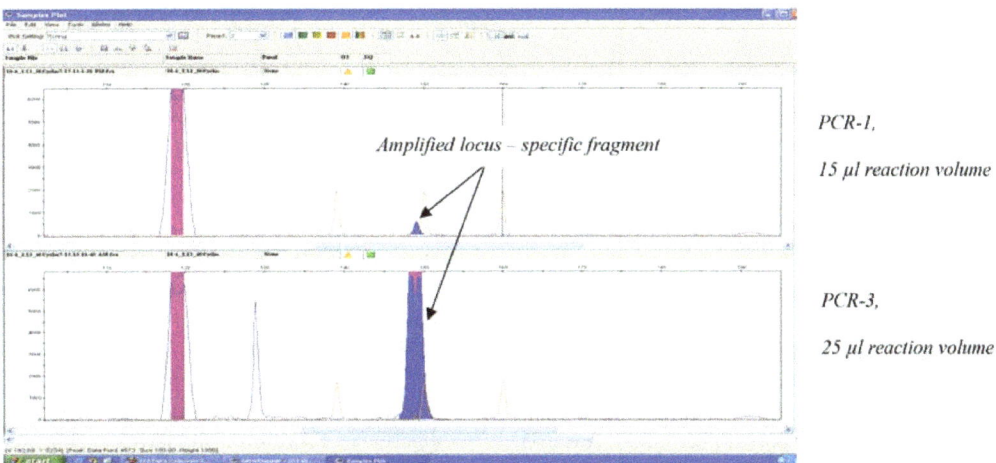

Figure 4. Electropherograms of the products obtained after two different PCR amplifications of bruce30 locus in 10^{-6} dilution of *B. abortus* DNA. Amplified locus was detected with both PCR protocols, but unspecific fragments were present when modified (PCR-3) protocol was used (lower electropherogram)

Real time PCR and genotyping - clinical samples

Brucella spp. DNA was detected in the eleven samples of genomic DNA extracted from the tissues. Obtained *Cq* values varied, indicating different *Brucella* concentrations in the tested samples (Table 3). *Brucella* DNA was detected in seven tissues from which *Brucella* could not be cultivated, although (as expected) with higher *Cq* values. Finally, MLVA-16 profiles were successfully obtained for all samples. There were some reproducibility problems when sample with highest *Cq* value (1-AL) was tested – some of the loci required more than one attempt for obtaining visible signal. This could be explained with low amount of DNA in the 1-AL sample, which was very close to the lower limit of detection of the system.

highly-discriminatory methods for its typing, play important role in the system of eradication.

As previously reported (11), real time PCR targeting *IS711* segment of *Brucella* spp. is a highly sensitive assay and a good candidate for direct testing of clinical samples. In our study, analytical sensitivity of the *IS711* real time PCR assay was 4.2 ng, which is comparable with findings of other authors (11, 37, 38) and proves the robustness of the implemented assay. Theoretically, if we take into account average genome sizes of *Brucella* members, *IS711* real time PCR assay could detect only few bacterial cells. The excellent lower limit of detection is a result of application of real time PCR technology, as well as of the presence of more *IS711* copies throughout the *Brucella* spp. genome.

Table 3. Clinical samples in which *Brucella* DNA was detected by IS711 rt-PCR and MLVA-16 profiles were determined using the described protocols

Sample ID	*Cq* value using *IS711* rt-PCR	ISOLATION (Farrell's medium)	Animal Host	Year
70	18.6	POSITIVE	sheep	2010
4	23.8	POSITIVE	sheep	2010
5	26.0	POSITIVE	sheep	2010
69	27.6	POSITIVE	sheep	2010
689	31.0	negative	sheep	2010
388	34.0	negative	goat	2010
652	35.2	negative	sheep	2010
10_ab	35.6	negative	sheep	2013
11/1	31.8	negative	sheep	2013
2-AL	34.8	negative	cattle	2014
1-AL	36.1	negative	cattle	2014

DISCUSSION

Confirmation of *Brucella* spp. infections is very important for successful control of brucellosis in animals. This is especially evident when the eradication programme is in its late stage and the prevalence of disease significantly decreased (4). In this case, rapid confirmation of suspected infections and successful trace-back of its origin and routes, provide significant support to progress towards complete disease eradication. Hence, the selection of proper laboratory methods for rapid, sensitive and specific detection of *Brucella* spp., as well as

Although the study was not designed to compare the performances of molecular detection and isolation, it confirmed the superior *Brucella* spp. detection capability of the *IS711* real time PCR, compared to the isolation when different clinical samples were tested (Table 3). Our results support the conclusion of other authors (39, 40), that isolation itself is not sufficient for confirmation of infected animals during epidemiological investigations. Therefore, we have established a diagnostic flowchart for *Brucella* spp. detection/ identification based on real time PCR, in addition to isolation on selective media (Fig. 5).

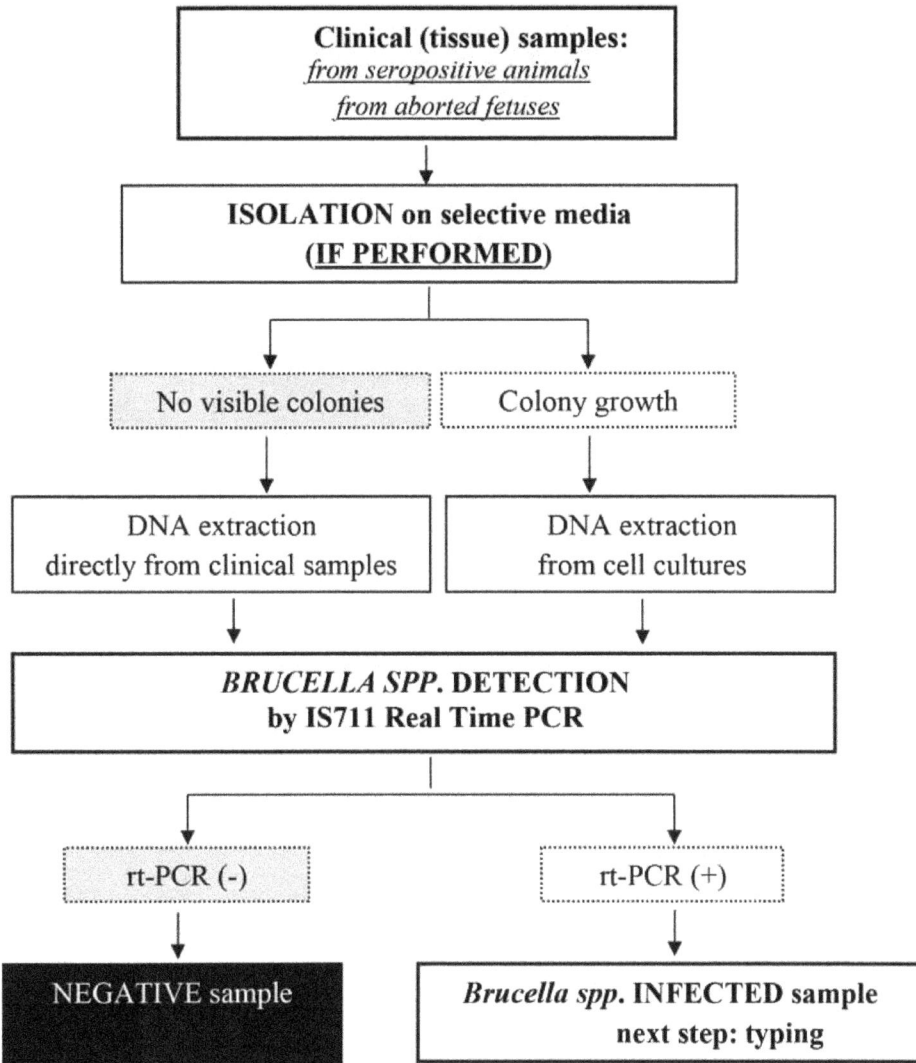

Figure 5. Diagnostic flowchart for *Brucella* spp. detection

Whenever *Brucella* spp. is isolated, all molecular tests for species determination and subspecies typing usually perform well, because a high concentration of bacterial DNA is extracted from colonies. In other words, the analytical sensitivity of molecular methods is not an issue when *Brucella* spp. has been isolated from clinical samples. However, if *Brucella* spp. is not isolated, but is present in the clinical samples in small numbers which are detectable by the *IS711* real time PCR, species and genotype of detected strain could be determined only if highly sensitive technologies are implemented.

The MLVA-16 typing system that we implemented had equal analytical sensitivity with the above mentioned real time PCR for *Brucella* spp. detection (Fig. 3), meaning that MVLA-16 allelic profiles could be obtained for all detected

Brucella spp. strains. This theoretical conclusion was practically evaluated with the successful genotyping of all clinical samples from Table 3. Moreover, quantitative capabilities of the real time PCR technology provide precise quantization of *Brucella* DNA loads in the clinical samples, which is very important for selection of the most appropriate MLVA PCR protocol and successful genotyping. Taking into account that DNA sample obtained from the infected tissue contains huge amounts of host DNA, concentration of *Brucella* DNA could not be measured using the common spectrometric method.

As a summary of all results from the study, we established a diagnostic flowchart for molecular typing of *Brucella* spp. strains (Figure 6) detected using the laboratory approach given in Figure 5.

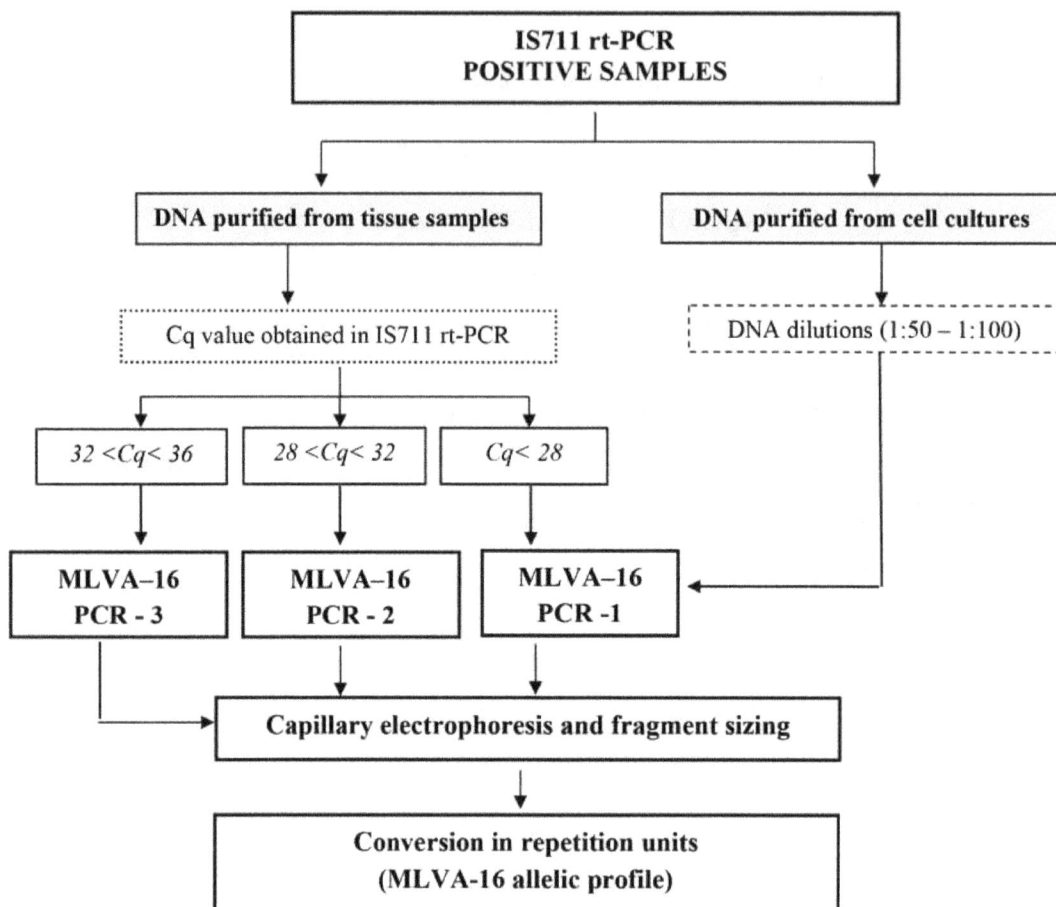

Figure 6. Diagnostic flowchart for genotyping detected *Brucella* spp. strains using MLVA-16

The described testing strategy enables highly sensitive *Brucella* spp. detection, and successful molecular characterization of detected strains. Its application could improve the effectiveness in infection confirmation and provide significant contribution in the accurate evaluation of epidemiological situations.

ACKNOWLEDGEMENT

The authors would like to acknowledge the Joint FAO/IAEA Division and Technical Cooperation Programme of IAEA for the continuous scientific and professional technical support, contributing to the successful upgrading of existing and implementation of new molecular techniques at FVMS.

REFERENCES

1. Scholz, H.C., Vergnaud, G. (2013). Molecular characterisation of Brucella species. Rev. Sci. Tech Off. int. Epiz., 32 (1): 149-162.

2. Whatmore, A. (2011). Current understanding of the genetic diversity of Brucella, an expanding genus of zoonotic pathogens. Infec. Genet. Evol., 9(6): 1168–1184
http://dx.doi.org/10.1016/j.meegid.2009.07.001
PMid:19628055

3. World Health Organization (2005). The control of neglected zoonotic diseases; a route to poverty alleviation. Zoonoses and Veterinary Public Health, WHO, Geneva, Switzerland.

4. European Commission, Directorate General for Health and Consumers (2009). Working Document on Eradication of Bovine, Sheep and Goats Brucellosis in the EU.SANCO/6095/2009. Available at: *http://ec.europa.eu/food/animal/diseases/eradication/eradication_bovine_sheep_goats_brucellosis_en.pdf. last access on 14/7/2015*

5. Scientific Committee on Animal Health and Animal Welfare (2001). Brucellosis in sheep and goat. SANCO.C.2/AH/R23/2001. Available at: *http://ec.europa.eu/food/fs/sc/scah/out59_en.pdf. last access on* 14/7/2015

6. Garin-Bastuji, B., Blasco, J.M., Martın, C., Albert, D. (2006). The diagnosis of brucellosis in sheep and goats, old and new tools. Small Ruminant Research 62, 63–70.
http://dx.doi.org/10.1016/j.smallrumres.2005.08.004

7. Poester, F.P, Nielsen, K., Samartino, L.E, Yu, W. L. (2010). Diagnosis of brucellosis. Open Vet. Sci. J., 4, 46-60.
http://dx.doi.org/10.2174/1874318801004010046

8. World Organization for Animal Health – OIE (2014). Chapter 8.4. Infection with Brucellaabortus, B. melitensis and B. suis. In Terrestrial Animal Health Code. OIE, Paris, 2012.

9. Hornitzky, M., Searson, J. (1986). The relationship between the isolation of Brucella abortus and serological status of infected, nonvaccinated cattle. Aust. Vet. J., 63, 172–174.
http://dx.doi.org/10.1111/j.1751-0813.1986.tb02966.x
PMid:3094489

10. Fekete, A., Bantlem, J.A., Hallingm, S.M., Sanborn, M.R. (1990). Preliminary development of a diagnostic test for Brucella using polymerase chain reaction. J. Appl. Bacteriol., 69, 216-227.
http://dx.doi.org/10.1111/j.1365-2672.1990.tb01512.x

11. Bounaadja, L., Albert, D., Chenais, B., Henault, S., Zygmunt, M.S., Poliak, S., Garin-Bastuji, B. (2009). Real-time PCR for identfication of Brucella spp.: A comparative study of IS711, bcsp31 and per target genes. Vet. Microbiol., 137, 156–164.
http://dx.doi.org/10.1016/j.vetmic.2008.12.023
PMid:19200666

12. Leal-Klevezas, D.S. et al. (1995). Single-step PCR for detection of Brucella spp. from blood and milk of infected animals, J. Clin. Microbiol., 12, 3087.

13. Ouahrani-Bettache, S., Soubrier, M.P., Liautard, J.P. (1996). IS6501-anchored PCR for the detection and identification of Brucella species and strains. J. Appl. Bacteriol., 81, 154–160.
http://dx.doi.org/10.1111/j.1365-2672.1996.tb04493.x
PMid:8760325

14. Rijpens, N.P.,Jannes, G., Van Asbroeck, M., Rossau, R., Herman, L.M. (1996). Direct detection of Brucella spp. in raw milk by PCR and reverse hybridization with 16S-23S rRNA spacer probes. Appl. Environ. Microbiol., 62(5): 1683-1688.
PMid:8633866   PMCid:PMC167942

15. Romero, C.,Gamazo, C., Pardo, M., López-Goñi, I. (1995). Specific detection of Brucella DNA by PCR. J. Clin. Microbiol., 33(3): 615-617.
PMid:7538508   PMCid:PMC227999

16. Yu, W.L., Nielsen, K. (2010). Review of detection of Brucella spp. by polymerase chain reaction. Croat. med. J., 51(4): 306–313.
http://dx.doi.org/10.3325/cmj.2010.51.306
PMid:20718083   PMCid:PMC2931435

17. Bricker, B.J., Halling, S.M. (1994). Differentiation of Brucella abortus bv.1, 2, and 4, Brucella melitensis, Brucella ovis, and Brucella suis bv.1 by PCR. J. Clin. Microbiol., 32, 2660 –2666.
PMid:7852552   PMCid:PMC264138

18. Bricker, B.J., Halling, S.M. (1995). Enhancement of the Brucella AMOS-PCR assay for differentiation of Brucella abortus vaccine strains S19 and RB51. J. Clin. Microbiol., 33, 1640-1642.
PMid:7650203   PMCid:PMC228233

19. Lopez-Goni, I., Garcia-Yoldi, D., Marin, C.M., de Miguel, M.J., Muñoz, P.M., Blasco, J.M., Jacques, I., Grayon, M., Cloeckaert, A., Ferreira, A.C., Cardoso, R., Corrêa de Sá, M.I., Walravens, K., Albert, D., Garin-Bastuji, B. (2008). Evaluation of a multiplex PCR assay (bruce-ladder) for molecular typing of all Brucella species, including the vaccine strains. J. Clin. Microbiol.,46, 3484-3487.
http://dx.doi.org/10.1128/JCM.00837-08
PMid:18716225   PMCid:PMC2566117

20. García-Yoldi, D., Marín, C.M., de Miguel, M.J., Muñoz, P.M., Vizmanos, J.L., López-Goñi, I. (2006). Multiplex PCR assay for the identification and differentiation of all Brucella species and the vaccine strains Brucella abortus S19 and RB51 and Brucella melitensis. Rev1. Clin Chem., 52(4): 779-781.
http://dx.doi.org/10.1373/clinchem.2005.062596
PMid:16595839

21. Probert, W.S., Schrader, K.N., Khuong, N.Y., Bystrom, S.L., Graves, M.H. (2004). Real-time multiplex PCR assay for detection of Brucella spp., B.abortus, and B. melitensis. J. Clin. Microbiol., 42, 1290–1293.
http://dx.doi.org/10.1128/JCM.42.3.1290-1293.2004
PMid:15004098 PMCid:PMC356861

22. Al Dahouk, S., Le Flèche, P., Nöckler, K. et al. (2007). Evaluation of Brucella MLVA typing for human brucellosis. J. Microbiol. Meth., 69, 137–145.
http://dx.doi.org/10.1016/j.mimet.2006.12.015
PMid:17261338

23. Bricker, B.J., Ewalt, D.R., Halling, S.M. (2003). Brucella "HOOF Prints": strain typing by multilocus analysis of variable number tandem repeats (VNTRs). BMC Microbiol., 3, 15.
http://dx.doi.org/10.1186/1471-2180-3-15
PMid:12857351 PMCid:PMC183870

24. Le Flèche, P., Jacques, I., Grayon, M., Al Dahouk, S., Bouchon, P., Denoeud, F., Nockler, K., Neubauer, H., Guilloteau, L.A., Vergnaud G. (2006). Evaluation and selection of tandem repeat loci for a Brucella MLVA typing assay. BMC Microbiol., 6, 9.
http://dx.doi.org/10.1186/1471-2180-6-9
PMid:16469109 PMCid:PMC1513380

25. Whatmore, A.M., Perrett, L.L., Macmillan, A.P. (2007). Characterisation of the genetic diversity of Brucella by multilocus sequencing. BMC Microbiol., 7, 34.
http://dx.doi.org/10.1186/1471-2180-7-34
PMid:17448232 PMCid:PMC1877810

26. Ferreira, A.C., Chambel, L., Tenreiro, T., Cardoso, R. et al. (2012). MLVA16 typing of Portuguese human and animal Brucella melitensis and Brucella abortus isolates. PLoS One 7, e42514.
http://dx.doi.org/10.1371/journal.pone.0042514
PMid:22905141 PMCid:PMC3419166

27. Garofolo, G., Di Giannatale, E., De Massis, F., Zilli, K., Ancora, M., et al. (2013): Investigating genetic diversity of Brucella abortus and Brucella melitensis in Italy with MLVA-16. Infect. Genet. Evol.19, 59–70.
http://dx.doi.org/10.1016/j.meegid.2013.06.021
PMid:23831636

28. Her, M., Kang, S.I., Cho, D.H., Cho, Y.S., Hwang, I.Y., et al. (2009). Application and evaluation of the MLVA typing assay for the Brucella abortus strains isolated in Korea. BMC Microbiol., 9, 230.
http://dx.doi.org/10.1186/1471-2180-9-230
PMid:19863821 PMCid:PMC2774859

29. Jiang, H., Fan, M., Chen, J., Mi, J., Yu, R., et al. (2011). MLVA genotyping of Chinese human Brucella melitensis biovar 1, 2 and 3 isolates. BMC Microbiol., 11, 256.
http://dx.doi.org/10.1186/1471-2180-11-256
PMid:22108057 PMCid:PMC3233519

30. Jiang, H., Wang, H., Xu, L., Hu, G., Ma, J., et al. (2013). MLVA genotyping of Brucella melitensis and Brucella abortus isolates from different animal species and humans and identification of Brucella suis vaccine strain S2 from cattle in China. PLoS One, 8, e76332
http://dx.doi.org/10.1371/journal.pone.0076332

31. Kang, S.I., Heo, E.J., Cho, D., Kim, J.W., Kim, J.Y., et al. (2011). Genetic comparison of Brucella canis isolates by the MLVA assay in South Korea. J. Vet. Med. Sci.73, 779–786.
http://dx.doi.org/10.1292/jvms.10-0334

32. Kiliç, S., Ivanov, I.N., Durmaz, R., Bayraktar, M.R., et al. (2011). Multiple-locus variable-number tandem-repeat analysis genotyping of human Brucella isolates from Turkey. J. Clin. Microbiol. 49, 3276–3283.
http://dx.doi.org/10.1128/JCM.02538-10
PMid:21795514 PMCid:PMC3165627

33. Marianelli, C., Petrucca, A., Pasquali, P., Ciuchini, F., Papadopoulou, S., Cipriani, P. (2008). Use of MLVA-16 typing to trace the source of a laboratory-acquired Brucella infection. J. Hosp. Infect. 68, 274–276.
http://dx.doi.org/10.1016/j.jhin.2008.01.003
PMid:18289724

34. Menshawy, A.M., Perez-Sancho, M., Garcia-Seco, T., Hosein, H.I., García, N., Martinez, I., Sayour, A.E., Goyache, J., Azzam, R.A., Dominguez, L. (2014). Assessment of genetic diversity of zoonotic Brucella spp. recovered from livestock in Egypt using multiple locus VNTR analysis. Biomed. Res. Int., 2014:353876.

35. Mick, V., Le Carrou, G., Corde, Y., Game, Y., Jay, M. et al. (2014). Brucella melitensis in France: Persistence in wildlife and probable spillover from alpine ibex to domestic animals. PLoS ONE, 9(4): e94168.
http://dx.doi.org/10.1371/journal.pone.0094168
PMid:24732322 PMCid:PMC3986073

36. Bosilkovski, M. (2015). Brucellosis: It is not only Malta! In A. Sing (Ed.), Zoonozes – Infections Affecting Humans and Animals (pp. 287-316). Springer Science+Business Media Dordrecht.
ISBN 978-94-017-9456-5.
http://dx.doi.org/10.1007/978-94-017-9457-2_11

37. Newby, D.T., Hadfield, T.L., Roberto, F.F. (2003). Real-time PCR detection of Brucella abortus: a comparative study of SYBR green I, 59-exonuclease, and hybridization probe assays. Appl. Environ. Microbiol., 69, 4753–4759.
http://dx.doi.org/10.1128/AEM.69.8.4753-4759.2003
PMid:12902268 PMCid:PMC169142

38. Redkar, R., Rose, S., Bricker, B., Del Vecchio, V. (2001). Real-time detection of Brucella abortus, Brucella melitensis and Brucella suis. Mol. Cell. Probes, 15, 43–52.
http://dx.doi.org/10.1006/mcpr.2000.0338
PMid:11162079

39. Hinić, V., Brodard, I., Thomann, A., Holub, M., Miserez, R., Abril, C. (2009). IS711-based real-time PCR assay as a tool for detection of Brucella spp. in wild boars and comparison with bacterial isolation and serology. BMC Vet. Res., 5, 22.
http://dx.doi.org/10.1186/1746-6148-5-22
PMid:19602266 PMCid:PMC2719624

40. Ilhan, Z., Aksakal, A., Ekin, I.H., Gulhan, T., Solmaz, H., Erdenlig. S. (2008). Comparison of culture and PCR for the detection of Brucella melitensis in blood and lymphoid tissues of serologically positive and negative slaughtered sheep. Lett. Appl. Microbiol., 46(3): 301–306.
http://dx.doi.org/10.1111/j.1472-765X.2007.02309.x
PMid:18179446

6

BILIARY CLEARANCE OF BROMOSULFOPHTHALEIN IN HEALTHY AND KETOTIC HOLSTEIN COWS

Kirovski Danijela[1], Sladojević Željko[2], Šamanc Horea[3]

[1]Department of Physiology and Biochemistry, Faculty of Veterinary Medicine, University of Belgrade, 11000 Belgrade, Serbia

[2]Veterinary Station ,, Veterina system Sladojević ", 78400 Gradiška Bosna and Herzegovina, Republic of Srpska

[3]Department of Farm Animal Disease, Faculty of Veterinary Medicine, University of Belgrade, 11000 Belgrade, Serbia

ABSTRACT

Ketosis is a metabolic disorder closely associated with liver lipidosis. Numerous tests have been developed to detect hepatic dysfunction in dairy cows. Bromosulfophthalein (BSP) clearance is established as a sensitive index of hepatic function. The objective of this study was to examine the difference of biliary excretion of BSP between ketotic and healthy Holstein cows and to correlate this excretion with other indicators of liver dysfunction. Twenty puerperal Holstein cows divided in two groups (10 cows each) were involved in the study. The first group included healthy and the second group ketotic cows. Blood samples were taken 10 days after parturition. Concentrations of total protein, albumin, total bilirubin, Ca, P, total lipids, urea and glucose were determined. Immediately after blood sampling, BSP test was performed. Blood samples were taken 5 and 45 minutes after injection, and the percentage of retained pigment in the sample obtained at minute 45 was calculated. Blood albumin and glucose concentrations were significantly higher in healthy then ketotic cows. Total bilirubin concentration was significantly higher in ketotic than healthy cows. BSP excretion was significantly higher in ketotic compared to healthy cows. There was a significant positive correlation between BSP values and total bilirubin concentrartions in both healthy and ketotic cows and a significant negative correlation between BSP values and glucose concentrartions in both healthy and ketotic cows. In conclusion, biliary clearance of BSP may be used as a reliable method for the detection of hepatic dysfunction associated with clinical symptoms of ketosis in dairy cows.

Key words: Holstein cows, BSP test, ketosis

INTRODUCTION

Dairy cows are highly susceptible to developing ketosis. Ketosis is a metabolic disorder caracterized by alterations in the metabolism of carbohydrates and lipids. High milk productive, stressed, and cows with hormonal disbalance are predisposed to this disorder which is usually combined with hypoglycemia, hyperketonemia and ketonuria (10).

Corresponding author: Prof. Kirovski Danijela, DVM, PhD
E-mail address: dani@vet.bg.ac.rs
Present address: Faculty of Veterinary Medicine, University of Belgrade, Studentski Trg 1, 11000 Belgrade, Serbia

During early lactation the mammary gland has a priority in nutrient supply, even in the case of clinical ketosis (7, 19). In hypoglicemic ketotic cows the mammary gland uses glucose in the same quantity as the mammary gland in cows with normal glycemia. It indicates that in most critical phases of lactation, when the metabolic processes are on the edge of developing into the ketotic state, the regulatory role of hormones and gluconeogenetic capacity of the liver are of crucial importance (15). The liver capacity to synthesize sufficient quantities of glucose for metabolic needs is most important during pregnancy and lactation. During this period the gluconeogenetic capacity of the liver is disrupted mainly by fatty liver. Fatty liver is a consequence of enhanced and uncontrolled lipid mobilization from body reserves (4). Earlier studies indicate that in ketotic cows fatty liver is very frequent and is crucial for the outcome of the disease. Some authors indicate that cows with severe hepatosteatosis develop ketosis more often than cows with mild fatty liver. Nevertheless it may be supposed that ketosis is a metabolic disorder closely associated with liver lipidosis and that those two diseases are the two most important metabolic disorders during early lactation (6). This is the reason why researchers are still focused on pathomorphological changes in the liver and metabolic tests that can serve as valid indicators of its functional state. Numerous tests have been developed to detect hepatic dysfunction in dairy cows (12). Among others, bromosulfophthalein (BSP) clearance is established as a sensitive index of hepatic function (5, 9).

Bromsulphalein (BSP) test is rarely used in veterinary medicine, especially for monitorinig the excretory capacity of the liver in ketotic cows. For normal pigment excretion, liver blood circulation, hepatocyte function and passage of bile canalicules should be preserved (3, 13). If the liver is healthy, only traces of the total pigment remained in the blood serum 45 minutes after BSP injection. According to Heidrich et al. (8) BSP test is acceptable in cattle to detect liver demage, although greater deviations in pigment retention can be expected in severe liver damages, only.

The objective of this study is to examine the difference of BSP excretion between ketotic and healthy Holstein cows and to correlate these variables to some other indicators of liver dysfunction.

MATERIALS AND METHODS

Twenty puerperal (10 days after calving) Holstein cows were involved in the study. These were divided in two groups (n = 10). The first group of cows included healthy animals and the second group included cows with clinical symptoms of ketosis. The cows were defined as clinically ketotic if they had signs of inappetence, ruminal atony, depression

and their urinary ketone body levels were higher than 17.2 mmol/L. Urine samples were qualitatively determined for ketone bodies using a Rothera test. Rothera's test detects acetone and aceto-acetate but not betahydroxybutyric acid (10). The intensity of the ring color was classified into N (negative), +1, +2 and +3 based on the color reaction of the sodium nitroprusside (SNP) test with a known amount of acetone in aqueous solution at 0 mmol (N), 1 to 3.4 mmol (+1), 3.5 to 17.2 mmol (+2), more than 17.2 mmol (+3), respectively (13). Cases with secondary ketosis (i.e. ketosis that appeared to be secondary to other conditions) were not included in this study.

Blood samples from all cows were taken from the jugular vein just before BSP testing. Separated blood sera were stored at -20°C until use. Concentrations of total protein, albumin, total bilirubin, Ca, P, total lipids, urea and glucose were measured by photometric method using the biochemical analyzer (VetScreen, Biochemical Systems, Italy).

Commercial bromosulphphotalein (Phenoltetra-bromphtalein-dinatriumsulphonat, Darmstadt; 5 % solution) was used for the BSP test. Five mg of BSP per kg of body weight was slowly injected into the jugular vein. One and forty five minutes later blood samples from the contralateral jugular vein were taken. The concentration of BSP in the serum was determined spectrophotometrically. Percent of BSP retention in blood sera 45 minutes after injection was calculated as follows: BSP (%) = A45/A5 x 100 (A45-absorbance measured at wavelength 570 nm in blood samples obtained 45 minutes after injection; A5- absorbance measured at wavelength 570 nm in blood samples obtained 1 minute after injection)

RESULTS

Results for concentrations of main biochemical indicators of hepatic function in healthy and ketotic cows, as well as BSP retention are presented in Table 1.

Table 1. Concentrationas of main biochemical parameters (X ± SD) and BSP excretion (%) in healthy and ketotic cows

Parameter	Healthy cows	Ketotic cows	Signif. of diff. between groups
Total protein (g/L)	75,83 ± 4,99	73,44 ± 7,95	n.s
Albumin (g/L)	37,50 ± 4,15	31,39 ± 6,09	p < 0,05
Total bilirubin (mmol/L)	7,21 ± 3,64	18,01 ± 8,69	p < 0,01
Ca (mmol/L)	2,18 ± 0,20	2,19 ± 0,23	n.s
P (mmol/L)	1,61 ± 0,20	1,58 ± 0,30	n.s
Total lipids (mmol/L)	4,15 ± 0,78	3,67 ± 0,90	n.s
Urea (mmol/L)	3,84 ± 0,63	3,35 ± 1,07	n.s
Glucose (mmol/L)	2,57 ± 0,33	1,79 ± 0,40	p < 0,001
BSP (%)	4,20 ± 2,40	24,90 ± 11,10	p < 0,001

Blood albumin and glucose concentrations were significantly higher in healthy compared to ketotic cows ($p < 0.05$ and $p < 0.001$, respectively) while total bilirubin concentration was significantly higher in ketotic compared to healthy cows ($p < 0.01$). In healthy cows BSP was cleared rapidly from the circulation. When 45 minutes expired, only traces of pigment were present in the sera of healthy cows, while 24.90 ± 11.10 % of the pigment was retained in the blood of ketotic cows. As shown in Table 1, BSP excretion was significantly higher in ketotic compared to healthy cows ($p < 0.001$).

Corelation coefficients between BSP excretion values and main biochemical indicators of hepatic functions of healty and ketotic cows are presented in Table 2.

Table 2. Correlation bettwen BSP excretion (%) and main biochemical parameters in healthy and ketotic cows

Healthy cows	Coeficinet of correlation	Significance
Total protein	-0.130	n.s
Albumin	-0.250	n.s
Total bilirubin	0.760	p < 0.01
Urea	-0.500	n.s
Glucose	-0.816	p < 0.01
Ketotic cows		
Total protein	-0.400	n.s.
Albumin	-0.580	n.s
Total bilirubin	0.800	p < 0.01
Urea	-0.220	n.s.
Glucose	-0.740	p < 0.01

There was a significant positive correlation between BSP values and total bilirubin concentrartions in both healthy ($r = 0.760$; $p < 0.01$) and ketotic cows ($r = 0.800$; $p < 0.01$) and a significant negative correlation between BSP values and glucose concentrations in both healthy ($r = -0.816$; $p < 0.01$) and ketotic cows ($r = -0.740$; $p < 0.01$).

DISCUSSION

Our results for biochemical parametars that are valuable biomarkers of liver function in dairy cows (albumin, total bilirubin and glucose), indicate that synthetic processes in liver are impaired in ketotic cows. Namely, glucose concentration which is good indicator of gluconeogenetic capacity of liver (11) is significantly lower in ketotic cows. Albumin is synthetasied in liver (2) and therefore its concentration was significantly lower in ketotic compared to healthy cows. Total bilirubin concentration is wellknown indicator of fatty liver in dairy cows (1). Total bilirubin concentration was significantly higher in ketotic than healthy cows indicating liver dysfunction in diseased cows. Percent of BSP retaained in blood serum 45 minutes after application of pigment was significantly higher in ketotic cows indicating on slower uptake, conjugation and/or excretion of pigment throught biliary canalicus in ketotic cows. Namely, several investigators (9) have noted a time lag between the uptake of BSP by the liver and its eventual secretion into the bile. They suggested that clearance of the pigment by the liver involves three independent processes: uptake, conjugation and secretion. As known, BSP is mainly taken up by the liver through the organic anion transporting polypeptide families, conjugated with reduced glutathione (GSH) within the hepatocytes by the glutathione-S-transferase (GST), and subsequently excreted into bile by the multidrug resistance associated protein 2 (16), similarly to bilirubin. Impaired clearance of BSP could result from interference with any one or any combination of these processes (14). Our results that indicate on significant positive correlation between BSP retention and total bilirubin concentrations both in ketotic and healthy cows are in accordance with other authors (17). Some authors indicated that elevation of BSP metabolites may be apparent long before any rise in serum bilirubin or aspartate aminotransferase became evident (18). This preferential appearance could be entirely a concentration effect. On the other hand, it is suggested that secretion at the cellular level may involve metabolic processes, some of which are specifically inhibited by metabolic products of damaged liver, and this inhibition produces a "metabolic" obstruction. Due to strong positive correlation between BSP % and bilirubinemia,

it has been suggested that measurement of BSP retention where hyperbilirubinemia exists does not give futher infomration about the liver function. Anyway, the sensitivity of the BSP test may depend on administration of large amounts of the pigment, sufficient to load the various systems involved in its metabolism. This process may be helpful in the detection of slight hepatic functional defects which are not reflected by changes in ie. serum bilirubin or aspartate aminotransferase levels. Since BSP is an exogenous substance, alteration of serum levels by its endogenous production, such as occurs with bilirubin, is not a complicating factor. In addition, BSP and bilirubin may reflect different functions of the liver: mercaptide synthesis and secretion by BSP and glucuronide and sulfate formation by bilirubin. The BSP test becomes in part a measure of a specific biochemical reaction in the liver. Under certain circumstances this reaction may be specifically inhibited while other liver functions proceed. Additionally, there is strong negative correlation between glucose concentrations and BSP excretion indicating that there is some interaction in gluconeogenetic pathways and BSP uptake, conjugation and/or excretion in dairy cows.

CONCLUSION

Based on the obtained results it may be concluded that biliary clearance of bromosulfophthalein may be used as a reliable method for the detection of hepatic dysfunction associated with clinical symptoms of ketosis in dairy cows. Additionally, total bilirubin and glucose concentrations may be good indicators of impaired liver function in puerperal cows.

ACKNOWLEDGEMENTS

This work was supported by Ministry of Science and Technology, Republic of Serbia, Project Grant No 46002.

REFERENCES

1. Acorda, JA., Yamada, H., Ghamsari, SM. (1995). Comparative evaluation of fatty infiltration of the liver in dairy cattle by using blood and serum analysis, ultrasonography, and digital analysis. Vet Q. 1995 Mar;17(1):12-4.

2. Bell, AW., Burhans, WS., Overton, TR., (2000). Protein nutrition in late pregnancy, maternal protein reserves and lactation performance in dairy cows. Proc Nutr Soc. Feb; 59(1):119-26.

3. Berk, PD., Bradbury, M., Zhou, SL., Stump, D., Han, NI. (1996). Characterization of membrane transport processes: lessons from the study of BSP, bilirubin, and fatty acid uptake. Semin Liver Dis. May; 16(2):107-20. Review.

4. Bobe, G., Young, JW., Beitz, DC. (2004). Invited review: pathology, etiology, prevention, and treatment of fatty liver in dairy cows. J Dairy Sci. Oct; 87(10):3105-24. Review.

5. Bordas, JM., Bruguera, M., Rodes, J., Teres, J. (1969). Hepatic clearence of bromosulphalein (BSF) in jaundice. Rev Esp Enferm Apar Dig. Jan;28(1):57-92. Review.

6. Gerloff, BJ. (2000). Dry cow management for the prevention of ketosis and fatty liver in dairy cows. Vet Clin North Am Food Anim Pract. Jul;16(2):283-92.

7. Grummer, RR., Mashek, DG., Hayirli, A. (2004). Dry matter intake and energy balance in the transition period. Vet Clin North Am Food Anim Pract. Nov; 20(3):447-70. Review.

8. Heidrich, HJ., Huhn, JE., Lupke, H. (1962). Ergebnisse der leberfunktionspufung bei der ketose des rindes. W.T.M. 49., 1, 84-92.

9. Ju-Hee, O., Se-Eun, P., Chang-Koo, S., Young-Joo, L. (2009). Biliary clearance of bromosulfophtalein in anesthetized and freely moving conscious rat. Biopharmaceutics and drug disposition, 30, 94-98.

10. Kaneko, J. (1989). Clinical biochemistry of domestic animals, Academic Press, Davis California, 4th Edition: 87-93.

11. LeBlanc, S. (2010). Monitoring metabolic health of dairy cattle in the transition period. J Reprod Dev. Jan; 56 Suppl: (29-35). Review.

12. Rukkwamsuk, T., Wensing, T., Geelen, MJ. (1999). Effect of fatty liver on hepatic gluconeogenesis in periparturient dairy cows. J Dairy Sci. 82(3):500-5.

13. Šamanc, H. (1985). Effects of ACTH on some biochemical and cellular blood components in puerperal ketotic cows. PhD thesis, University of Belgrade.

14. Šamanc, H., Kirovski, Danijela., Stojić, V., Stojanović, D., Vujanac, I., Prodanović, R., Bojković-Kovačević, S. (2011). Application of metabolic profile test in the prediction and diagnosis of fattz liver in Holstein cows. Acta Veterinaria Beograd, 61, 6, 543-553.

15. Sato, T. (1997). Indocyanine green and sulfobromophthalein tests. Nihon Rinsho. 55 Suppl 2:177-9. Review.

16. Soto, A., Foy, BD., Frazier, JM. (2002). Effect of cadmium on bromsulfophthalein kinetics in the isolated perfused rat liver system. Toxicol Sci; 69: 460-469.

17. Steen, A., Grønstøl, H., Torjesen, PA. (1997). Glucose and insulin responses to glucagon injection in dairy cows with ketosis and fatty liver. Zentralbl Veterinarmed A. 44(9-10):521-30.

18. Takikawa, H. (2002). Hepatobiliary transport of bile acids and organic anions. J Hepatobiliary Pancreat Surg 9: 443-447.

19. Torres, AM., MacLaughlin, M., Quaglia, NB., Stremmel, W. (2003). Role of BSP/bilirubin binding protein on p-aminohippurate transport in rat kidney. Mol Cell Biochem Mar; 245 (1-2): 149-56.

20. Vaubourdolle, M., Gufflet, V., Chazouilleres, O., Giboudeau, J., Poupon, R. (1991). Indocyanine green-sulfobromophthalein pharmacokinetics for diagnosing primary biliary cirrhosis and assessing histological severity. Clin Chem. 37 (10 Pt 1): 1688-90.

21. Xia, C., Wang, Z., Xu, C., Zhang, HY. (2012). Concentrations of plasma metabolites, hormones, and mRNA abundance of adipose leptin and hormone-sensitive lipase in ketotic and nonketotic dairy cows. J Vet Intern Med. 26(2):415-7.

7

DETECTION OF HEPATITIS E VIRUS IN FAECES AND LIVER OF PIGS COLLECTED AT TWO SLOVENIAN SLAUGHTERHOUSES

Lainšček Raspor Petra[1], Toplak Ivan[2], Kirbiš Andrej[1]

[1]Institute for Food Hygiene and Bromatology,
University of Ljubljana, Veterinary Faculty, Ljubljana, Slovenia
[2] Institute for Microbiology,
University of Ljubljana, Veterinary Faculty, Ljubljana, Slovenia

ABSTRACT

In recent years there have been numerous reports from different parts of the world describing hepatitis E virus (HEV) as a zoonotic agent, but the clinical cases in humans are still reported only sporadically. Domestic pigs represent the main reservoir of the HEV. Until recently it was believed that the HEV was transmitted only by faecal-oral route, but it has been proved that eating raw or undercooked pork meat and offal can cause acute HEV infection in human. This has triggered the alarm and many developed countries have already done a few studies to assess the percentage of infected pigs.

In this study the situation regarding the risk factor of HEV among pigs that enter the food chain in Slovenia was evaluated. At two different slaughterhouses 87 faeces and liver samples were collected from pigs within two age groups. 32 faeces and liver samples were collected from 3 months old pigs and 55 faeces and liver samples from 6 months old pigs. Animals were brought to the slaughterhouse from different farms located at the north eastern part of Slovenia, where the majority of the pig population is located. Collected samples were analysed with real-time RT-PCR method. Nucleic acids of HEV was found in 6 faeces samples from the younger age group (3 months of age), which represents 19% of examined samples. All liver samples from 3 months old pigs were negative. All samples of faeces and liver from 6 month old pigs were negative. The results were comparable with those from other European countries, where 7-30% of swine faeces samples were found HEV positive.

Key words: hepatitis E virus, pigs, slaughterhouse, undercooked pork meat, zoonosis

INTRODUCTION

Hepatitis E virus is a non-enveloped RNA virus with a polyadenylated, single stranded RNA genome. The genome has three open reading frames (1, 2). It has been classified in the genus *Hepevirus* in the family *Hepeviridae*. Based on the genome sequence analysis the virus is grouped into 4 genotypes, named genotype 1, 2, 3 and 4, that differ by their geographical distribution and host range. Genotype 1 and 2 cause infection only in humans, while genotype 3 and 4 infect also pigs and other mammals (3).

Antibodies for hepatitis E virus have been found in many animal species like pigs, cattle, sheep, goats, horses, cats, dogs, mice and rats. Most data is known about pigs, since they have been mainly investigated (4).

At first, HEV was only causing concerns in developing countries, their biggest problem regarding hepatitis E virus spread was poor sanitation. But lately infections have become a problem also in industrialized countries. It has been proved that eating raw or undercooked swine meat or offal can cause infection in humans (4).

Clinical symptoms in people infected with HEV are typical for hepatitis; abdominal pain, nausea, vomiting, followed by icterus and dark urine (5, 6). In most cases the disease disappears by itself in a few weeks, but if the patient has a history of

Corresponding author: Lainšček Raspor Petra, DVM
E-mail address: Petra.RasporLainscek@vf.uni-lj.si
Present address: Veterinary Faculty University of Ljubljana, Gerbiceva 60, 1000 Ljubljana, Slobenia

hepatic problems it can cause acute liver failure. It affects young to middle age adults and can be fatal in pregnant women, where the mortality is as high as 20% (6).

On the other hand, the symptoms in infected animals are non-existent, except for some hepatocyte necrosis and sometimes slightly enlarged mesenteric lymph nodes (7).

Although most of death cases related to HEV occur in developing countries, the interest in the disease in recent years has been growing in the developed countries. Many of the European countries have been collecting data about the infection status in pigs. From what has been published, we can estimate that approximately 20-40% of domestic pigs up to 6 months old are infected (8).

The situation in Slovenia has been quite poorly inspected so far, we have some data about the condition on a few Slovenian farms, but none from the slaughterhouses (9, 10). Since pigs that enter the slaughterhouse are the ones that end up on the consumers table, we were curious about the infection percentage of those pigs.

be divided into two groups: younger age group – 3 months old pigs and older age group – 6 months old pigs. In total, 87 samples of faeces and 87 samples of liver were collected: 32 from the younger age group and 55 from the older age group. Faeces were sampled directly on the line from the colon of individual pigs. At the same time, a part of liver from the same pig was taken and stored in a separate sterile plastic centrifuge tube. Tubes where then put in a coolbox until being stored in a deep freezer at minus 70°C.

In the laboratory, 1g of samples were homogenized in 5 ml RPMI 1640 (Gibco, Invitrogen) with a homogenizer (IUL masticator). After homogenization, the suspensions of samples were centrifuged for 15 min at $2500 \times g$. The supernatant was recovered and used for the extraction of total RNA. Total viral RNA was extracted from samples using QIAamp® Viral RNA Mini Kit (Qiagen, Germany) according to manufacturer's instructions. For HEV RNA detection in samples rapid and sensitive real-time RT-PCR assay for the detection of four genotypes of HEV was used (11).

MATERIALS AND METHODS

From November 2012 to March 2013, samples of pig faeces and liver were collected at two different slaughterhouses in Slovenia. Pigs originated from 17 different farms, all of them located in the north eastern part of Slovenia (municipalities Ptuj, Gornja Radgona, Destrnik, Ljutomer, Murska Sobota, Tišina, Cerkvenjak, Benedikt, Ključarovci, Lokavec-Sv.Ana, Trate). Pigs that were sampled can

RESULTS

The results of real-time RT-PCR method in 3 months old pigs showed positive results (with cycle threshold value between 33,08 and 41,76) in six faeces samples, while all 32 pigs were negative in liver (Table 1).The results of 55 samples from the older age group (6 months old) were all negative in faeces and liver using real-time RT-PCR for HEV RNA detection (Table 2).

Table 1. Real-time RT-PCR results of fecal and liver samples, 3 months old pigs

	No. of samples	No. of positive samples	Percentage of positive samples (%)
Liver	32	0	0
Faeces	32	6	19

Table 2. Real-time RT-PCR results of fecal and liver samples, 6 months old pigs

	No. of samples	No. of positive samples	Percentage of positive samples (%)
Liver	55	0	0
Faeces	55	0	0

DISCUSSION

The majority of pigs that are brought to the slaughterhouses in Slovenia are around 6 months old. Since these are the animals that end up on the consumer's plate, we decided first to collect samples from this age group and have a look at the situation. All 55 samples of faeces and liver were negative for the presence of HEV RNA. The results did not come as a huge surprise to us: they were not much different from what was found in other European countries, although we didn't expect all the results to be negative. Because the number of samples in this study was rather small these results may not necessarily represent the real situation and further study on larger number of samples should be done.

While searching through the articles and gathering information about the infection of pigs in other countries, we came to the conclusion, that viral RNA is much more frequently found in younger animals. According to the literature the peak of viremia in pigs is from the first to the third month of age (12). As mentioned earlier, pigs slaughtered in Slovenia for consumption are mostly older, but there is also small percent of pigs that are slaughtered younger, at the age of 3 months.

From the 32 samples of faeces 19% (6 samples) were detected as positive in this study. These results are comparable with previous observations on samples collected between 2010 and 2011, when 25,2 % of faeces samples were detected as HEV positive in real-time RT-PCR in pigs between 2 and 4 month old (9).

All 32 liver samples from this study were negative for the presence of HEV RNA. The problem when collecting liver samples is that the HEV infection in liver is focal, so the chances of sampling the right part of the liver are much smaller (13). This could explain why the samples from animals that were tested positive in faeces were at the same time detected as negative for the presence of viral RNA in liver.

Finding viral RNA in faeces of slaughtered animals is alarming in many ways.

The most important is the possibility of cross-contamination of the meat during the evisceration. If such contaminated meat is not properly cooked, it is possible that the virus remains active and it can cause infection in human (12).

There is also a high risk of infection for the workers that are regularly exposed to infected animals. It has been proven that people which are in contact with pigs every day, like workers in a slaughterhouse, have higher prevalence of hepatitis E virus-specific antibodies (14).

Finally, there is also a risk of environmental pollution in case of not properly cleaned effluent.

REFERENCES

1. Vivek, C., Shikha, T., Manjula, K., Shahid, J. (2008). Molecular biology and pathogenesis of hepatitis. E virus. J Biosci., 33, 451-464.

2. Vasickova, P., Psikal, I., Kralik, P., Widen, F., Hubalek, Z., Pavlik, I. (2007). Hepatitis E virus: a review. Vet Med (Praha), 52, 365-384.

3. Song, Y. J. (2010). Studies of hepatitis E virus genotypes. Indian J Med Res., 132, 487-488.

4. Meng, X. J. (2010). Recent advances in hepatitis E virus. J Viral Hepat., 17, 153-161.

5. Chandra, V., Taneja, S., Kalia, M., Jameel, S. (2008). Molecular biology and pathogenesis of hepatitis E virus. J Biosci., 33, 451-464.

6. Teshale, E. H., Hu, D. J., Holmberg, S. D. (2010). The two faces of hepatitis E virus. Clin Infect Dis., 51, 328-34.

7. Lee, Y. H., Ha, Y., Ahn, K. K., Chae, C. (2009). Localisation of hepatitis E virus in experimentally infected pigs. Vet J., 179, 417-421.

8. Berto, A., Backer, J. A., Mesquita, J. R., Nascimento, M. S. J., Banks, M., Martelli, F., Ostanello, F., Angeloni, G., Di Bartolo, I., Ruggeri, F.M., Vasickova, P., Diez-Valcarce, M., Hernandez, M., Rodriguez-Lazaro, D., van der Poel, W.H.M. (2012). Prevalence and transmission of hepatitis E virus in domestic swine populations in different European countries. BMC Res Notes, 5, 190.

9. Toplak, I., Rihtarič, D., Jamnikar Ciglenečki, U., Hostnik, P., Grom, J. (2012). High diversity of hepatitis E virus detected in pig fecal samples in Slovenia. 9th International Congress of Veterinary Virology, Madrid, 2012. ESVV 2012. One world, one health, one virology. Madrid: European Society for Veterinary Virology, 163-164.

10. Naglič, T. (2010). Virus hepatitisa E pri domačih prašičih in v površinskih vodah v Sloveniji. Diploma thesis. University of Ljubljana, Biotechnical faculty.

11. Jothikumar, N., Cromeans, T.L., Robertson, B.H., Meng X.J., Hill, V.R. (2006). A broadly reactive one step real-time RT-PCR assay for rapid and sensitive detection of hepatitis E virus. J Virol Methods, 131, 65-71.

12. Pavio, N., Meng, X.-J., Renou, C. (2010). Zoonotic hepatitis: animal reservoirs and emerging risks. Vet Res., 41, 46.

13. Di Bartolo, I., Ponterio, E., Castellini, L., Ostanello, F., Ruggeri Franco, M. (2011). Viral and antibody HEV prevalence in swine at slaughterhouse in Italy. Vet Microbiol., 149, 330-338.

14. Krumbholz, A., Mohn, U., Lange, J., Motz, M., Wenzel, J., Jilg, W., Walther, M., Zell, R. (2012). Prevalence of hepatitis E virus-specific antibodies in humans with occupational exposure to pigs. Med Microbiol Immunol., 201, 239-244.

8

INFLUENCE OF THE SEASON ON THE METABOLIC PROFILE IN CHIOS SHEEP

Igor Dzadzovski[1], Irena Celeska[2], Igor Ulchar[2],
Aleksandar Janevski[1], Danijela Kirovski[3]

*[1]Farm Animal Health Department, Faculty of Veterinary Medicine Skopje,
Ss. Cyril and Methodius University, Skopje
[2]Department of Pathophysiology, Faculty of Veterinary Medicine Skopje,
Ss. Cyril and Methodius University, Skopje
[3]Department of Physiology and Biochemistry, Faculty of Veterinary Medicine,
University of Belgrade*

ABSTRACT

Chios is a breed of sheep selected for milk production, with metabolic features typical for a dairy sheep breed. The energy requirements of pregnant sheep is increase in the last weeks of gestation. Metabolic imbalance in the late pregnancy in sheep, usually cause a metabolic disorder known as pregnancy toxemia. Additionally, a pregnant sheep exposed to low environmental temperatures has increased energy demands, due to its adaptation to undesirable environmental conditions. The aim of this study was to compare the metabolic profile of Chios sheep exposed to different environmental conditions.Two groups of ewes were instigated. First group included 8 pregnant ewes with clinical signs of pregnancy toxemia exposed to cold stress during the winter season. The second group included 8 non-pregnant, clinically healthy ewes, that were examined during the non-breeding period, in the spring season. Blood samples were taken and serum concentrations of glucose, beta-hydroxybutirate (BHBA), total protein, albumin, urea, creatinine, triglyceride and cholesterol, as well as activity of AST and ALP were determined. Pregnant ewes exposed to cold stress had significantly lower levels of glucose and total protein, and significantly higher levels of BHBA, albumin and AST in the serum compared to non-pregnant ewes that were in optimal environmental conditions. There was no significant difference between the serum levels of urea, creatinine, cholesterol, triglycerides and ALP among the groups. In conclusion, low environmental temperature and poor feeding during the winter season caused metabolic distress in pregnant ewes during the early winter season.

Key words: sheep, season, metabolic profile

INTRODUCTION

Ruminants have different carbohydrate metabolism compared to non-ruminant animals. Namely, dietary glucose in sheep and other ruminants is converted into short-chain volatile fatty acids in the rumen, so the main source of blood glucose is gluconeogenesis in the liver (1), with gluconeogenesis evident even in the fetal sheep liver (2). This also causes blood glucose concentrations to be lower than in non-ruminant animals, and predispose the animal to a negative energy balance (NEB), when energy demands arise. In pregnant ewes, the increased fetal demand is not combined with increaseed endogenous glucose production, so maternal tissues manifest a relative energy deficit, compared with non-pregnant ewes (3). This energy deficit causes mobilization of fatty acids from the adipose tissue which are utilized in the liver, leading to increased level of ketone bodies, especially beta-hydroxibutirate (BHBA) (4). This condition could progress into a very severe metabolic disorder - pregnancy toxemia (5), a disease manifested with neural signs due to the

Corresponding author: Prof. Igor Ulchar, PhD
E-mail: iulcar@fvm.ukim.edu.mk
Address: Faculty of Veterinary Medicine – Skopje
Ss. Cyril and Methodius University in Skopje
Lazar Pop-Trajkov 5/7, 1000 Skopje, R. of Macedonia

fact that glucose is the only energy source for the brain (6). There are various factors which have an impact on energy metabolism and contribute to the development of a negative energy balance (NEB). Those are food intake, starvation (7,8), hormonal status (9,10,11,12,13,14), age and gender (15), twin-bearing (16) and cold stress (17). Pregnancy in sheep commonly occurs during the winter season when animals might be exsposed to cold stress. Exposure to low enviromental temperatures decreases insulin secretion (17). In the condition of a disturbed energy balance, some biochemical parameters in the serum, which are indicators of metabolic disorder and hepatic insufficiency could be changed. These parameters could also be changed due to exposure of animals to extreme enviromental temperatures, as was found in cattle (18). Therefore, the aim of this study was to determine possible seasonal variations of biochemical parameters in Chios sheep.

MATERIAL AND METHODS

Multiparous Chios ewes from one flock in Pelagonia, a region in R. of Macedonia, were chosen for the study. One group of ewes (n=8) were chosen during the early winter season (December), when cows were exposed to cold stress, while the other group (n=8) was chosen during the spring season(May). Ewes examined during the winter season were pregnant and manifested clinical signs

of pregnancy toxemia (inappetence, ataxia, lethargy, weight loss) and ewes investigated during the spring season were non-pregnant and clinically healthy. During the winter period, the flock was exposed to enviromental low temperature and consumed frozen low quality roughage hay, that caused many lesions in the oral mucosa. According to the data from the flock farm, ewes were not treated for endoparasites. Blood samples were taken from each animal included in study, by venepunction from *v. jugularis*. Biochemical parameters that were measured in the blood samples were glucose, BHBA, total protein, albumin, urea, creatinine, triglycerides (TG), cholesterol, AST and ALP. Glucose, total protein, albumin, triglyceride, cholesterol were determined by standard "end point" methods according to the manufacturer's instructions Human, Germany. AST, ALP (Human, Germany) and BHBA (Randox, United Kingdom) were measured by kinetic methods according to the manufacturer's instructions, on semiautomatic photometer STAT Fax 3300 (Awareness Technology, Inc, USA).

RESULTS

The obtained results for concentrations of glucose, BHBA, total protein, albumin, urea, creatinine, triglycerides and cholesterol, and for activity of AST and ALP in examined ewes are shown in Table 1.

Table 1. Concentrations (X±SE) of some biochemical parameters in ewes during different seasons. P values indicate the seasonal effect

Parameter	Pregnant ewes during the winter season	Non-pregnant ewes during the spring season	P value
	mean	mean	n.s
glucose (mmol/L)	1.74 ±0.17	2.96±0.14	< 0.01
BHBA (mmol/L)	1.35±0.05	0.69±0.07	< 0.001
total protein (g/L)	57.56±1.89	68.23±1.25	< 0.01
albumin (g/L)	41.30±2.08	32.05±0.91	< 0.01
urea (mmol/L)	5.47±0.44	5.95±0.50	n.s
creatinine (μmol/L)	116.88±5.76	109.82±6.51	n.s
triglycerides (mmol/L)	0.46±0.13	0.27±0.03	n.s
cholesterol (mmol/L)	2.19±0.21	1.57±0.11	n.s
AST (U/L)	191.49±25.71	95.86±7.09	< 0.05
ALP (U/L)	196.55±26.42	128.35±9.09	n.s

According to the results, the group of pregnat ewes during the winter session had significantly lower level of glucose and total protein (1.74 ± 0.17 mmol/L, and 57.56 ± 1.89 g/L, respectivey) than non-pregnant ewes during spring session (2.96 ± 0.14 mmol/L, and 68.23 ± 1.25 g/L, respectively) (p < 0.01), and significantly higher level of albumin (41.30 ± 2.08 g/L vs. 32.05 ± 0.91 g/L, respectively) (p < 0.01). BHBA levels were significantly higher in pregnant ewes during the winter season (1.35 ± 0.05 mmol/L) than in non-pregnant ewes during the spring season (0.69 ± 0.07 mmol/L) (p < 0.001), and also this was found in levels of AST (191.49 ± 25.71 U/L in pregnant ewes vs. 95.86 ± 7.09 U/L in non-pregnant ewes) (p < 0.05). There were no significant differencies in values of urea, creatinine, triglycerides, cholesterol and ALP between two groups.

DISCUSSION

Pregnant ewes have high energy demands due to intensive fetal growth during the last few weeks of pregnancy (14). Pregnant sheep exposed toextremly low environmental temperatures have to increase generation of heat for maintaining body temperature. This could be obtained by intake of a high-energy diet (19). Due to increased energy demands of pregnant ewes, adaptation to environmental conditions could be compromised, especially if cold exposure is accompanied with fasting. Common metabolic disorder in late pregnancy in sheep, especially in sheep with two or more lambs, known as gravidity toxemiais usually caused by metabolic imbalance and environmental stress (5).

Many investigations with sheep exposed to cold (17, 19, 20, 21, 22) have shown that extremly low enviromental temperature may causes hyperglycemia, due to decreased secretion of insulin from the pancreas (21). This is opposite toour results, which showed significant hypoglycemia in sheep with pregnancy toxemia during the winter season, when animals were exposed to extrimely low enviromental temperature and decreased feed intake. Contrary to this, during the spring period animals showed normoglycemia, which is in accordance with the results obtained on sheep exposed to normal enviromental conditions (17). There was significant difference (p<0.001) in the glucose level between ewes exposed to cold stress (1.74 ± 0.79 mmol/L) and ewes not exposed to cold stress (2.96 ± 0.44 mmol/L). This finding obviously differs from results of others, probably because the latter included fattering breeds of sheep Suffolk (17, 19, 20), Suffolk-Hampshire-Rambouilet crossbred (21),

Corridale-Suffolk crossbred (22), respectively. This suggests possible significant differences in energy metabolism in dairy and fattering breeds of sheep. In pregnant ewes gluconeogenesis does not increase with increased fetal demand, which may causes energy deficit of maternal tissues. This is not a case in non-pregnantewes (3). Low concentration of serum glucose inpregnant ewes is probably the consequence of inappropriate gluconeogenesis in the liver from glucogenoplastic precursors, like propionate that originate from rumen fermentation. Food deprivation, which was evident in pregnant ewes during the winter season, causes lack of propionate precursors for glucose production. Biochemical pathways are further complicated with inappropriate beta-oxidation of acetate and butyrate leading to increased production of acetil-Co-A by hepatocytes. This product is a precursor for aceto-acetyl-Co-A. Aceto-acetyl-Co-A is a primordial molecule for ketone bodies with high effect on acido-base status. This molecule is converted into a very unstable molecule acetoacetate. Reduction of acetoacetate produces BHBA, while irreversible decarboxilation of acetoacetate produces aceton molecules. Excessive concentration of serum BHBAcannot be utilized by extrahepatic tissue, and therefore the serum level of BHBA remainshigh. Significantly marked hyperketonemia was noticed in pregnant (1.35 ± 0.27 mmol/L), but not in non-pregnant sheep (0.69 ± 0.21 mmol/L), though it was not as high as found by other authors (24). The difference in BHBA concentrations between pregnant and non-pregnant sheep was significant (p<0.001), due to decreased alimentary energy resources in pregnant sheep. BHBA is an indirect indicator of negative energy balance, and season variation during the late spring period showed lower serum concentration as a result of better energy supply.

Insufficient energy derived by carbohydrate metabolism causes lipolysis, but energy derived from free fatty acids cannot be adequatelly used in Krebs cycle, because of a lack of oxalacetate, derived from glycogenic precursors. The hepatic capacity for metabolizing of non-esterified fatty acids (NEFA) released from adipose tissue is overloaded. Physiologicaly, NEFA can be reesterified in triglycerides which are included in the formation of VLDL for secretion in blood. Sheep have a very low capacity for production of VLDL (24), especially breeding and non-breeding sheep compared with sheep in lactation (13), and thereby not capable to produce enough VLDL in condition of compromised lipid metabolism in hepatocites. In that case, TG can not be removed from hepatocytes, remaining in the hepatocytes causing hepatic insufficency. In our study, this was evident by higher serum activity of AST (191.49 ± 117.84 U/L) in pregnant ewes which suffered from severe liver impairment and had decreased liver capacity to maintain gluconeogenesis, compared to non-pregnant ewes (128.35 ± 27.27 U/L) (p<0.05). AST is a liver enzyme that enhances the process of transamination, with oxalacetate, a main metabolite in Krebs cycle, as a final product. As a cytosol enzyme with many isoformes it can easily passthe hepatocyte membrane,so increased serum activity of AST indicates an over loaded hepatocyte activity. Thus, in our study the liver was affected by metabolic distress during the critical period and further complicated by lack of alimentary glycogenic precursors. Homeostatic regulatory mechanisms are disrupted, because of neuro-endocrinological requirements in the period of late gestation and lambing. This critical period in the sheep is further complicated with low environmental temperature and high metabolic energy demand. Variations in environmental conditions during the cold season reflects on the energy metabolism, presented through biochemical parameters. So environmental stress, inappropriate feeding management and inappropriate dehelmintisation decompensate liver function and capacity to survive the critical period. Stress hormones, such as high values of serum cortisol level, further enhance the catabolic processes in the extra mammary tissue and skeletal muscles, affecting the body condition score. It is known that pregnancy toxemia is accompanied with increased cortisol level (24).

Particularly, serum protein fractions pattern could give information about dehydration, plasma volume expansion and hepatic function. Particularly, serumprote infractions pattern could give information about dehydration, plasma volume expansion and hepatic function.

Another indicator of liver dysfunction are serum proteins levels, especially albumin, which decrease during hepatic insufficiency. In our study, the albumin level was significantly higher during the winter period in pregnant sheep (41.30 ± 9.53 g/L) compared with non-pregnant sheep (32.05 ± 2.73 g/L) (p<0.001), but in fact this was probably pseudo hyperalbuminemia, as the result of dehydratation, which is related with changes in particular serum protein fractions (25). Dehydraton of sheep appears as a result of the osmotic activity of ketone bodies, because they are very strong acids causing keto-acidotic condition. Lack of water consumption also is one of the main reason for dehydration. Serum concentration of total proteins (68.23 ± 3.76 g/L) showed significantly higher values in non-pregnant sheep during the late spring period, because of regular alimentary protein precursors supply, compared to underfed pregant sheep (57.65 ± 5.44 g/L). Status of proteinemia clearly revealed appropriate synthesis and utilization when amino acids precursors are supplied from alimentary recourses. Statistically significant lower concentration of total proteins (p<0.001) in pregnant ewes during the winter period is a result of proteolysis, caused by energy deficit.

There was no significant difference between serum concentrations of urea, creatinine, cholesterol and ALP in pregnant sheep during the winter period (5.47 ± 2.04 mmol/L; 116.88 ± 26.41 µmol/l; 2.19 ± 1.00 mmol/L, 196.55 ± 121.10 U/L, respectively), and non-pregnant sheep during the spring period (5.95 ± 1.51 mmol/L; 109.82 ± 19.54 µmol/l; 1.57 ± 0.35 mmol/L; 128.35 ± 27.27 U/L respectively), and these values were all within physiological ranges (26). Also, serum concentrations of triglycerides (0.46 ± 0.60 mmol/L) in pregnant sheep showed mild decrease of values, probably due to reesterification of triglycerides in hepatocytes, but it was not statistically significant compared with non-pregnant sheep (0.27 ± 0.10 mmol/L).

CONCLUSION

Metabolic pathways in pregnant ewes were not able to overcome the negative energy balance during the winter period. On the contrary, the spring period favorably affected the energy status of Chios sheep. During the winter period, the Chios sheep were in an inadequate energy status during late pregnancy and lambing when poor feeding management occurred. Glucose and BHBA concentrations could be reliable indicators of negative energy balance and gravidity toxemia in Chios sheep.

REFERENCES

1. Wang, J., Zhu, X., Chen, C., Li, X., Gao, Y., Li, P., Zhang, Y., Long, M., Wang, Z., Liu, G. (2012). Effect of insulin-like growth factor-1 (IGF-1) on the gluconeogenesis in calf hepatocytes cultured in vitro. Mol Cell Biochem, 362, 1-2, 87-91.
   http://dx.doi.org/10.1007/s11010-011-1130-9
   PMid:22015655

2. Thorn, S.R., Sekar, S.M., Lavezzi, J.R., O'Meara, M.C., Brown, L.D., Hay Jr., W.W., Rozance, P. J. (2012). A physiological increase in insulin suppresses gluconeogenic gene activation in fetal sheep with sustained hypoglycemia. Am J Physiol Regul Integr Comp Physiol 303: R861-R869
   http://dx.doi.org/10.1152/ajpregu.00331.2012

3. Raoofi, A., Jafarian, M., Safi, S., Vatankhah, M. (2013). Fluctuations in energy-related metabolites during the peri-parturition period in Lori-Bakhtiari ewes. Small Rum Res. 109, 1, 64-68. http://dx.doi.org/10.1016/j.smallrumres.2012.06.012

4. Moallem, U., Rozov, A., Gootwine, E., Honig, H. (2012). Plasma concentrations of key metabolites and insulin in late-pregnant ewes carrying 1 to 5 fetuses. JAS, 90, 1, 318-324. http://dx.doi.org/10.2527/jas.2011-3905

5. Radostits O, Gay C, Hinchcliff K., Constable P. (2006). Veterinary Medicine - A textbook of the diseases of cattle, horses, sheep, pigs and goats, 10th Edition. Saunders Ltd.

6. Duehlmeier, R., Fluegge, I., Schwert, B., Ganter, M. (2013). Insulin sensitivity during late gestation in ewes affected by pregnancy toxemia and in ewes with high and low susceptibility to this disorder. J Vet Intern Med. 27, 2, 359-366. http://dx.doi.org/10.1111/jvim.12035 PMid:23397990

7. Verbeek, E., Waas, J.R., Oliver, M.H., McLeay, L.M., Ferguson, D.M., Matthews, L.R. (2012). Motivation to obtain a food reward of pregnant ewes in negative energy balance: Behavioural, metabolic and endocrine considerations. Hormones and Behavior, 62, 2, 162-172. http://dx.doi.org/10.1016/j.yhbeh.2012.06.006 PMid:22789465

8. Cal-Pereyra, L., Benech, A., González-Monta-a, J.R., Acosta-Dibarrat, J., Da Silva, S,. Martína, A. (2015). Changes in the metabolic profile of pregnant ewes to an acute feed restriction in late gestation. N Z Vet J. 63 (3): 141-146. http://dx.doi.org/10.1080/00480169.2014.971083 PMid:25275560

9. Sosa, C., Forcada, F., Meikle, A., Abecia, J.A. (2013). Increase in ovine plasma cortisol at oestrus and its relation with the metabolic status during the sexual cycle in sheep Biological Rhythm Research, 44, 3, 445-449. http://dx.doi.org/10.1080/09291016.2012.704793

10. Plested, P.C., Taylor, E., Brindley, D.N., Vernon, R.G. (1987). Interactions of insulin and dexamethasone in the control of pyruvate kinase activity and glucose metabolism in sheep adipose tissue. Biochem. J. 247 (2), 459-465. PMid:3322264 PMCid:PMC1148430

11. Vernon, R.G., Taylor, E. (1988). Insulin, dexamethasone and their interactions in the control of glucose metabolism in adipose tissue from lactating and nonlactating sheep. Biochem. J. 256 (2), 509-514. PMid:3066347 PMCid:PMC1135439

12. Vernon R.G., Finley, E. (1988). Roles of insulin and growth hormone in the adaptations of fatty acid synthesis in white adipose tissue during the lactation cycle in sheep. Biochem. J. 256 (3), 873-878. PMid:2465000 PMCid:PMC1135497

13. Emmison, N., Agius, L. Zammit, V.A. (1991). Regulation of fatty acid metabolism and gluconeogenesis by growth hormone and insulin in sheep hepatocyte cultures - Effects of lactation and pregnancy. Biochem. J. 274 (1), 21-26. PMid:2001235 PMCid:PMC1149914

14. Regnault, T.R.H., Oddy, H.V., Nancarrow, C., Sriskandarajah, N. Scaramuzzi, R.J. (2004). Glucose-stimulated insulin response in pregnant sheep following acute suppression of plasma non-esterified fatty acid concentrations. Reprod Biol Endocrinol, 2:64 PMid:15352999 PMCid:PMC519029 http://dx.doi.org/10.1186/1477-7827-2-64

15. Kiran, S., Bhutta, A.M., Khan, B.A., Durrani, S., Ali, M., Ali, M., Iqbal, F. (2012). Effect of age and gender on some blood biochemical parameters of apparently healthy small ruminants from Southern Punjab in Pakistan. Asian Pac J Trop Biomed. 2 (4): 304–306. PMCID: PMC1283008 http://dx.doi.org/10.1016/S2221-1691(12)60028-8

16. Rumball, C.W.H., Harding, J.E., Oliver, M.H., Bloomfield, F. H. (2008). Effects of twin pregnancy and periconceptional undernutrition on maternal metabolism, fetal growth and glucose-insulin axis function in ovine pregnancy. J Physiol 586 (5), 1399-1411. http://dx.doi.org/10.1113/jphysiol.2007.144071

17. Sasaki, Y., Takahashi, H. (1980). Insulin Secretion in Sheep Exposed to Cold. J. Physiol., 306, 323-335. http://dx.doi.org/10.1113/jphysiol.1980.sp013399

18. Ulcar I., Celeska I. (2010). Seasonal variations of serum biochemical parameters in dairy cows. Abstracts of Days of Veterinary Medicine 2010, 28-30 October 2010, Ohrid. Mac. Vet. Rev.33 (2), 30

19. Sano, H., Matsunobu, S., Abe, T., Terashima, Y. (1992). Combined Effects of Diet and Cold Exposure on Insulin Responsiveness to Glucose and Tissue Responsiveness to Insulin in Sheep. J. Anim. Sci. 70 (11), 3514-3520. PMid:1459914

20. Sasaki, Y., Takahashi, H. (1983). Insulin response to secretagogues in sheep exposed to cold. J Physiol. 334: 155-167. http://dx.doi.org/10.1113/jphysiol.1983.sp014486

21. Terashima, Y., Tucker, R.E., Deetz, L.E., Degregorio, R.M., Muntifering, R.B., Mitchell, G.E. Jr. (1982) Plasma magnesium levels as influenced by cold exposure in fed or fasted sheep. J Nutr. 112(10): 1914-1920. PMid:6750054

22. Sano, H., Takebayashi, A., Kodama, Y., Nakamura, K., Ito, H., Arino, Y., Fujita, T., Takahashi, H., Ambo, K. (1999). Effects of feed restriction and cold exposure on glucose metabolism in response to feeding and insulin in sheep. J Anim Sci.77(9):2564-2573. PMid:10492466

23. Leat, W.M., Kubasek, F.O., Buttress N. (1976). Plasma lipoproteins of lambs and sheep. Q J Exp Physiol Cogn Med Sci. 61 (3): 193-202.
http://dx.doi.org/10.1113/expphysiol.1976.sp002353

24. Henze, P., Bickhardt, K., Fuhrmann, H., Sallmann, H.P. (1998). Spontaneous pregnancy toxaemia (ketosis) in sheep and the role of insulin. Zentralbl Veterinarmed A. 45 (5): 255-266.
http://dx.doi.org/10.1111/j.1439-0442.1998.tb00825.x
PMid:9719756

25. Piccione, G., Alberghina, D., Marafioti, S., Giannetto, C., Casella, S., Assenza, A., Fazio, F. (2012). Electrophoretic serum protein fraction profile during the different physiological phases in Comisana ewes. Reprod Domest Anim.47(4): 591-595.
http://dx.doi.org/10.1111/j.1439-0531.2011.01925.x
PMid:21988675

26. Pernthaner, A., Baumgartner, W., Jahn, J., Plautz, W., Angel, T. (1993) The hematologic parameters, concentrations of minerals and metabolic products and activities of enzymes in sheep. Berl Munch Tierarztl Wochenschr. 106 (3): 73-79.
PMid:8471013

9

THE INFLUENCE OF NUTRITION (DIET TREATMENT) IN STREPTOZOTOCIN – INDUCED DIABETIC RATS

Chrcheva-Nikolovska Radmila [1], Sekulovski Pavle[1], Jankuloski Dean[1], Angelovski Ljupco[1]

[1]*Faculty of Veterinary Medicine, Ss Cyril and Methodius University, Lazar PopTrajkov 5-7, 1000 Skopje, Republic of Macedonia;*

ABSTRACT

The present study was designated to evaluate the effect of special antidiabetic diet treatment upon oxidative stress parameters in the initial stages of the development of diabetes. Male Wistar strain rats were used as an experimental model, divided into five groups: group 1, control rats; group 2, antidiabetic diet group; group 3, rats with induced diabetes mellitus – diabetic control; group 4, rats with induced diabetes mellitus and diet food, and group 5, rats with induced diabetes mellitus and insulin treatment.

A significant decrease in superoxide dismutase (SOD) and total glutathione (GSH) activities were observed in the liver of diabetic rats when compared with control animals. There was simple evidence that elevation in glucose concentration depress natural antioxidant defense such as SOD and GSH. The observed decrease in SOD activity could result from inactivation by H_2O_2 or by glycation of the enzyme, which have been reported to occur in diabetes. The possible source of oxidative stress in diabetes includes shifts in redox balance resulting from altered carbohydrate and lipid metabolism, increased generation of reactive oxygen species, and decreased level of antioxidant defences such as GSH and SOD. The plasma level of aminotransferases (ALT, AST), creatine kinase (CK), lactate dehydrogenase (LDH) and urea were significantly increased after induction of diabetes, in all groups under treatment. In contrast, rats fed special diet food, have shown slight different, but not significant changes. The decrease in total protein and albumin fraction may be due to microproteinuria and albuminuria, which are important clinical markers of diabetic nephropathy, and/or may be due to increased protein catabolism.

The findings of the present study suggest that special diet formula useful for prevention of progressive hyperglycaemia in age induced diabetes in dogs, could not restore the imbalance of cellular defence mechanism provoked by streptozotocin.

Key words: oxidative stress, liver, hyperglycemia, diabetic rats, diet supplement

INTRODUCTION

Diabetes mellitus is accepted to be the most commonest endocrine disease, which are multi-systemic disorders resulting from the deficiency in the secretion or action of the pancreatic hormone-insulin, which in turn produces profound abnormalities of metabolism (1). Diabetes mellitus is known also in dogs, cats, rats and probably occurs in most mammals, although it is only likely to be diagnosed in laboratory animals (2). At present, there no internationally accepted criteria for the classification of canine diabetes. No laboratory test is readily available to identify the underlying cause of diabetes in dogs, and diagnosis is generally made late in the disease course. If the criteria established for human diabetes are applied to dogs, at least 50% of diabetic dogs would be classified as type 1, because this proportion has been shown to have antibodies against β cells. The reminder probably has other specific type of diabetes that results from pancreatic destruction or chronic insulin resistance (3).

The pathogenesis of diabetes mellitus and the possibility of its management by oral administration of hypoglycaemic agents have stimulated greater

Corresponding author: Ass. Radmila Chrcheva-Nikolovska , MSc

e-mail address: rnikolovska@fvm.ukim.edu.mk
Present address: Food institute, Faculty of Veterinary medicine-Skopje, "Ss. Cyril and Methodius" University in Skopje
Lazar Pop- Trajkov 5-7, 1000 Skopje, R. Macedonia

interest in recent years. Nutrition is one of the most respective factors that had a great influence on maintenance of normal activity in the body determining his health condition. In diabetes mellitus, chronic hyperglycaemia produces multiple biochemical sequels, and diabetes-induced oxidative stress could play a role in the symptoms and progression of the disease (4). Oxidative stress in cells and tissue results from the increased generation of reactive oxygen species and/or from decreases in antioxidant defence potential (5). Several hypotheses have been put forth to explain the genesis of free radicals in diabetes. These include autoxidation processes of glucose, the non-enzymatic and progressive glycation of proteins with the consequently increased formation of glucose-derived advanced glycosylation end products, and enhanced glucose flux through the pathway (6,7,8). According to the hypothesis of, normalizing the increased mitochondrial concentration of reactive oxygen species (ROS), prevents all major pathways for diabetes-induced damage.

The possible hypoglycaemic and antioxidant effect of special-designed animal feed was investigated in order to have new information about the nutrition and its influence on some biochemical parameters, body mass and activities of enzymatic and nonenzymatic antioxidants in the control and diabetic rats, that where feed special or commercial laboratory feed.

MATERIAL AND METHODS

Experimental design

Thirty (30) White *Wistar* strain rats of male gender, 4 months old at the start of the experiment, were used. The animals were obtained from the animal facility of the Department of Physiology and Biochemistry of the Faculty of Natural Sciences and Mathematics, Skopje. Prior the experiment, they were given tap water and pellet diet (Filpaso, 52.11, Skopje, Republic of Macedonia). The components of the commercial feed as listed by manufacturer were: crude fat min. 5.7 % , crude proteins minimum 18 %, carbohydrates minimum 60 %, fibre maximum 4.5%, ash maximum 8 %.

Induction of diabetes in rats and Insulin treatment A single i.p. injection of 55 mg/kg streptozotocin (Sigma Aldrich Chemie, GmbH, Deutschland) dissolved immediately before administration in freshly prepared 50 mM citrate buffer (pH 4.0) was

given to STZ, STZ+Ins. and STZ+Diet rats on day 0. The injections were given after 12 hours of food deprivation. Control animals received an equivalent volume of citrate buffer. The group under insulin treatment received subcutaneous initial dose of 4 to 8U (Novo Rapid, Flex Pen, 2880 Bagsvaerd, Denmark) followed by 1 to 2 U daily to obtain euglicemia. The diabetic and normal animals were kept in the cages separately and their body weight, the levels of serum glucose in all animals were measured and then these quantities were compared.

Dietary characteristics of Purina Veterinary Diets® DCO® brand Canine formula provides complete and balanced nutrition for maintenance of the adult dog and has been formulated to achieve the following characteristics: High level of complex carbohydrates; Increased fibre including soluble fibre; Moderate total dietary fat and calories and high omega 6:3 ratio. The components of the special Purina feed as listed by manufacturer were: crude protein minimum 21%; crude fat minimum 10%; crude fibre maximum. 10%; moisture maximum 12%; Carbohydrate maximum 46%.

*Chemical composition of the special feed: Whole grain corn, dried beet pulp, poultry by-product meal, corn gluten meal, pearled barley, animal fat preserved with mixed-tocopherols (form of Vitamin E), pea fibre, animal digest, calcium phosphate, dried whey, potassium chloride, fish oil, salt, calcium carbonate, L-Lysine monohydrochloride, choline chloride, Vitamin E supplement, zinc sulphate, ferrous sulphate, niacin, manganese sulphate, Vitamin A supplement, calcium pantothenate, thiamine mononitrate, copper sulphate, riboflavin supplement, Vitamin B-12 supplement, pyridoxine hydrochloride, folic acid, Vitamin D-3 supplement, calcium iodide, biotin, menadione sodium bisulphite complex (source of Vitamin K activity), sodium selenite. *15% - a source of fibre.*

Animals were divided into 5 groups as follows:

C -control group: control group of rats (n=6)

Diet - group: healthy rats with diet food *ad libitum* (6);

STZ - group: rats with induced diabetes mellitus – diabetic control (6);

STZ+Diet - group: rats with induced diabetes mellitus and diet food (6);

STZ+Ins. - group: rats with induced diabetes mellitus and insulin (6).

The whole procedure was in accordance with National Institutes of Health guidelines for the care and use of experimental animals. At overnight fast of 12 hours, the animals were sacrificed by exsaquination under ketamine: xylazine anaesthesia (90 mg/kg i.p. and 10 mg/kg, i.p. respectively). For plasma separation, blood samples were collected into tubes with anticoagulant solution. Tissue samples were removed immediately, flash frozen, measured and stored in −80°C until further analysis. Liver tissue, heart, aorta and testes were harvested between 10-12 AM, except for those animals, which died during the experiment.

Plasma biochemical assay - Biochemical parameters were measured in heparinised plasma of rats at the start and the end of the experiment by a photometric clinical chemistry analyser (Olympus, AU 400) using routine clinical chemical assays. Blood samples were collected into tubes after an overnight fast of 12 hours, and centrifuged at 1450 × g at 4°C for 10 minutes.

Tissue antioxidant analysis - *Superoxide dismutase activity* Liver SOD (EC 1.15.1.1) activity was assayed with a method of Winterbourn and co workers (1975), with SOD determination kit (RA20408, Fluka, Biochemika, Steinheim, Germany).

Glutathione reductase activity Liver glutathione reductase (GSSG-Red; EC 1.6.4.2) activity was analysed with a glutathione reductase assay kit (GRSA 114K4000, Sigma-Aldrich, Steinheim, Germany) according to the method of Dolphin et al. (23).

Tissue glutathione content Liver glutathione (GSH) content was measured with a glutathione assay kit (CS0260, Sigma-Aldrich, Steinheim, Germany) according to method described by Akerboom et al. (24).

Protein quantification - The protein content in different tissues was measured according to Lowry et al (25).

Statistical analysis - Statgrafics (version No 5.0) was used for determination of statistical significance using analysis of variance and post-hoc analysis as appropriate. A p<0.05 value was considered significant.

RESULTS

Eighteen hours after STZ administration, and daily thereafter, the animals were weighed, urinalysis were performed for glucose and ketones using Forty-eight hours after STZ administration, all animals that had been treated with STZ displayed glucosourea, hyperglycemia, hypoinsulinemia (data not shown) and a moderate loss of body weight.

After streptozotocin injection, glucose concentration was measured using tail vein blood samples obtained from rats after overnight food deprivation. A glucose level >14mmol/L was considered indicative of diabetes, approximately 48 hours after the experimental groups start with insulin administration (group STZ+Ins.), and fed with diet feed (STZ+Diet.). Blood glucose concentrations were determined from blood samples obtained from the tail vein from all animals (MediSense, Bedford, Mass., USA). The blood glucose concentrations and body weights were monitored weekly throughout the course of the study.

A single intravenous injection of 55 mg/kg dose of Streptozotocin in adult Wistar rats, made pancreas swell and at the end of the experiment it caused degeneration in Langerhans islet beta cells and provoked experimental diabetes mellitus within 3-4 days. Streptozotocin induced one type of diabetes which is similar to diabetes mellitus with non-ketosis hyperglycaemia in some animal species. Three days after degeneration of beta cells, diabetes was induced in all animals.

The effects of a *Purina Veterinars Diets Colitis Canine Formula DCO* are presented:

Table 1. Biochemical data in plasma of control and diabetic rats

Variables	(1th week)	(6 th week)	(6 th week)	(6 th week)	(6 th week)
	Control	Diet	STZ	STZ+Diet	STZ+Ins.
Glucose mM/L	4,4 ± 0,7	4,8 ± 0,3	14 ± 4,4**	12,0 ± 0,6**	6,0 ± 0,4*
Urea mM/L	4,8 ± 1,6	6,6 ± 2,4	9,9 ± 0,4**	8,8± 2,3**	7,0 ± 1,2*
Creatinin µM/L	62,8 ± 8,0	58,2 ± 4,8	77,1 ± 1,6 **	62,8 ± 8,0	64,8 ± 9,7
AST U/L	73,7 ± 15,3	111,4 ± 24,3	142,1±18,6*	210,4 ± 73,6 **	120,8±11,2*
ALT U/L	44,6 ± 4,3	58,8 ± 18,3	158,9 ± 8,6**	130,0 ± 33,4**	98,8 ± 13,9*
CK U/L	321, 7 ± 139,9	456,0 ± 153,8	890,2 ± 143,1**	808,1 ± 160,1**	508,3 ± 157,0*
LDH U/L	1263,1 ± 444,8	1985,2 ± 620,0	4o21,8 ± 1096,4**	3838,8 ± 1058,1**	1941,6 ± 587,2*
tot. Proteins g/L	75,5 ± 3,9	76,9 ± 3,5	78,6±4,3	78,5±5,9	76,3±5,4
Albumins g/L	33,1 ± 2,2	32,1 ± 1,8	26,9±0,4	28,8±3,1	35,7±1,5
Uric acid µM/L	119,2 ± 21,0	103,1 ± 21,3	117,3 ± 19,8	125,8 ± 47,0	72,6 ± 25,8

The biochemical parameters were also analyzed in the normal, diabetic untreated rats, rats with diet food, diabetic treated rats with diet food and diabetic treated rats with insulin. The streptozotocin injected rats developed diabetes as indicated by increased fasting blood glucose values, which were 3 to 3.5 fold higher in STZ groups: $4,4 \pm 0,7$ in control, 14 ± 4.4 in STZ rats and 12.0 ± 0.6 in group STZ + diet fed. Significant reduction of glucose level, were registered in STZ group treated with insulin. The activities of serum AST, ALT and LDH were increased in treated animals compared to control animals, which are AST $210.4 \pm 73,6$; ALT 130.0 ± 33.4; CK 808.1 ± 160.1 and LDH $3838,8 \pm 1058,1$ in treated group compared with AST $73,7 \pm 15,3$; ALT $44,6 \pm 4,3$; CK 321.7 ± 139.9 and LDH $1263.1 \pm 444,8$ in control group.

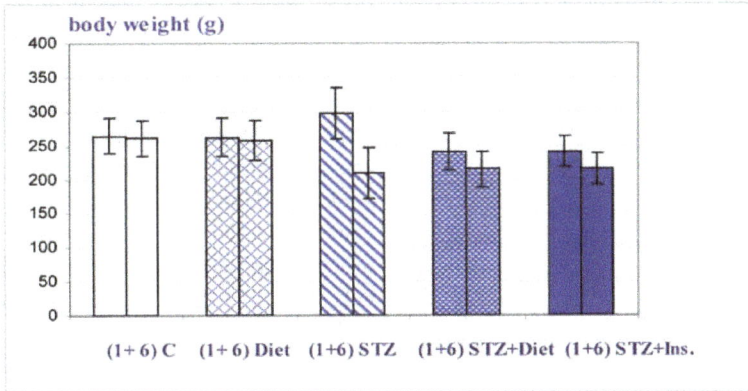

Figure 1. Changes in body weight in control and diabetic rats

The weights of diabetic rats were significantly lower as compared with those in the control group: diabetic animals weighed 210 ± 31 g at the end of experiment, while control animals weight 261.03 ± 29 g at the end of 8th week. Consumption of water, food and serum glucose increases in diabetic animals in comparison with normal rats, followed by decreased in the body weight.

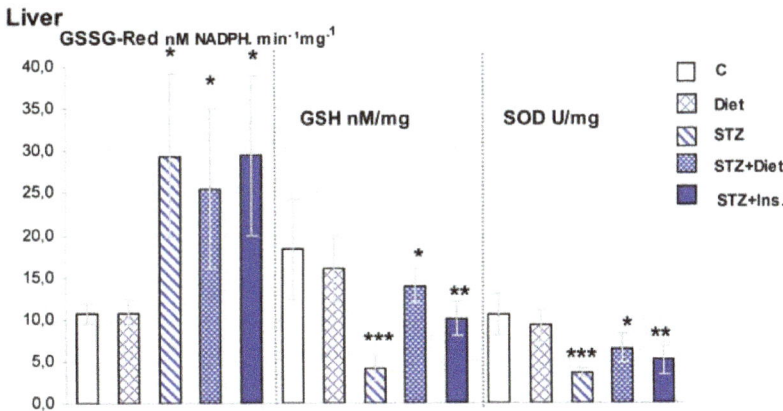

GSSG-red (nM NADPH.min^{-1}mg^{-1})		SOD (U/mg)	GSH (nM/mg)
STZ:C	p<0.05 (177%)	p<0,001(-65,67%)	p<0.001(-77,21%)
STZ+Diet.:C	p<0.05 (139%)	p<0,05 (-38.17%)	p<0.05 (-23,76%)
STZ+Ins.:C	p<0.05 (177%)	p<0,01(-51,48%)	p<0.01 (-45,34%)

Figure 2 and **Table 2.** Oxidation parameters in liver tissue of control and diabetic male rats *significant changes in total glutathione content, activity of glutathione reductase and superoxide dismutase compared with control group, *p< 0.050; ** p<0.01; *** p<0.001.

Fig. 2 demonstrates a significant interaction between glutathione level and glutathione reductase activity in liver tissue. The analyzed results marked that the glutathione content in liver tissue of diabetic animals, was decreased for 77,21 % for group STZ and 24% for STZ+Diet, and decreased for 45,34% for STZ+Ins. Significant enhancements in glutathione reductase activity were achieved in all diabetic groups. In parallel, tissue activity of superoxide dismutase (SOD) within diabetic group tended to decline up to the sixth week compared with respective control.

DISCUSSION

STZ is widely used in studies of experimental diabetes because it selectively destroys the pancreatic β-cell. Researchers around the world have used STZ to create experimental diabetes because it is a simple, inexpensive and available method. Streptozotocin induces one type of diabetes which is similar to diabetes mellitus with non-ketosis hyperglycaemia in some animal species (9).

We performed our experiments 3 days after STZ treatment, considering that this is an adequate interval to address the time point of cell necrosis when STZ is used. In this sense, Doi K., (1975) (10) has determined that 48 h after injection, rats were completely diabetic and microscopic examinations showed pyknosis, degranulation and marked degeneration of β-cells. Hyperglycaemia, hypoinsulinemia, polyphagia, polyuria and polydipsia accompanied by weight loss were seen in adults rats within three days of Streptozotocin treatment and, within one week to ten days, the amounts of the relevant factors were almost stable, which indicates irreversible destruction of Langerhans islets cells moreover. The glucose level was 3 to 3.5 fold higher in the diabetic groups according to baseline during the 6 weeks treatment.

The biochemical parameters were also analyzed in the normal, diabetic untreated rats, diabetic treated rats with diet food and diabetic rats treated with insulin. The streptozotocin injected rats developed diabetes as indicated by increased fasting blood glucose values, followed with decrease in body weight. We marked a slight but significant increase in the level of glucose in group under STZ + insulin administration. This observation is in agreement

with the studies reported by Stephen and Ezekiel (2006) (11).

Since muscle and liver dysfunction is frequently associated with diabetes mellitus, many clinical reports have indicated that serum enzymes activities derived from the muscle and liver such as lactate dehydrogenase (LDH), creatine kinase (CK) and γ glytamil transferase (GGT), are elevated. The plasma level of ALT, AST, CK, LDH and urea were significantly increased after induction of diabetes, in all groups under treatment, in contrast, rats fed special diet food, have shown slight, but not significant changes. The decrease in total protein and albumin fraction may be due to microproteinuria and albuminuria, which are important clinical markers of diabetic nephropathy, and/or may be due to increased protein catabolism (Table 1). This result is consistent with results obtained by Bakris G.L. (1997) (12). Parameters of kidney function, such as urea and creatinine, were slightly reduced after fed with special diet food. This seems to be in accordance with many publishing data (13), describing the effects of different types of mostly antioxidants on markers of artificially induced diabetes. In parallel, the weights of diabetic rats were significantly lower as compared with those in the control group (Fig. 2), which are consistent with results of Kakkar et al. (1998) (14).

In both type 1 and type 2 diabetes mellitus the late diabetic pathological complications are mostly due to excessive elevated production of reactive oxygen species over the capacity of their removal by internal enzymatic and non-enzymatic mechanisms (15). Therefore, additional numerous dietary artificial or natural antioxidants may be of great importance in such cases (16). Figure 2 shows the activity of enzymatic antioxidants such as SOD, GSH and GSSG-Red in the liver of normal, STZ-diabetic animals, Diet, STZ+Diet, and STZ+Ins. group of animals. There were significant reductions in the activity of SOD and GSH in the liver of diabetic rats while the activity of GSSG-Red increased in the liver in diabetic rats. GSH is known to protect the cellular system against the toxic effects of lipid peroxidation. There is also sample evidence that elevation in glucose concentration may depress natural antioxidant defense such as SOD and GSH, SOD scavenges the superoxide radical by converting it to H_2O_2 and molecular oxygen. The activity of SOD was found to be lower in diabetic control rats (17). The observed decrease in SOD activity could result from inactivation by H_2O_2 or by glycation of the enzyme, which have been reported to occur in diabetes (18). The possible source of oxidative stress in diabetes includes shifts in redox balance resulting from altered carbohydrate and lipid metabolism, increased generation of reactive oxygen species, and decreased level of antioxidant defences such as GSH and SOD (19).

CONCLUSION

Hyperglycemia, hypoinsulinemia, polyphagia, polyuria and polydipsia accompanied by weight loss were seen in adults rats within three days of Streptozotocin treatment and, within one week to ten days, the amounts of the relevant factors were almost stable, which indicates irreversible destruction of Langerhans islets cells moreover. Researchers around the world have used STZ to create experimental diabetes because it is a simple, inexpensive and available method.

The role of dietary management in diabetes mellitus is to provide a proper balance of total nutrients while meeting the special dietary needs of the patient. Complex carbohydrates and dietary fiber help to delay the absorption of glucose from the intestinal tract and minimize postprandial fluctuation of glucose. Soluble fiber in the diet may also prolong gastrointestinal transit time, allow greater water absorption, and promote the production of short chain fatty acids which nourish the intestinal mucosa. The findings of the present study suggest that special diet formula useful for prevention of progressive hyperglycaemia in aged depended diabetes in dogs, could not restore the imbalance of cellular defence mechanism provoked by streptozotocin. However, these diabetic induced alteration in ROS production, might be prevented if longer period of supplementation of this hypoglycaemic and antioxidant diet is applied.

REFERENCES

1. Leninger, A.L. (1982): Principles of Biochemistry. New York. Worth Publishers, 712-714.

2. Stewart, M. (1991): Animal Physiology.Holder and Stough Ltd., 313-7.

3. Rand, J.S., Fleeman, L.K., Farrow, H.A., Appleton , D.J. Lederer, R. (2004): Canine and Feline Diabetes mellitus: Nature or Nurture? Amer.Soc. for Nutriton. Scien. 2072S-2080S

4. Guigliano, D.,Ceriello A., Paolissi G.,(1996): Oxidative stress and diabetic vascular complications. Diabets Care, 19: 257-267

5. Gumieniczek, A., Hopkala H., Wojtowich Z., Nikolajuk J. (2002): Changes in antioxidant status of heart muscule tissue in experimental diabetes in rabbits. Acta Biochim. Pol. 49: 529-535

6. Subbiah, R., Karuran, S., Sorimuthu, S. (2005): Antioxidant effect of aloe vera gel extract in streptozotocin-induced diabetes in rats. Pharmacological Reports, 57: 90-96

7. Oberley, L.W.,(1988): Free radicals and diabetes. Free Radical Biol Med., 5:113-124

8. Tiwari, A.K., Rao, J.M. (2002): Diabetes mellitus and multiple therapeutic approaches of phytochemicals: present status and future prospects.Curr Sci, 83:30-38

9. Akbarzadeh A., Norouzian D., Mehrabi M.R., Jamshidi S., Farhangi A., Allah Verdi, Mofidian S.M.A and Rad L., (2007): Induction of diabetes by streptozotocin in rats, Indian Journal of Clinical Biochemistry,22(2):60-64

10. Doi, K. (1975): Studies on the mechanism of the diabetogenic activity of streptozotocin and on the ability of compounds to block the diabetogenic activity of streptozotocin. Nippon Naibunpi Gakkai Zasshi, 51:129-147

11. Stephen, O.A., Ezekiel, A., (2006): Morphological changes and Hypoglycemic Effects of Annona Muricata Linn.(annonaceae) leaf Agueous Extract on pancreatic B-cells of Streptozotocin-treated diabetic rats Caxton-Martins, Afr.J.Biomed.Res.9: 173-187

12. Bakris G.L., (1997): Diabetic neurophaty. Postgrad Med, 89 -93

13. Ulicna, O., Vancova, O., Bozek, P., Carsky, J., Sekekova, K., Br, P., Nakano, M., Greksak, M. (2006): Rooibos Tea (Aspalathus linearis) partially prevents oxidative stress in streptozotocin-induced diabetic rats. Physiol. Res.55:157-164

14. Kakkar, R., Mantha SV., Radhi J., Prasad K, (1998): Increased oxidative stress in rats liver and pacreas during progression of streptozotocin-induced diabetes.Clinical Science, 94: 623-632

15. Bonnefont-Rousselot, D. (2002): Glucose and reactive oxygen species. Curr. Opin. Nutr. Metab. Care 5:561-568

16. Ruhe, R.C., McDonald R.B. (2001): Use of antioxidant nutrients in the prevention and treatment of type 2 diabetes. J. Am. Coll. Nutr. 20:363S-369S

17. McCord, J.M., Keele B.B., Fridovich I., (1976): An enzyme based theory of obligate anaerobiosis. The physiological functions of superoxide dismutase. Proc. Natl. Acad. Sci. USA, 68:1024-1027

18. Sozmen, E.Y., Sozmen, B., Delen, Y., Onat, T. (2001): Catalase/superoxide dismutase (SOD) and catalase/paraoxonase (PON) ratios may implicate poor glycemic control. Arch. Med. Res., 32: 283-287

19. Baynes, J.W. (1991): Role of oxidative stress in the development of complications in diabetes. Diabetes. 40:405-412

20. Valko, M., Rhodes, C.J., Moncol, J., Izakovic, M., Mazur, M. (2006): Free radicals, metals and antioxidants in oxidative stress-induced cancer. ChembioInt. 160: 1-40.

21. Vecera, R., Skottova, N., Vana, P., Kazdova, L., Chmela, Z., Svagera, Z., Walterova, D., Urlichova, J., Simanek, V. (2003): Antioxidant status, Lipoprotein profile and liver lipids in rats fed on high-cholesterol diet containing currant oil rich in n-3 and n-6 polyunsaturated fatty acids. Physiol. Res. 52: 177-187.

22. Winterbourn, C.C., Hawkins, R.E., Brian, M., and Carrell, R.W.(1975) The estimation of red cell superoxide dismutase activity. J. Lab. Clin. Med. 85: 337-341

23. Dolphin, D., Poulson, R., and Avramovic, O., (eds.) (1989), in Glutathione: Chemical, Biochemical and Metabolic Aspects, Vols. A and B, J. Wiley and Sons.

24. Akerboom, T.P., and Sies, H. (1981) Assay of glutathione, glutathione disulfide, and glutathione mixed disulfides in biological samples. Methods Enzymol., 77, 373-382.

25. Lowry, O.H., N.J. Rosebrough, A.L. Farr, and R.J. Randall (1951) Protein Measurement with the Folin Phenol Reagent. J. Biol. Chem. 193:265-275

10

FATTY ACID COMPOSITION OF OSTRICH (*STRUTHIO CAMELUS*) ABDOMINAL ADIPOSE TISSUE

Daniela Belichovska[1], Zehra Hajrulai-Musliu[2], Risto Uzunov[2],
Katerina Belichovska[3], Mila Arapcheska[4]

[1]Faculty of Ecological Resources Management, MIT University in Skopje
[2]Food Institute, Faculty of Veterinary Medicine
Ss. Cyril and Methodius University in Skopje
[3]Institute for Animal Biotechnology, Faculty of Agricultural Sciences and Food
Ss. Cyril and Methodius University in Skopje
[4]Faculty of Biotechnical Sciences, St. Kliment Ohridski University in Bitola

ABSTRACT

Fatty acid composition of foods has a great impact on nutrition and health. Therefore, the determination and knowledge of the fatty acid composition of food is very important for nutrition. Due to the high nutritional characteristics of ostrich meat and its products, the research determining their quality is of topical interest. The aim of the present investigation was the determination of fatty acid composition of ostrich adipose tissue. The content of fatty acids was determined according to AOAC Official Methods of Analysis and determination was performed using a gas chromatograph with a flame-ionization detector (GC-FID). The results are expressed as a percentage of the total content of fatty acids. The method was validated and whereupon the following parameters were determined: linearity, precision, recovery, limit of detection and limit of quantification. The repeatability was within of 0.99 to 2.15%, reproducibility from 2.01 to 4.57%, while recovery ranged from 94.89 to 101.03%. According to these results, this method is accurate and precise and can be used for analysis of fatty acids in foods. It was concluded that the content of saturated fatty acids (SFA) accounted 34.75%, of monounsaturated fatty acids (MUFA) 38.37%, of polyunsaturated fatty acids (PUFA) 26.88%, of total unsaturated fatty acids (UFA) 65.25% and of desirable fatty acids (DFA) (total unsaturated + stearic acid) 70.37% of the analysed samples. The ratio polyunsaturated/saturated fatty acids accounted 0.77. The most present fatty acid is the oleic ($C18:1n9c$) with 28.31%, followed by palmitic ($C16:0$) with 27.12% and linoleic ($C18:2n6c$) acid with 25.08%. Other fatty acids are contained in significantly lower quantities.

Key words: ostrich, adipose tissue, fatty acids, validation, GC-FID

INTRODUCTION

In recent decades the interest for ostrich farms in the world has been growing. Great interest in breeding ostriches has appeared also in the Republic of Macedonia over the past decade. According to our regulations, ostriches belong to farm breeding game (15). Otherwise, besides the major ostrich products (dietetic meat and highly esteemed skin)

Corresponding author: Assoc. Prof. Zehra Hajrulai Musliu, PhD
E-mail address: zhajrulai@fvm.ukim.edu.mk
Present address: Faculty of Veterinary Medicine
Lazar Pop Trajkov 5/7, 1000 Skopje, Macedonia

the by-products, including fat are also utilized in the industry as well.

Fats (extra-muscular) in the ostrich carcass are deposited in the abdominal cavity, breast and back (18). Their quantity, composition and properties vary depending on the type of animal (2, 4), genotype (8), diet (7, 12) age (9), sex (4) etc.

On a live weight basis, 5.2% of the live animal is fat, while carcass contains 9.2% knife separable fat (6). The content of abdominal fat accounted for 4.3% (11), or 5.5% (13). Ostrich fat is used in the food industry as an ingredient of processed meat (8, 10). It is also sold locally, where it is used in cooking, as a source of lard (8), for production of oil which is used in cosmetics (3, 16) and as a supplement to pet food, mainly dogs and cats (10). Today, the production of ostrich meat and oil is constantly increasing. Ostrich oil is a source of various commercial products including moisturizing creams, body lotion, soap and lipbalm (5). Ostrich oil is a high quality oil with high similarity to human skin lipids (19).

The age and the diet of ostriches are in correlation with the fatty acid composition of fat (9). PUFA high content of ostrich adipose tissue could be a source of essential fatty acids in human and animal diets (10). Ostrich fat has a more advantageous composition of fatty acids than porcine (4), beef, sheep and chicken fat (2).

In recent times consumers are becoming increasingly aware of the importance of food and nutrition for their health. Emphasis is placed on the content of cholesterol and fat or fatty acid composition after it was revealed that some aspects of these components may be a risk factor in cardiovascular disease (17). Knowledge of the quality properties of fat, especially of the fatty acid profile, provides a real view about its quality. Fats which contain more unsaturated fatty acids are appreciated.

Given that our knowledge of ostrich fat is still limited, the aim of this study was to examine the content of fatty acids in abdominal ostrich fat.

MATERIAL AND METHODS

The research was performed on abdominal adipose tissue of seven South African Black ostriches (*Struthio camelus* var. *domesticus*), bred in Republic of Macedonia. Ostriches were reared on a farm in Demir Kapija and were fed with 40% alfalfa and 60% mixture of maize, barley, soya bean, sunflower meal, bran, salt, limestone and vitamins. The birds were slaughtered at the age of 13 to 14 months. The content of fatty acids was determined in seven samples which were frozen and stored into polyethylene bags for 21 days at a temperature of 21°C and then slowly thawed.

Analysis of samples

The fatty acids composition was determined according to AOAC Official Method 996.06 (2005). 30 g abdominal adipose tissue was minced and

homogenized, then 0.1 g from the homogenized sample was dissolved in 3.0 ml chloroform and 3.0 ml diethyl ether. The mixture was transferred into a 10 ml glass vial and then evaporated to dryness in 40°C water bath under nitrogen stream. The conversion into fatty acid methyl esters (FAMEs) was achieved by adding 2.0 ml 7% BF_3 reagent and 1.0 ml toluene. The vial was heated in oven at 100 °C for 45 min. Every 10 min the vial was shook gently. After heating, the vial was cooled down to room temperature (20-25°C) and 5.0 ml distilled water, 1.0 ml hexane and 1.0 g sodium sulfate anhydrous were added. The sample was shaken on vortex for 1 min. When the layers were separated, the top layer was transferred into another vial containing 1.0 g sodium sulfate anhydrous. Determinations of FAMEs were carried out on a GC-FID 5890 (Agulent-USA).

Preparation of standards

The individual fatty acid methyl ester standards (FAMEs): myristic acid (C14:0), myristoleic acid (C14:1), pentadecanoic acid (C15:0), palmitic acid (C16:0), palmitoleic acid (C16:1), heptadecanoic acid (C17:1), stearic acid (C18:0), oleic acid (C18:1n9c), linoleic acid (C18:2n6c), conjugated linoleic acid (CLA) were purchased from Sigma (Sigma-Aldrich, Germany). Individual FAMEs standards were used for preparation of stock standard mixture (50 mg/ml) from which six working standards (0.5 – 30.0 mg/ml) were prepared by diluting with n-hexane. Furthermore, from these six working standards calibration curves were produced. For construction of the calibration curve, the aforementioned working standards were analyzed in triplicate. Identification and contents of the fatty acids were carried out by comparing sample FAME peak retention times and peak area with those obtained for FAME mix standard.

Gas chromatograph (GC) analyses

Analyses of the FAMEs were performed on a GC-FID 5890. The analysis was carried out using a column HP88 (J&W 112 -8867; 250°C; 60m x 250mm x 0.2 mm, Agilent, USA). In Table 1 the column temperature parameters are given.

Table 1. Column temperature parameters

	Rate °C/min	Temperature °C	Hold Time min	Run Time min
Initial	/	70	1	1
Ramp 1	5	100	2	9
Ramp 2	10	175	2	18.5
Ramp 3	3	220	5	38.5

Table 2. Linearity of the method

Fatty acids	Retention time (min)	Coefficient of correlation (r^2)
Myristic	20.000	0.99991
Myristoleic	20.851	0.99990
Pentadecanoic	22.016	0.99879
Palmitic	22.759	0.99994
Palmitoleic	23.500	0.99877
Margaroleic	24.479	0.99886
Stearic	25.794	0.99992
Oleic	26.575	0.99983
Linoleic	27.796	0.99998
Conjugated linoleic	29.330	0.99994

Injector and detector temperatures were kept at 250°C and 300°C, respectively. Helium was used as a carrier gas at a flow rate of 1.4 mL/min with split ratio 200:1 and nitrogen was used as a make up gas at a flow rate of 23 mL/min. 1 μL volume of each sample was injected two times into GC-FID for separation and identification of the FAMEs.

Method validation

A guideline for validation of chromatographic methods was used for validation of the method (20). Within the validation procedure linearity, precision and recovery, limit of detection (LOD) and limit of quantification (LOQ) were investigated.

About the data obtained from the examination of the fatty acid profile, arithmetic mean ($\overline{x}$), standard deviation (SD) and coefficient of variation (CV) were calculated.

RESULTS

Linearity

The linearity of the method was estimated by performing of 3 replicates of FAME mix standard solution in a range from 0.5 to 30.0 mg/ml at six concentration levels. Table 2 indicates the retention time and coefficient of correlation (r^2) for fatty acids.

Limit of detection and limit of quantification

The results for LOD and LOQ were calculated from the mean noise value (analysed in six blanks) multiplied by 3 and 10 respectively. In Table 3 values for LOD and LOQ are presented.

Table 3. Limit of detection and limit of quantification

Fatty acids	LOD (μg/ml)	LOQ (μg/ml)
Myristic	0.04	0.17
Myristoleic	0.05	0.14
Pentadecanoic	0.10	0.24
Palmitic	0.05	0.21
Palmitoleic	0.09	0.24
Margaroleic	0.03	0.10
Stearic	0.07	0.24
Oleic	0.09	0.31
Linoleic	0.06	0.28
Conjugated linoleic	0.04	0.23

Table 4. Repeatability, reproducibility and accuracy of the method

Fatty acids	Repeatability (n=6) RSD, %			Reproducibility (n=9) RSD, %			Recovery %
	Sample			Sample			
	1	2	3	1	2	3	
C14:0	1.94	1.71	1.35	3.15	3.28	2.94	95.7
C14:1	1.15	1.43	1.37	2.99	3.14	3.56	97.1
C15:0	1.23	1.10	1.22	2.01	2.15	2.07	94.9
C16:0	1.44	1.36	1.35	2.97	3.01	3.44	98.1
C16:1	0.99	1.14	1.41	3.46	3.42	3.01	97.5
C17:1	1.71	1.46	1.52	3.47	3.36	3.45	94.5
C18:0	1.12	1.41	0.99	2.96	2.84	3.01	101
C18:1n9c	1.47	1.52	1.31	3.14	3.36	3.27	97.5
C18:2n6c	1.22	1.37	1.15	3.71	4.13	4.01	98.1
CLA	1.77	2.01	2.15	4.43	4.57	4.07	96.1

Precision and accuracy of the method

The precision of the method was evaluated through repeatability and reproducibility and the results are expressed as the relative standard deviation (RSD, %) (Table 4). Repeatability of the method was established by six fold analyses of three different samples in one day, while the reproducibility was established by three fold analyses of three different samples in three consecutive days. The recovery (%) of the method was established by spiking a sample with a standard working solution at one concentration level (10.0 mg/ml), and assaying it in triplicate (Table 4). Accuracy of the method was verified through the recovery.

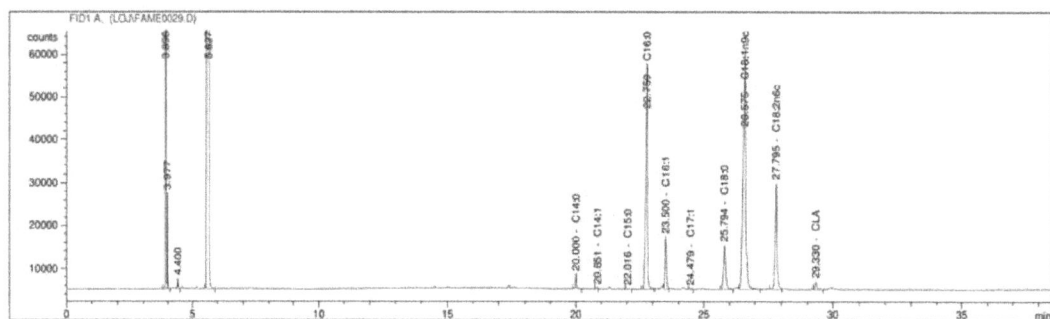

Figure 1. Chromatogram from fatty acid composition in abdominal adipose tissues of ostrich

The fatty acid profile of ostrich fat

The fatty acid composition of the abdominal ostrich fat is presented in Table 5. The results of the examination showed that oleic (28.31%) acid was

Table 5. Mean ($\overline{x}$), standard deviation (SD) and coefficient of variation (CV) for fatty acid composition (% of total fatty acids present) in abdominal ostrich fat (n=7)

Fatty acids		$\overline{x}$	SD	CV
Designation	Trivial name			
C14:0	Myristic	2.16	0.15	6.94
C14:1	Myristoleic	0.20	0.03	15.0
C15:0	Pentadecanoic	0.35	0.10	28.6
C16:0	Palmitic	27.1	1.10	4.06
C16:1	Palmitoleic	9.73	1.50	15.4
C17:1	Margaroleic	0.13	0.02	15.4
C18:0	Stearic	5.12	1.12	21.9
C18:1n9c	Oleic	28.3	2.01	7.10
C18:2n6c	Linoleic	25.1	1.07	4.27
CLA	Conjugated linoleic	1.80	0.20	11.1

presented with the highest percentage, followed by palmitic (27.12%) and linoleic (25.08%) acid. Palmitoleic (9.73%), stearic (5.12%) and myristic (2.16%) acid participated with a significantly lower percentage. Other fatty acids were found in insignificant quantities and will not be discussed.

In the total content of fatty acids (Table 6), MUFA were contained in the greatest amount (38.37%), followed by SFA (34.75%) and least present were PUFA (26.88%). Total UFA participated with 65.25% and DFA with 70.37%. The ratio of polyunsaturated to saturated fatty acids amounted 0.77.

(7), and depending on the genotype from 30.3% to 30.6% (8). Frontczak et al. (4) obtained a lower value (24.98%). Content of stearic acid was nearest to the values (5.34%) (4) and 4.8 to 5.6% (8), and a slightly higher content (6.26%) was found by Sales and Franken (1996) (16) and Hoffman et al. (7) (6.93 to 9.71%).

The abundant MUFA were oleic (28.31%) and palmitoleic (9.73%). These values were higher than those (19.38 to 22.77% and 5.39 to 9.07%) reported by Hoffman et al. (7), while Hoffman et al. (8), Frontczak et al. (4) and Sales and Franken (16) obtained higher values of oleic acid (30.1 to 33.7%,

Table 6. Total fatty acids (%) and ratio between them in ostrich fat (n=7)

Fatty acids	$\overline{X}$	SD	CV
Saturated (SFA)	34.8	2.47	7.11
Monounsaturated (MUFA)	38.4	3.56	9.28
Polyunsaturated (PUFA)	26.9	1.27	4.72
Unsaturated (UFA)	65.3	4.83	7.40
Desirable (DFA)*	70.4	5.95	8.45
PUFA/SFA	0.77	0.02	2.60

* DFA - desirable fatty acids (total unsaturated + stearic acid)

DISCUSSION

Determination of fatty acids is usually carried out by gas chromatography, but in special cases it may be necessary to process separations with high pressure liquid chromatography (HPLC). The highest value of HPLC is for volatile fatty acids (short chain fatty acids), for preparative scale separations or for studying isotopically labeled fatty acids. A rapid and simple method for volatile fatty acids by HPLC analysis with ultraviolet detection has been reported (22). In this study we analyzed biological samples which contain long chain fatty acids in the range from C14 to C24, by using (GC-FID) method as more suitable.

The results of the present study show that in abdominal ostrich fat oleic, palmitic and linoleic acid were presented with highest concentration, followed by palmitoleic, stearic and myristic. A similar sequence of quantitative presence of fatty acids in abdominal ostrich fat was found by other authors as well (4, 8, 16). Such an order was found also in breast ostrich fat (12, 19).

From SFA the mostly present was palmitic (Table 5). Sales and Franken (16) found a similar value (28.44%). Depending on the diet, the content of palmitic acid ranged from 32.50% to 33,47%

42.76% and 36.94%, respectively). Close values for palmitoleic acid (9.2 to 10.5%) were found by Hoffman et al. (8), while Frontczak et al. (4) and Sales and Franken (16) determined lower values (5.89%, 8.44%, respectively).

The concentration of linoleic acid (25.08%), determined in present study was higher than the values reported in the literature (4, 7, 8, 16).

In terms of the total fatty acids content (Table 6), Hoffman et al. (8) reported higher values for MUFA (42.4 to 43.9%) and SFA (37.9 to 40.7%) and lower for PUFA (16.9 to 18.8%).

Frontczak et al. (4) found a higher value for MUFA (51.54%), and lower for SFA (31.26%) and PUFA (17.14%). Hoffman et al. (7) suggested that in the abdominal fat pads SFA dominated (46.71 to 48.92%), followed by MUFA (28.23 to 29.84%) and PUFA (22.28 to 23.52%). The UFA value of 65.25% was slightly lower than that of Frontczak et al. (4) (68.66%).

To assess the nutritional quality of ostrich fat, PUFA/SFA ratio was determined, as well as the content of DFA. Stearic acid, one of the dominant saturated fatty acids has health promotional benefit, i.e. reduces blood cholesterol (14). The value of DFA (70.37%) in the present study, was somewhat lower than the published by Frontczak et al. (4) (74.02%)

and higher than those of Hoffman et al. (8) (64.1 to 67.7%). PUFA/SFA ratio of 0.77 is in compliance with the recommended value (> 0.4) of WHO (21).

The content of the certain fatty acids in the abdominal fat of the African Black ostrich reared in Republic of Macedonia is within the frame of the data published by other authors, but in the present study a slightly higher percentage of PUFA was determined than in the results of other authors. The high content of the unsaturated fatty acids indicates that abdominal ostrich fat has high nutritional value.

CONCLUSION

In abdominal ostrich adipose tissue monounsaturated fatty acids dominate (38.37%). The content of saturated (34.75%) and polyunsaturated (26.88%) is lower. Desirable fatty acids are present in high percentage (70.37%). The oleic (28.31%), palmitic (27.12%) and linoleic (25.08%) are the dominant fatty acids. The ratio of polyunsaturated to saturated fatty acids is in compliance with those recommended by the World Health Organization (> 0.4).

In general, ostrich fat is characterized by a high content of unsaturated fatty acids, unlike other animal fat, so it can be considered as a healthy food and used in different ways in the human diet.

REFERENCES

1. AOAC. (2005). Official Methods of Analysis of AOAC International, 18th Edition. Gaithersburg, MD, USA.

2. Basuny, A.M.M., Arafat, S.M., Nasef, S.L. (2011). Utilization of ostrich oil in foods. Int. Res. J. Biochem. Bioinfor., 2, 199-208.

3. Escobar, S. (2003). Processing of the fat in commercial oil of ostrich.
http://www.world-ostrich.org/download/ostoilen.pdf.

4. Frontczak, M., Krysztofiak, K., Bilska, A., Uchman, W. (2008). Characteristics of fat from African ostrich Struthio camelus. Food Sci. Technol., 11, 420- 428.

5. Grompone, A.M., Irigaray, B., Gil, M. (2005). Uruguayan nandu (Rhea americana) oil: A comparison with emu and ostrich oils. J. Am. Oil Chem. Soc., 82, 687-689.
http://dx.doi.org/10.1007/s11746-005-1130-1

6. Harris, S.D., Morris, C.A., May, S.G., Jackson, T.C., Lucia, L.M., Hale, D.S., Miller, R.K., Keeton, J.T., Savell, J.W., Acuff, G.R. (1994). Ostrich Meat Industry Development. Final report to AOA. Texas Agricultural Extension Service, the Texas A&M University System, College Station, TX, USA.

7. Hoffman, L.C., Joubert, M., Brand, T.S., Manley, M. (2005). The effect of dietary fish oil rich in n – 3 fatty acids on the organoleptic, fatty acid and physicochemical characteristics of ostrich meat. Meat Sci., 70, 45-53.
http://dx.doi.org/10.1016/j.meatsci.2004.11.019
PMid:22063279

8. Hoffman, L.C., Brand, M.M., Cloete, S.W.P., Muller, M. (2012). The fatty acid composition of muscles and fat depots of ostriches as influenced by genotype. S. Afr. J. Anim. Sci., 42, 256-265.
http://dx.doi.org/10.4314/sajas.v42i3.7

9. Horbañczuk, J.O., Cooper, R.G., Jóźwik, A., Klewiec, J., Krzyżewski, J., Malecki, I., Chyliński, W., Wójcik, A., Kawka, M. (2003). Cholesterol content and fatty acid composition of fat from culled breeding ostriches (Struthio camelus). Anim. Sci. Pap. Rep., 21, 271-275.

10. Horbañczuk, J.O., Malecki, I., Cooper, R.G., Jóźwik, A., Klewiec, J., Krzyżewski, J., Khalifa, H., Chyliński, W., Wójcik, A., Kawka, M. (2004). Cholesterol content and fatty acid composition of two fat depots from slaughter ostriches (Struthio camelus) aged 14 months. Anim. Sci. Pap. Rep., 22, 247-251.

11. Morris, C.A., Harris, S.D., May, S.G., Jackson, T.C., Hale, D.S., Miller, R.K., Keeton, J.T., Acuff, G.R., Lucia, L.M., Savell, J.W. (1995). Ostrich slaughter and fabrication: 1. Slaughter yields of carcasses and effects of electrical stimulation on post-mortem pH. Poult. Sci., 74, 1683-1687.
http://dx.doi.org/10.3382/ps.0741683
PMid:8559734

12. Poławska, E., Jóźwik, A., Wójcik, A., Strzałkowska, N., Pierzchała, M., Tolik, D., Półtorak, A., Hoffman, L.C. (2013). Effect of dietary linseed and rapeseed supplementation on fatty acids profiles in the ostriches. Part 2. Fat. Anim. Sci. Pap. Rep., 31, 347-354.

13. Pollok, K.D., Hale, D.S., Miller, R.K., Angel, R., Blue-McLendon, A., Baltmanis, B., Keeton, J.T. (1997). Ostrich slaughter and by-product yields. American Ostrich, 4, 31-35.

14. Rhee, K. S. (1992). Fatty acids in meat and meat products. In: Fatty acids in foods and their health implications. (pp. 65-93).C.K. Chow (Ed.), New York: Marcel Dekker, Inc.

15. Rulebook for specific requirements for food of animal origin, Official Gazette of RM no. 115/2008.

16. Sales, J., Franken, L. (1996). Ostrich fat. Aust. Ostrich Assoc. J., 37, 39-45.

17. Sales, J., Marais, D., Kruger, M. (1996). Fat Content, caloric value, cholesterol content and fatty acid composition of row and cooked ostrich meat. J. Food Compos. Anal., 9, 85-89.
http://dx.doi.org/10.1006/jfca.1996.0010

18. Sales, J., Horba-czuk, J.O., Dingle, J., Coleman, R., Sensik, S. (1999). Carcass characteristics of emus (Dromaius novaehollandiae). Br. Poult. Sci., 40, 145-147. http://dx.doi.org/10.1080/00071669987999 PMid:10405052

19. Shahryar, H.A., Lotfi, A. (2012). Fatty acid composition of fat depot in 11 month old slaughtered ostriches, Struthio camelus L. Current Biotica, 6, 246-250.

20. Taverniers, I., De Loose, M., Van Bockstaele, E. (2004). Trends in quality in the analytical laboratory: Analytical method validation and quality assurance. Trends in analytical chemistry, 23, 535 – 552. http://dx.doi.org/10.1016/j.trac.2004.04.001

21. WHO/FAO. (2003). Diet Nutrition and the Prevention of Chronic Diseases. WHO, Geneve, 4-101 (cit. Poławska et al., 2013).

22. Stein, J., Kulemeier, J., Lembcke, B., Caspary, W.F. (1992). Simple and rapid method for determination of short-chain fatty acids in biological materials by high-performance liquid chromatography with ultraviolet detection. J Chromatogr., 576(1):53-61. http://dx.doi.org/10.1016/0378-4347(92)80174-O

11

FIN DAMAGE OF FARMED RAINBOW TROUT IN THE REPUBLIC OF MACEDONIA

Cvetkovikj Aleksandar[1], Radeski Miroslav[1], Blazhekovikj-Dimovska Dijana[2], Kostov Vasil[3], Stevanovski Vangjel[2]

[1]Veterinary Institute, Faculty of Veterinary Medicine,
University Ss. Cyril and Methodius in Skopje
[2]Fishery Department, Faculty of Biotechnical sciences,
University St. Kliment Ohridski in Bitola
[3]Fishery Department, Institute of Animal Science,
University Ss. Cyril and Methodius in Skopje

ABSTRACT

The aims of this study were to determine the prevalence of fin damage in farmed rainbow trout and to see whether the level of damage differed between different fish categories and farms. The study was field based and included the fin damage analysis and clinical description of the damaged fins. Fins were analyzed in two categories of fish [weight below 30g (min. 5g) and over 100g (max. 250g)]. Thirty fish per category were randomly selected, netted and each rayed fin was assessed and photographed (total of 5880 fins were analyzed in 840 fish from seven rainbow trout farms). The prevalence of fin damage was 100% and there was a large range in the level of damage which was mainly characterized by surface abrasions. Worst affected fins in both fish categories were dorsal and pectoral fins. Fin damage was present to a lesser degree in the smaller categories, but there was fin damage in the smallest fish examined. Pattern of damage was Dorsal Pectoral>Abdominal>Anal>Tail fin. Differences in fin damage in all surveyed farms indicate that some factor or group of factors specific to each farm influence the extent of damage. Fin damage is operational welfare indicator and future research should identify and explore the impact of the factors affecting fin damage and propose management practices that can minimize the level of fin damage. Additional knowledge is needed to identify whether fin damage is etiologically connected to different production system, handling procedures or another background.

Key words: rainbow trout, fin damage, fish welfare, welfare indicator

INTRODUCTION

The term "fin damage" includes visible changes and/or loss of fin tissue and it is a well known abnormality in many farmed and wild fish species, especially salmonids (1). It has been recognized and accepted as a common problem in farmed rainbow trout (*Oncorhynchus mykiss* Walbaum, 1792) for more than four decades (2). The presence

Corresponding author: Dr. Aleksandar Cvetkovikj, DVM, MSc, PhD
E-mail address: acvetkovic@fvm.ukim.edu.mk
Present address: Veterinary Institute, Faculty of Veterinary Medicine-Skopje, "Ss. Cyril and Methodius" University,
Lazar Pop-Trajkov 5-7, 1000 Skopje, R. Macedonia

of fin damage is so ubiquitous in some species that it can be used to distinguish the origin of the fish (farm or open water) (3). Damaged fins reduce the aesthetic appearance of the fish for both consumers and anglers, and potentially affect the survival of the fish for stocking open waters (4-6). Fin damage has been associated with the constantly increasing intensification of the farming process and was largely tolerated by the industry until it was highlighted as a welfare issue. Fish welfare is gaining more and more attention and fin damage has been highlighted as a fish welfare issue representing injury to live tissue that has blood vessels, nerves and nociceptors involved in the perception of pain (7-10). Latest studies of salmonid welfare included fin damage as an "operational welfare indicator" (2, 11-24) because as an external injury is evident and understandable, easily recognizable by fish farmers and welfare evaluators, and potentially easy to quantify (2).

Despite the extensive experimental work, there is little objective information on the prevalence and severity of fin damage on commercial farms. It has been documented that fin damage is widespread in the salmon and trout farms in the USA and Europe (4, 13, 25-30) and the severity can vary from superficial erosions to total loss of one or more fins (13, 29, 31-33).

There is no similar data about rainbow trout farmed in Republic of Macedonia, so the aims of this study were to determine if farmed rainbow trout experience fin damage, to compare the level of damage of all the rayed fins among different rainbow

trout categories, and to see whether the level of damage differed between farms. The collected data should help to identify risk factors that favor the process of fin damage.

MATERIALS AND METHODS

The study included seven trout farms with a total annual production of 650.000 kg of rainbow trout [~75% of the annual production of rainbow trout in Republic of Macedonia (V. Stevanovski, pers. comm.)]. The selection of the farms was based according to the scale of production and the willingness to participate in the study. All of the selected farms had their own hatcheries and were producing fish for consumption. The location of the farms is shown with dotted squares on Figure 1.

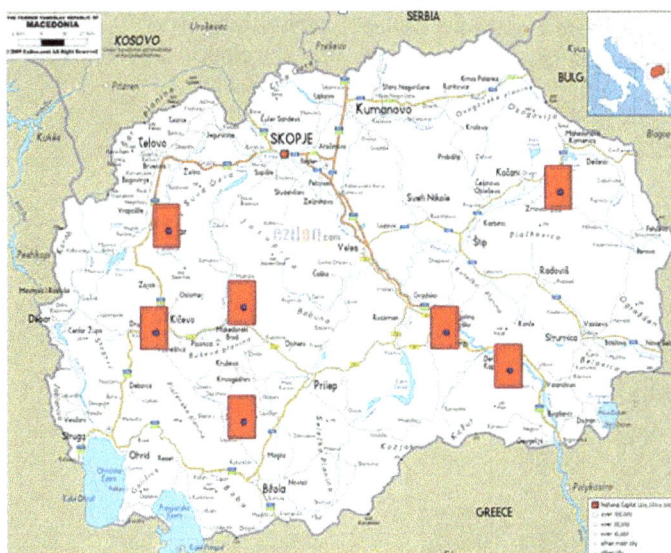

Figure 1. Map of Republic of Macedonia showing the locations of the selected trout farms (dotted squares). Source: http://www.ezilon.com/maps/europe/macedonia-maps.html

The study was field based and included the fin damage analysis and clinical description of the damaged fins. Before the onset of the fin damage analysis, the fish from the selected breeding units were clinically examined for signs of diseases.

Fins were analyzed in two categories of fish [weight below 30g (min. 5g) and over 100g (max. 250g)]. From the rearing units where these categories were present, 30 fish per category were

randomly selected, netted and each rayed fin [dorsal (D), caudal (C), anal (A), pectoral (P1) and pelvic (P2)] was assessed and photographed. To determine whether seasonal variations in the farming process affect the level of fin damage, the first assessment was carried out in late winter and early spring, and the second during the summer period in 2012. In total, 5880 fins from 840 fish were analyzed. All fins were scored by the same operator [A.Cvetkovikj].

Fin damage was analyzed using the validated quantitative macroscopic key described by Hoyle et al. (15). In brief, the analysis was based on rapid macroscopic description of all rayed fins in field conditions and included two parts. In the first part, based on a photographic key, the lack of fin tissue was quantified on a scale of 0 to 5 (0 - no damage; 5 - almost complete loss of fin). In the second part, based on the qualitative clinical descriptors, the injuries and lesions of the fins were classified as: damaged edges (surface abrasions); splits ("V" shaped tear between the rays); exposed rays (lack of soft tissue); hemorrhages (dark red spots with clearly defined margins); inflammation (presence of unnatural redness and swelling); healing and/or thickening (presence of white and smooth tissue with greater thickness compared to a normal fin) and side folding (as a consequence of re-growth).

The time needed for the assessment was 10-15 sec and was sufficient for analysis of the fin profile without compromising the welfare of the fish. After the analysis, the fish were returned to the same breeding unit.

Statistical analyses were performed using Daniel's XL Toolbox ver. 4.01 (http://xltoolbox. sourceforge.net), and all results were expressed as mean ± SE. To determine whether there are intra- or inter-farm statistical differences, all data were subjected to one-way analysis of variance (ANOVA). The results were considered statistically different at 0,01 significance level (p<0,01).

RESULTS

Prevalence of fin damage

Fin damage occurred throughout all the tested rainbow trout farms. The prevalence was determined from the presence of the clinical descriptors of fin damage. Fins were classified as "damaged" on all farms, in all rearing units, and the prevalence reached 100% in all fins (Graph. 1). Recording of damaged edge was consistent on every fin, so we excluded it when there was presence of another clinical descriptor.

The clinical descriptors are shown on Figure 2, 3, 4, 5, 6 and 7.

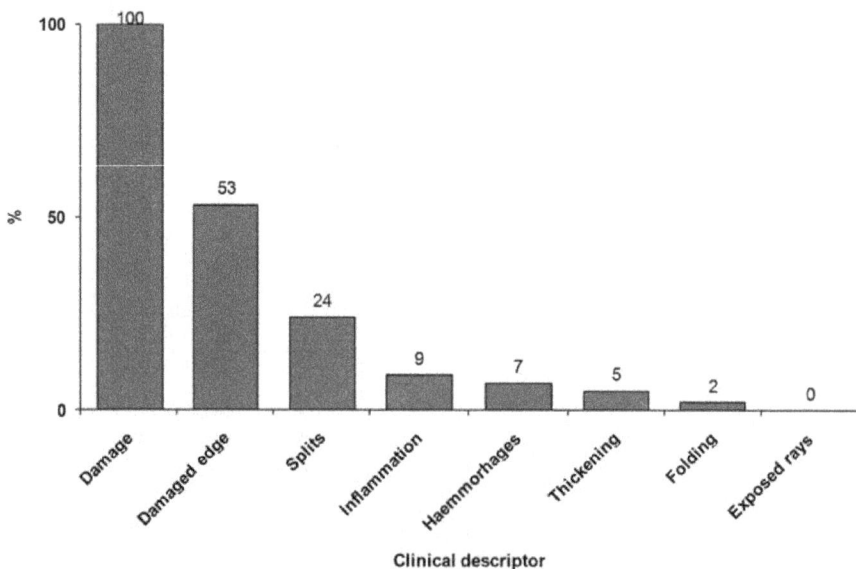

Graph. 1. Prevalence (%) of clinical descriptors of the fin damage observed in all analyzed fins (n=5880)

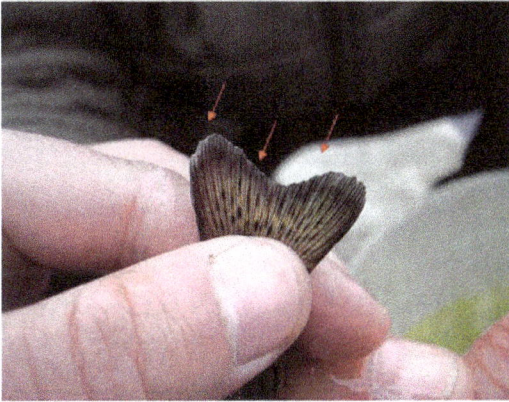

Figure 2. Damaged edge on caudal fin

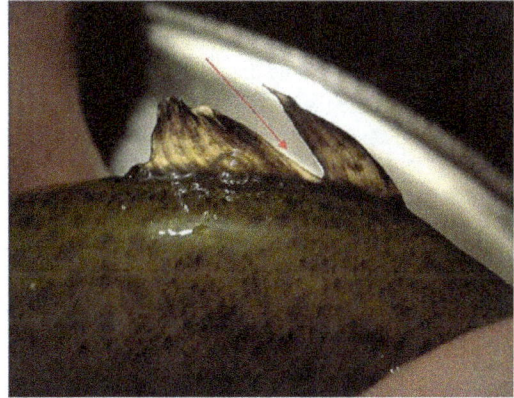

Figure 3. Split on dorsal fin

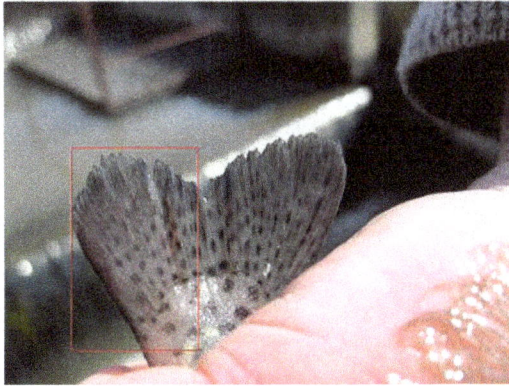

Figure 4. Inflammation of caudal fin

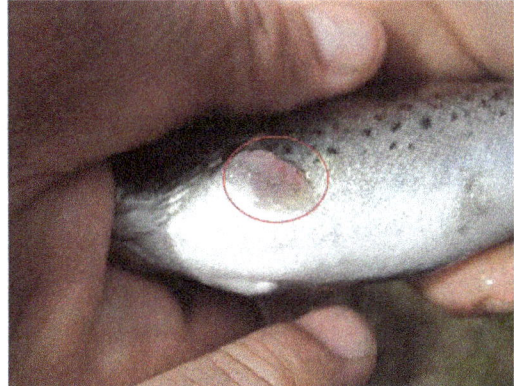

Figure 5. Hemorrhages on left pectoral fin

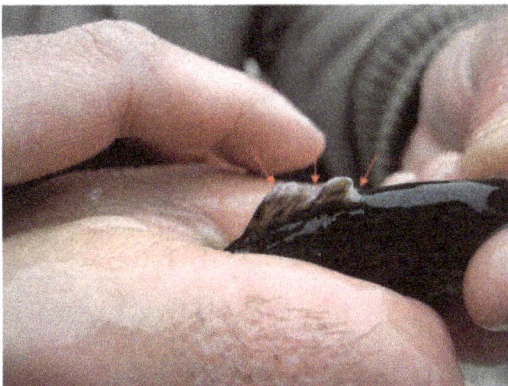

Figure 6. Thickening of dorsal fin

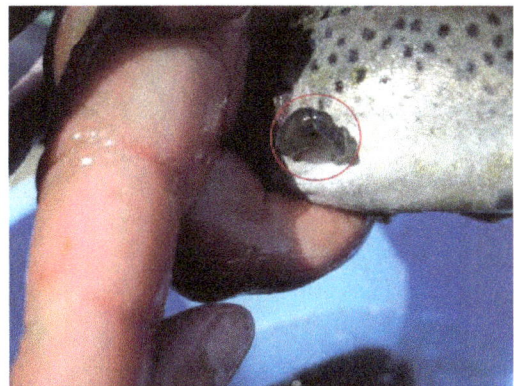

Figure 7. Folding of left pectoral fin

Level of fin damage

The results from the level of the fin damage are presented in Table 1. The data is presented as mean ± SE values of the level of damage calculated on 60 individual fish per category [ANOVA for seasonal variations showed non-significant differences ($p > 0.1$, data not shown) and we recalculated the results for 60 individual fish per category].

Table 1. Level of the fin damage and significance of the results between the different fish categories and fish farms

	Farm 1	Farm 2	Farm 3	Farm 4	Farm 5	Farm 6	Farm 7	p-level
Dorsal < 30g	3.63 ±0.06	2.53 ±0.13	3.02 ±0.15	2.30 ±0.11	1.50 ±0.09	2.35 ±0.12	2.13 ±0.15	p<0.001
Dorsal > 100g	4.27 ±0.06	3.23 ±0.12	4.07 ±0.09	2.77 ±0.12	2.10 ±0.09	2.72 ±0.13	3.32 ±0.15	p<0.001
p	p<0.001	p<0.001	p<0.001	p<0.001	p<0.001	p<0.01	p<0.001	
Caudal < 30g	1.43 ±0.06	1.30 ±0.06	1.37 ±0.06	1.33 ±0.06	1.03 ±0.02	1.13 ±0.04	1.07 ±0.03	p<0.001
Caudal > 100g	2.95 ±0.3	1.73 ±0.07	2.07 ±0.07	1.85 ±0.10	1.73 ±0.09	1.73 ±0.08	2.28 ±0.11	p<0.001
p	p<0.001	p<0.001	p<0.001	p<0.001	p<0.001	p<0.001	p<0.001	
Anal < 30g	1.73 ±0.07	1.67 ±0.09	1.52 ±0.09	1.47 ±0.06	1.10 ±0.04	1.73 ±0.08	1.33 ±0.06	p<0.001
Anal > 100g	3.60 ±0.10	1.85 ±0.08	2.37 ±0.09	2.07 ±0.11	1.80 ±0.10	2.03 ±0.09	2.40 ±0.11	p<0.001
p	p<0.001	p<0.001	p<0.001	p<0.001	p<0.001	p<0.01	p<0.001	
Pectoral left < 30g	2.10 ±0.13	2.02 ±0.12	1.78 ±0.09	1.82 ±0.09	2.10 ±0.08	2.03 ±0.09	1.73 ±0.17	p>0.05
Pectoral left > 100g	4.10 ±0.13	2.70 ±0.11	2.57 ±0.08	2.43 ±0.13	3.07 ±0.14	2.43 ±0.06	3.08 ±0.18	p<0.001
p	p<0.001	p<0.001	p<0.001	p<0.001	p<0.001	p<0.001	p<0.001	
Pectoral right < 30 g	2.07 ±0.14	2.03 ±0.12	1.80 ±0.10	1.83 ±0.10	2.07 ±0.07	2.02 ±0.09	1.70 ±0.12	p>0.05
Pectoral right > 100 g	4.12 ±0.13	2.67 ±0.09	2.53 ±0.08	2.47 ±0.14	3.10 ±0.10	2.40 ±0.08	3.05 ±0.17	p<0.001
p	p<0.001	p<0.001	p<0.001	p<0.001	p<0.001	p<0.01	p<0.001	
Pelvic left < 30 g	1.58 ±0.11	1.75 ±0.09	2.18 ±0.14	1.50 ±0.09	1.33 ±0.06	1.30 ±0.06	1.47 ±0.09	p<0.001
Pelvic left > 100 g	3.07 ±0.10	1.93 ±0.11	3.03 ±0.06	2.13 ±0.12	1.87 ±0.07	1.90 ±0.09	2.47 ±0.12	p<0.001
p	p<0.001	p<0.01	p<0.001	p<0.001	p<0.001	p<0.001	p<0.001	
Pelvic right < 30 g	1.57 ±0.10	1.77 ±0.11	2.20 ±0.14	1.53 ±0.09	1.43 ±0.08	1.33 ±0.07	1.43 ±0.09	p<0.001
Pelvic right > 100 g	3.05 ±0.10	1.97 ±0.10	3.07 ±0.13	2.15 ±0.12	1.97 ±0.08	1.93 ±0.09	2.43 ±0.11	p<0.001
p	p<0.001	p<0.01	p<0.001	p<0.001	p<0.001	p<0.001	p<0.001	

For the smaller fish category (<30g), the most damaged fin was the dorsal fin in the farm 1 (3.63±0.06) and the least damaged was the caudal fin in the farm 5 (1.03±0.02). Fins with the greatest level of damage were: dorsal and pectoral fins in the farms 1, 2, 4, 6 and 7; dorsal and pelvic fins in the farm 3 and pectorals and dorsal fin in the farm 5. The caudal fin was the least damaged in the all tested fish.

Fin damage was greater for the large fish than the small fish. For this category (>100g), the most damaged fin, as for the smaller ones, was the dorsal fin in the farm 1 (4.27±0.06), and the least

damaged was the caudal fin in the farms 2, 5 and 6 (1.73±0.07). Fins with the greatest level of damage were again the dorsal and pectoral fins in the farm 1, 2, 4, 6 and 7; dorsal and pelvic fins in the farm 3 and pectorals and dorsal fin in the farm 5. The caudal fin was also the least damaged in all the tested fish.

Although there was a large range in the fin grade, we observed complete fin loss for every fin, especially for the dorsal and pectoral fins.

The pattern of the fin damage and the summarized data on the level of the fin damage on the all farms are presented on Graph. 2 and Graph. 3.

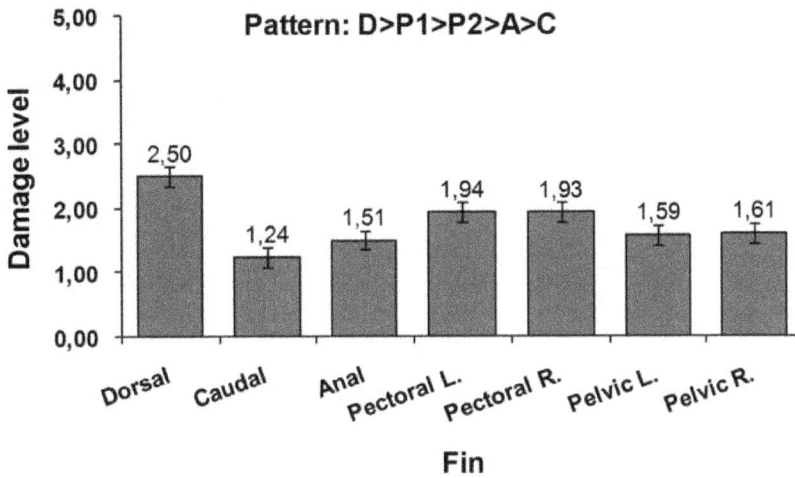

Graph. 2. Mean damage level on the separate fins for category < 30g in all the fish farms. Bars represent SE.

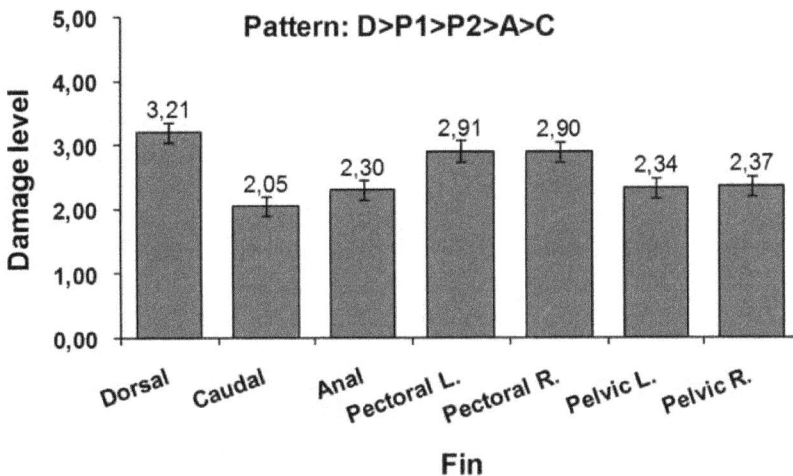

Graph. 3. Mean damage level on the separate fins for category > 100g in all the fish farms. Bars represent SE.

As it is shown in Table 1, as well as in Graph. 2 and Graph. 3, different fins were differently prone to fin loss, but the pattern of the fin damage, i.e. Dorsal > Pectoral > Pelvic > Anal > Caudal was consistent for both fish categories.

The data for the left and right pectoral and pelvic fins from both fish categories were correlated (Table 2). If one fin was damaged, in almost every case its pair was also damaged in the same way.

Table 2. Pearson's correlation coefficient

Pearson's	Pectoral right < 30g	Pectoral right > 100g	Pelvic right < 30g	Pelvic right > 100g
Pectoral left < 30g	0.987*			
Pectoral left > 100g		0.998*		
Pelvic left < 30g			0.990*	
Pelvic left > 100g				0.997*

* $p < 0.01$

DISCUSSION

The fin damage can be assessed in many different ways with different or similar pros and cons (9). The method used in this study by Hoyle et al. (15) was applied because it considers all types of fin damage and enabled us to quantify the fin damage in a very short period of time, without the need for anesthesia or euthanasia of the fish. The proposed five levels of damage gave an instant picture of the fin profile and can be used in future research of fish quality and welfare. The only difficulty is that it is still unknown what level and type of fin damage are acceptable in terms of welfare (11, 34-37).

The fin damage analysis showed 100% prevalence and all rayed fins were damaged to some extent. This is the first study in Republic of Macedonia that confirms the suggestions that fin damage is ubiquitous, agreeing with previous research that it is widespread in rainbow trout farms worldwide and that all rayed fins are prone to damage (4, 9, 13, 15, 25, 29, 30). During the study, we did not find any diseased fish and there was no mortality in all examined rearing units. From a

single point of view, this implies that damaged fins do not pose a serious threat to the production. This is expected, because fin damage is greatly tolerated in the expansive development of the salmonid culture over the past four decades (2).

The most damaged fins in both fish categories were the dorsal and pectoral fins. However, the severity of damage varied for the other fins that suggest that some fins were more prone to damage compared to others. Bosakowski and Wagner (25) made similar observations. The dorsal and pectoral fins were damaged even in the smallest fish examined (5g), which indicates that the damage occurred in the early life stages in the hatchery. These findings do agree with previous research (13, 38), even though the method used to assess fin damage was different. The other fins had higher level of damage in the larger fish category, which implies that the living conditions, factors that differ between farms and the ongrowing technology significantly affect the extent of damage. This is also supported by the ANOVA analysis that showed that the interfarm comparison of the level of damage of the pectoral fins in the small fish category was the only nonstatistically significant result. The overall fin damage was present to a lesser degree in the small fish categories. This finding supports the findings of Barrows and Lellis (39) and St-Hilaire et al. (13) that fin damage continues to increase throughout the entire farming process.

The severity of damage varied between fins and the pattern of the fin damage was consistent for both fish categories, although there were minor differences at a farm level. The pattern, with the exception of dorsal and pectoral fins, is not in accordance with other published research. Abbott and Dill (40) assessed tissue loss by subjective classification of the damage and found D>P1>C>P2>A in juvenile steelhead trout. Turnbull et al. (41) by assessing tissue damage from the length of the fin splits found D>P1>C>P2>A in Atlantic salmon parr. The following three studies assessed tissue loss by comparing the fin lengths of farmed fish with those of control (feral or wild) fish. Bosakowski and Wagner (4) found P1>D>A>P2>C in cutthroat trout and D>P1>A>P2>C in rainbow and brown trout; Pelis and McCormick (42) found P1>D>P2>A>C and D=P1>A>P2>C in two Atlantic salmon hatcheries and St-Hilaire et al. (13) found D>P1>C>A>P2 in rainbow trout. The different findings may be due to the different methodology used for the fin damage assessment, the causes of damage were different and were acting individually or in a combination, and/or different fins were differentially prone to different causes and factors affecting the process of fin damage. Generally, observation of fin damage can be divided in two major groups. First is fin damage as a result of bad handling and management of fish and second due to individual damage as a result of aggression, interactions among fish etc.

We didn't find any seasonal differences in the level of fin damage in both fish categories. This is in accordance with previous research (43) and this finding further emphasizes the importance of farm practices in the process of fin damage.

The almost perfect correlation between the left and right-paired fins implies that a similar process affects the level of damage of these fins. This finding is also in accordance with previous research of St-Hilaire et al. (13).

The lack of the fin damage of wild trout and trout reared in isolation indicates that farm conditions (e.g. rearing unit surface; handling and transport; water quality; sunburn; feed quality) initiate the damage (38). Therefore, fin damage is considered as a phenomenon in the farmed trout. Differences in fin damage in all surveyed farms indicate that some factor or group of factors specific to each farm influence the extent of damage (e.g. temperature; stocking density; water current; feed ration and distribution). Future research should identify and explore the impact of the factors affecting fin damage and propose management practices that can minimize the level of fin damage.

The primary function of the fins is locomotion and posture control. Having in mind the behavioral welfare aspects of fin damage, it can be easily proposed that fin damage could affect its primary function during routine swimming and feeding behavior (44). There are some experimental data that show that reduction of the pectoral fin area had no effect upon the swimming capacity of the fish (45, 46). The authors suggest that fish make behavioral compensations to adjust for the reduced fin size. However, the complete loss (amputation) of pectoral fins reduces the ability of station-holding of Atlantic salmon parr (47). The evidence that damaged fins do not affect the behavioral performance is scarce and additional studies are needed to demonstrate whether fish do compensate for the behavioral changes due to fin damage.

Severe fin damage is indicative of bad fish health and acts as fish quality indicator (13, 15, 18). Therefore, the difference in the fin damage level indicates that it may be possible to improve the fin profile on rainbow trout farms, which would benefit both the welfare of the fish and the aesthetic quality of table fish.

REFERENCES

1. Latremouille, D.N. (2003). Fin erosion in aquaculture and natural environments. Rev Fish Sci, 315–335.

2. Ellis, T., Hoyle, I., Oidtmann, B., Turnbull, J., Jacklin T.E., Knowles, T. (2009). Further development of the "Fin Index" method for quantifying fin erosion in rainbow trout. Aquaculture, 289, 283–288.

3. Butler, J.R.A., Cunningham, P.D., Starr, K. (2005). The prevalence of escaped farmed salmon, *Salmo salar* L., in the River Ewe, Western Scotland, with notes on their ages,

weights and spawning distribution. Fish Manag Ecol, 12, 149–159.

4. Bosakowski, T., Wagner, E.J. (1994a). Assessment of fin erosion by comparison of relative fin length in hatchery and wild trout in Utah. Can J Fish Aquat Sci, 51, 636–641.

5. Larmoyeux, J.D., Piper, R.G. (1971). A promising method of reducing eroded fin condition in hatchery trout. Am Fish U.S. Trout News, 16 (3), 8–9.

6. Rønsholdt, B., McLean, E. (1999). Quality characteristics of fresh rainbow trout as perceived by the Danish processing industry. Aquacult Int, 7, 117–127.

7. Farm Animal Welfare Council (1996). Report on the welfare of farmed fish. *FAWC*, Surbiton, Surrey.

8. Chervova, L.S. (1997). Pain sensitivity and behaviour of fishes. J Ichthyol, 37, 98–102.

9. Ellis, T., Oidtmann, B., St-Hilaire, S., Turnbull, J., North, B., MacIntyre, C., Nikolaidis, J., Hoyle, I., Kestin, S., Knowles, T. (2008). Fin erosion in farmed fish. In: Branson, E. (Ed.), Fish Welfare (pp. 121–149). Blackwell, Oxford.

10. Sneddon, L.U., Braithwaite, V.A., Gentle, M.J. (2003). Do fishes have nociceptors? Evidence for the evolution of a vertebrate sensory system. Prod R Soc Lond B: Biol, 270, 1115–1121.

11. Turnbull, J., Bell, A., Adams, C., Bron, J., Huntingford, F. (2005). Stocking density and welfare of cage farmed Atlantic salmon: application of multivariate analysis. Aquaculture, 243, 121–132.

12. North, B.P., Turnbull, J.F., Ellis, T., Porter, M.J., Migaud, H., Bron, J., Bromage, N.R. (2006). The impact of stocking density on the welfare of rainbow trout (*Oncorhynchus mykiss*). Aquaculture, 255, 466–479.

13. St-Hilaire, S., Ellis, T., Cooke, A., North, B.P., Turnbull, J.F., Knowles, T., Kestin, S. (2006). Fin erosion on commercial rainbow trout farms in the UK. Vet Rec, 159, 446–450.

14. Adams, C.E., Turnbull, J.F., Bell, A., Bron, J.E., Huntingford, F.A. (2007). Multiple determinants of welfare in farmed fish: stocking density, disturbance and aggression in salmon. Can J Fish Aquat Sci, 64, 336–344.

15. Hoyle, I., Oidtmann, B., Ellis, T., Turnbull, J., North, B., Nikolaidis, J., Knowles, T.G. (2007). A validated macroscopic key to assess fin damage in farmed rainbow trout (*Oncorhynchus mykiss*). Aquaculture, 270, 142–148.

16. Rasmussen, R.S., Larsen, F.H., Jensen, S. (2007). Fin condition and growth among rainbow trout reared at different sizes, densities and feeding frequencies in high temperature recirculated water. Aquacult Int, 15, 97–107.

17. Noble, C., Kadri, S., Mitchell, D.F., Huntingford, F.A. (2008). Growth, production and fin damage in cage-held 0+ Atlantic salmon pre-smolts (*Salmo salar L.*) fed either a) ondemand, or b) to a fixed satiation–restriction regime: data from a commercial farm. Aquaculture, 275, 163–168.

18. Person-LeRuyet, J., Bayo, N.L., Gros, S. (2007). How to assess fin damage in rainbow trout, *Onchorynchus mykiss*? Aquat Living Resour, 20, 191–195.

19. Person-LeRuyet, J., Labbe, L., Bayon, N.L., Severe, A., Roux, A.L., Delliou, H.L., Quemener, L. (2008). Combined effects of water quality and stocking density on welfare and growth of rainbow trout (*Oncorhynchus mykiss*). Aquat Living Resour, 21, 185–195.

20. Good, C., Davidson, J., Welsh, C., Brazil, B., Snekvik, K., Summerfelt, S. (2009). The impact of water exchange rate on the health and performance of rainbow trout *Oncorhynchus mykiss* in water recirculation aquaculture systems. Aquaculture, 294, 80–85.

21. Roque d'Orbcastel, E., Person-Le Ruyet, J., Le Bayon, N., Blancheton, J.P. (2009). Comparative growth and welfare in rainbow trout reared in recirculated and flow through rearing systems. Aquacult Eng, 40, 79–86.

22. Canon Jones, H.A., Hansen, L.A., Noble, C., Damsgard, B., Broom, D.M., Pearce, G.P. (2010). Social network analysis of behavioural interactions influencing fin damage development in Atlantic salmon (*Salmo salar*) during feed-restriction. Appl Anim Behav Sci, 127, 139–151.

23. Canon Jones, H.A., Noble, C., Damsgard, B., Pearce, G.P. (2011). Social network analysis of

the behavioural interactions that influence the development of fin damage in Atlantic salmon parr (*Salmo salar*) held at different stocking densities. Appl Anim Behav Sci,133, 117–126.

24. Canon Jones, H.A., Noble, C., Damsgard, B., Pearce, G.P. (2012). Investigating the influence of predictable and unpredictable feed delivery schedules upon the behaviour and welfare of Atlantic salmon parr (*Salmo salar*) using social network analysis and fin damage. Appl Anim Behav Sci, 138, 132-140.

25. Bosakowski, T., Wagner, E.J. (1994b). A survey of trout fin erosion, water quality, and rearing conditions at state fish hatcheries in Utah. J World Aquacult Soc, 25, 308–316.

26. Sedgwick, S.D. (1985). Trout Farming Handbook. Fishing News Books, Farnham.

27. Peters, G. (1990). Problems concerning animal protection laws in connection with mass culture of fishes. Dtsch tieräztl Wschr, 97, 157-160.

28. North, B.P. (2004). Effects of stocking density on the welfare of farmed rainbow trout (*Oncorhynchus mykiss*). PhD thesis, Institute Of Aquaculture,University of Stirling

29. Turnbull, J.F., Richards, R.H., Robertson, D.A. (1996). Gross, histological and scanning electron microscopic appearance of dorsal fin rot in farmed Atlantic salmon, *Salmo salar* L., parr. J Fish Dis, 19, 415–427.

30. Poppe, T.T. (2000). Husbandry diseases in fish farming - an ethical challenge to the veterinary profession. Norsk Vet Tids, 2, 91–96.

31. Heimer, J.T., Frazier, W.M., Griffith, J.S. (1985). Post-stocking performance of catchable size hatchery rainbow trout with and without pectoral fins. N Am J Fish Man, 5, 21–25.

32. Kindschi, G.A., Shaw, H.T., Bruhn, D.S. (1991a). Effect of diet on performance, fin quality, and dorsal skin lesions in steelhead. J App Aquacult, 1, 113–120.

33. Lellis, W.A., Barrows, F.T. (1997). The effect of diet on dorsal fin erosion in steelhead trout (*Oncorhynchus mykiss*). Aquaculture, 156, 233–244.

34. Ashley, J.P. (2007). Fish welfare: Current issues in aquaculture. Appl Anim Behav Sci, 104, 199–235.

35. Ellis, T., North, B., Scott, A.P., Bromage, N.R., Porter, M., Gadd, D. (2002). The relationships between stocking density and welfare in farmed rainbow trout. J Fish Biol, 61, 493–531.

36. Huntingford,F.A.,Adams,C.,Braithwaite,V.A., Kadri, S., Pottinger, T.G., Sandøe, P., Turnbull, J.F. (2006). Current issues in fish welfare. J Fish Biol, 68, 332–372.

37. Huntingford, F. (2008). Animal welfare in aquaculture. In: Culver, K., Castle, D. (Eds.), Aquaculture Innovation and Social Transformation 17, 21–33.

38. Kindschi, G.A., Shaw, H.T., Bruhn, D.S. (1991b). Effects of baffles and isolation on dorsal fin erosion in steelhead trout, *Oncorhynchus mykiss* (Walbaum). Aquacult Fish Manage, 22, 343–350.

39. Barrows, F.T., Lellis, W.A. (1999). The effect of dietary protein and lipid source on dorsal fin erosion in rainbow trout, *Oncorhynchus mykiss*. Aquaculture, 180, 167–175.

40. Abbott, J.C., Dill, L.M. (1985). Patterns of aggressive attack in juvenile steelhead trout (*Salmo gairdneri*). Can J Fish Aquat Sci, 42, 1702–1706.

41. Turnbull, J., Adams, C., Richards, R., Robertson, D. (1998). Attack site and resultant damage during aggressive encounters in Atlantic salmon (*Salmo salar* L.) parr. Aquaculture, 159, 345–353.

42. Pelis, R.M., McCormick, S.D. (2003). Fin development in stream- and hatchery-reared Atlantic salmon. Aquaculture, 220, 525–536.

43. Macintyre, C., (2008). Water quality and welfare assessment on United Kingdom trout farms. PhD thesis. Institute Of Aquaculture, University Of Stirling

44. Barthel,B.L.,Cooke,S.J.,Suski,C.D.,Philipp,D.P. (2003). Effects of landing net mesh type on injury and mortality in a freshwater recreational fishery. Fish Res, 63, 275–282.

45. Higham,T.E.,Malas,B.,Jayne,B.C.,Lauder,G.V. (2005). Constraints on starting and stopping: behavior compensates for reduced pectoral fin area during braking of the bluegill sunfish Lepomis macrochirus. J Exp Biol, 208, 4735–4746.

46. Wagner, C.P., Einfalt, L.M., Scimone, A.B., Wahl, D.H. (2009). Effects of fin-clipping on the foraging behavior and growth of age-0 muskellunge. N Am J Fish Manage, 29, 1644–1652.

47. Arnold, G.P., Webb, P.W., Holford, B.H. (1991). The role of the pectoral fins in station-holding of Atlantic salmon (Salmo salar L.). J Exp Biol, 156, 625–629.

12

AIR QUALITY MEASUREMENTS IN LAYING HENS HOUSING

Mirko Prodanov[1], Miroslav Radeski[2], Vlatko Ilieski[3]

[1]*Food Institute, Faculty of Veterinary Medicine Skopje*
University "Ss. Cyril and Methodius" in Skopje
[2]*Veterinary Institute, Faculty of Veterinary Medicine Skopje,*
University "Ss. Cyril and Methodius" in Skopje
[3]*Institute for Reproduction and Biomedicine, Faculty of Veterinary Medicine*
Skopje, University "Ss. Cyril and Methodius" in Skopje

ABSTRACT

Ensuring good environmental conditions of the poultry houses can be costly for the farmers, but without it losses due to poor bird health and performance due to poor air quality can be much more detrimental to net returns. The goal of this study was to investigate the variations in air quality in various areas inside the laying hen house. Ten houses with laying hen conventional battery cages were measured for O_2, H_2S, CO, NH_3 temperature, relative humidity, CO_2, airflow and luminance. The results of the physical measures showed that temperatures in the houses were between 15.31–25.6°C, the relative humidity 48.03-81.12%, while the luminance rarely exceeded 8 lux. As for the gasses, the values for NH_3 rarely exceeded 8 ppm, although at some measuring points it reached 26 ppm. O_2 was generally at 20.9 %, and the levels of CO_2 were very low. No presence of H_2S and CO was detected. In this study it was concluded that the measurement of the air quality in a house can vary depending of the places this measures are taken. Multiple measurement points are important because they may make the staff aware of the problems connected to low ventilation and culmination of harmful gases. The air quality in different positions in the houses is of great importance not only for the animal welfare, but also for the safety of the staff.

Key words: laying hens, ammonia, temperature, air quality

INTRODUCTION

In intensive poultry housing systems, laying hens should be kept in good environmental conditions, ensuring good care, in order to ensure that laying hens are performing to their maximum yield capacities within their genetic potential (1, 13). Maintaining a proper ventilation can be costly for the farmers, but without it poor bird health and performance due to poor air quality can be much more detrimental to net returns. A part of the environmental conditions is the areal environment (8). The areal conditions in

Corresponding author: Mirko Prodanov, DVM, MSc.
E-mail address: m.prodanov@fvm.ukim.edu.mk
Present address: Food Institute, Faculty of Veterinary Medicine Skopje
University "Ss. Cyril and Methodius" in Skopje
Str. Lazar Pop- Trajkov 5-7, 1000 Skopje, R. Macedonia

the poultry houses depend on physical (temperature, relative humidity, luminance, ventilation and dust) and chemical factors (compound of the air such as ammonia, carbon dioxide and oxygen) (1, 2).

In poultry houses, harmful gases like ammonia, carbon dioxide, methane, hydrogen sulfide and nitrous oxide, are generated by the hens and their waste (1, 2). These gases may accumulate and reach toxic levels which may cause risk to the health of both chickens and the workers, therefore an adequate ventilation must be maintained. Levels of CO_2 such as 12000 ppm were observed to have effect on weight loss in broilers (3). For the CO level of 1500 ppm in the air can cause death in an hour (4, 5, 6). Levels of ammonia as low as 20 ppm have been shown to increase the susceptibility of chicken to diseases (7). Although poor aerial conditions normally don't cause disease directly, they do reduce the chickens' immune defenses, therefore making them more susceptible to existing viruses and pathogens (8).

The most common air contaminant in the poultry facilities is ammonia. The concentration varies depending on many factors, among which are manure handling, temperature, humidity and ventilation rate of the facility. Hens exposed to high levels of ammonia can show reduction in feed consumption, feed efficiency, weight gain, and egg production (8-12).

In the process of regulating temperature, relative humidity and gases, ventilation is of great importance. In laying hen houses the recommended optimal temperature is 18°C (13). The measures of performance such as body weight, consumption of feed and water, feed intake, egg production, and egg weight, have been correlated with the environmental temperature (14). It is possible that under heat stress, a reduction of egg production occurs due to the alterations in the respiratory pattern (15).

It is advised that the optimal relative humidity in laying hen houses should be between 50-70% (16). If the relative humidity drops below the advised levels increases of mortality, and in some cases respiratory diseases can accrue (16).

The goal of this study was to investigate the variations of air quality, except dust levels, in various areas inside the laying hen houses.

MATERIAL AND METHODS

Ten houses with laying hen conventional battery cages were measured for the air quality. Seven of the houses were completely closed with no windows and had tunnel ventilation type. Two of the houses (G1, G2) had windows which were open in order to increase the ventilation and a fan at each corner that was sucking air out of the house, and one house (D)

had fans pumping air out of the house on one side and openings on the other side where fresh air was entering the house. Detailed information about the houses are given in Table 1.

All the measurements were taken in October and November in the period between 9 a.m. and 12 a.m. when the eggs were collected. The measuring was performed inside the houses at 9 points at multiple cage heights. The points of measurements were: 3 at the corridor next to the left wall, 3 at the corridor in the middle of the batteries, and 3 points at the corridor next to the right wall. At each corridor, measurements were taken at the beginning, at the middle and at the end of the battery. The measurements of O_2, CO and NH_3 were done with a portable detector MultiRAE (RAE systems, US) and temperature, relative humidity, CO_2, airflow and luminance was measured with TESTO measurement instrument (Testo Inc., US) with multiple sensor probes. For every house, an average value and the standard variation were calculated for each measure.

RESULTS

Summary of the results from the measurement of the physical parameters are shown in Table 2. The temperature in the houses was in the range between 15.31°C and 25.6°C with the highest standard deviation of 3.09°C. The deviation in temperature in a house depended on the heights of the battery and the air flow. The relative humidity was between 48.03% and 81.12% with the maximum standard deviation of 4.89%. The luminance was between 1.83 and 28.25 lux with maximal standard deviation

Table 1. Information about the houses where the study air quality measurements were performed

House	Hybride	Age (weeks)	Population	House size in meters (W x L x H)	Ventilation method	Manure menagement
House A	Dekalb brown	69	35600	10 x 70 x 4,20	Tunel	Belt
House B1	Lohmann white	30	13000	9 x 72 x 3,6	Tunel	Belt
House B2	Lohmann white	88	15000	9 x 72 x 3,6	Tunel	Belt
House C1	ISA Brown	48	11000	12,5 x 80 x 4,6	Side vents	Scraper
House C2	ISA Brown	30	11000	12,5 x 80 x 4,6	Tunel	Scraper
House D	Lohmann white	72	9800	8 x 50 x 4,20	Tunel	Belt
House F1	Lohmann white	53	54600	23 x 72 x 6,5	Tunel	Belt
House F2	Lohmann white	40	59300	23 x 72 x 6,5	Tunel	Belt
House G1	Lohmann white	52	22100	12 x 83,5 x 2,4	Modification	Scraper
House G2	Lohmann white	84	22100	12 x 83,5 x 2,4	Modification	Scraper

Table 2. Summary measured values for the physical parameters in the houses

Farm	Temperature (°C)				Relative humidity (%)				Luminance (lux)				Air flow (m/s)			
	average	min	max	stdev	average	min	max	stdev	average	min	max	stdev	average	min	max	stdev
House A	21.80	18.94	22.63	0.99	58.40	54.79	61.28	1.84	8.68	2.00	17.00	4.94	0.41	0.03	0.93	0.24
House B1	20.80	17.82	22.16	1.21	64.72	58.84	73.68	4.08	4.23	2.00	10.10	2.10	0.33	0.07	0.79	0.20
House B2	20.46	16.50	22.86	1.92	64.89	59.96	74.48	4.89	3.89	2.60	7.00	1.30	0.26	0.03	0.54	0.14
House C1	25.38	24.57	26.27	0.41	49.69	43.57	55.08	0.34	4.02	2.00	5.90	1.00	0.05	0.01	0.11	0.03
House C2	25.60	24.50	26.12	0.60	48.03	45.69	50.98	2.32	4.02	2.00	5.90	1.00	0.23	0.05	0.61	0.20
House D	24.47	21.40	25.40	1.52	81.12	78.70	84.00	1.80	1.83	1.00	2.00	0.41	0.36	0.12	1.06	0.37
House F1	22.36	19.00	25.45	1.89	69.52	61.26	76.92	4.29	6.66	1.90	20.60	4.85	0.35	0.03	1.06	0.29
House F2	16.45	12.96	19.23	2.16	64.00	56.64	74.64	4.33	4.60	1.20	12.60	2.74	0.22	0.07	0.37	0.15
House G1	16.49	15.00	19.23	1.02	48.50	39.13	54.99	3.85	28.25	2.00	362.00	83.69	0.24	0.03	0.73	0.18
House G2	15.31	13.27	16.89	1.08	49.98	43.05	53.52	2.86	5.83	2.00	16.80	4.04	0.51	0.04	1.25	0.38

Table 3. Summary of the measured values in the houses for the gasses

Farm	NH$_3$ (ppm)				O$_2$ (%)				CO$_2$ (ppm)			
	average	min	max	stdev	average	min	max	stdev	average	min	max	stdev
House A	1.04	0.00	3.00	0.85	20.80	19.40	20.80	0.54	1139.88	926.00	1322.50	123.88
House B1	0.94	0.00	1.00	0.20	20.90	20.90	20.90	0.00	1046.99	855.40	1211.40	92.87
House B2	0.39	0.00	1.00	0.50	20.90	20.90	20.90	0.00	930.64	556.70	1179.80	206.51
House C1	8.50	1.00	26.00	7.16	19.36	18.50	20.60	0.75	747.51	625.60	934.70	84.79
House C2	8.17	1.00	18.00	5.98	21.22	21.20	21.30	0.04	696.20	549.00	789.00	111.29
House D	6.33	4.00	12.00	3.01	20.90	20.90	20.90	0.00	750.00	725.00	771.00	18.90
House F1	5.04	1.00	11.00	2.68	19.96	19.50	20.50	0.31	1158.99	838.10	1436.10	195.28
House F2	1.44	0.00	3.00	0.64	20.09	19.40	20.90	0.53	1466.56	886.80	1832.10	321.39
House G1	8.00	2.00	17.00	4.68	20.90	20.90	20.90	0.00	840.28	620.50	1067.40	112.14
House G2	4.00	1.00	9.00	7.94	20.90	20.90	20.90	0.00	836.91	630.40	1092.20	138.15

83.69 lux. Different cages were getting different amounts of luminance. The ones that were the closest to the light source had higher value for luminance, as the lower cages got the lower value for luminance. In one of the houses one of the sides was allmost open, at this point values of 362 lux was measured. The airflow was between 0.05 m/s and 0.51 m/s with maximal standard deviation of 0.38 m/s.

Summary of the results from the measurement of the gases are shown in Table 3. The NH_3 was between 0.39 ppm and 8.17 ppm with the biggest standard deviation of 7.94 ppm. The O_2 was between 19.36% and 21.22% with the biggest standard deviation of 0.75%. The CO_2 was between 696.2 ppm and 1466.56 ppm with the biggest standard deviation 321.39 ppm. In all the farms, it was noted that there were blind spots of ventilation. In one of the houses there was a point where the air flow was at minimum as low as 0.01 m/s, and at this point the highest concentration of NH_3 (26 ppm) was measured. Also the amount of oxygen in most of the farms was at the level of 20.9%, which is same as fresh air. However in one of the farms an alarmingly low level (18.5%) of O_2 was measured. This was the same farm that had the lowest ventilation rate. CO and H_2S were not detected in any of the houses.

DISCUSSION

The average temperature in the farms did not vary more than 3°C below, and 8°C above the recommended values. The highest value measured was 26.27°C. Oarad et al. (17) stated that temperatures above 27°C can reduce the productive performance of the hens, and temperatures over 35°C can lead to pronounced decrease of feed consumption and egg shell thickness. According to Talukder (18) feed consumption and egg weight gradually decrease with relative humidity above 70%, which was the case only in one of the houses. Although the mean value exceeded 70% in 4 other houses the maximum values exceeded this relative humidity. As for the luminance it generally had low values which are reported to reduce the risk of pecking (19). However the variation between the values was dependent on the distance of the measuring point from the light source. In one of the houses, at one of the sides, the panel for the opening fell off and thus did not block any light, and the values were close to those of daylight. The highest level CO_2 measured in any of the houses was 1436 ppm and it was never close to concentrations that can be harmful for the health (3). The average levels of NH_3 in the houses did not exceeded 8 ppm.

However in one of the houses, at one measuring point, the NH_3 level reached 26 ppm, a concentration which has been recorded to have adverse effects on the health of the birds and the workers (9, 20, 21, 22).

During the measurements of the houses with the tunnel ventilation a pattern was noticed. The maximum values for temperature, relative humidity and the minimal values of airflow were recorded at the measurement points located at the back end of the houses, especially at the corners. At these measurement points the maximal values for the NH_3 were recorded, which is according to the literature where the levels of the NH_3 is dependent of temperature, relative humidity and airflow (23).

CONCLUSION

In this study it was concluded that the air quality in a house can differ depending of the places this measurements are taken. Multiple measurement points are important because they may make the staff aware of the problems connected to low ventilation and culmination of harmful gases. The air quality in different positions in the houses is of great importance not only to the animal welfare, but also to the safety of the staff. Although there was no repeated detection of gasses at levels that can be harmful in this study, it does give an insight to the places in the house where they are most likely to accrue.

REFERENCES

1. Kocaman, B., Yaganoglu, A.V., Yanar, M. (2005). Combination of fan ventilation system and spraying of oil-water mixture on the levels of dust and gases in caged layer facilities in Eastern Turkey. J Appl Anim Res. 27, 109-111.
http://dx.doi.org/10.1080/09712119.2005.9706551

2. Liang, Y., Xin, H., Li, H., Wheeler, E.F., Zajaczkowski, J.L., Topper, P.A., Gates, R.S., Casey, K.D., Behrends, B.B., Burnham, D.J., Zajaczkowski, F.J. (2005). Ammonia emissions from U.S. laying hen houses in Iowa and Pennsylvania. Transactions of the ASAE. 48 (5): 1927-1941.
http://dx.doi.org/10.13031/2013.20002

3. Reece, F.N., Lott, B.D. (1980). Effect of carbon dioxide on broiler chicken performance. Poult Sci. 59 (11): 2400-2402.
http://dx.doi.org/10.3382/ps.0592400
PMid:6780990

4. Stiles, G.W. (1936). Carbon monoxide poisoning in chickens. Poult Sci. 15(3): 270-272.
http://dx.doi.org/10.3382/ps.0150270

5. Breurec, J.Y., Valancony, V., Blevin, F., Baert, A., Charles, D., Arzel, Y., Presle, J.C., Curtes J.P. (1999). Carbon monoxide poisoning among poultry breeders. Indoor and Built Environment 8 (3): 193-198. http://dx.doi.org/10.1177/1420326X9900800312

6. Carlson, H.C., Clandinin, D. R. (1963). Carbon monoxide poisoning in chicks. Poultry Sci. 42 (1): 206-214. http://dx.doi.org/10.3382/ps.0420206

7. Anderson, D.P., Beard, C.W., Hanson, R.P. (1964). The adverse effects of ammonia on chickens including resistance to infection with New castle disease virus. Avian Dis. 8 (3): 369-379. http://dx.doi.org/10.2307/1587967

8. Quarles, C.L., Kling, H.F. (1974). Evaluation of ammonia and infectious bronchitis vaccination stress on broiler performance and carcass quality. Poul Sci. 53, 1592-1596. http://dx.doi.org/10.3382/ps.0531592

9. Charles, D.R., Payne, C.G. (1966). The influence of graded levels of atmospheric ammonia on chickens. Brit Poul Sci. 7 (3): 189-198. http://dx.doi.org/10.1080/00071668608415623 PMid:6007527

10. Wang, Y.M., Meng, Q.P., Guo, Y.M., Wang, Y.Z., Wang, Z., Yao Z.L., Shan T.Z. (2010). Effect of atmospheric ammonia on growth performance and immunological response of broiler chickens. J Anim Vet Adv. 22 (9): 2802-2806. http://dx.doi.org/10.3923/javaa.2010.2802.2806

11. Deaton, J.W., Reece, F.N., Lott, B.D. (1984). Effect of atmospheric ammonia on pullets at point of lay. Poult. Sci. 63 (2): 384–385. http://dx.doi.org/10.3382/ps.0630384 PMid:6709574

12. Deaton, J.W., Reece, F.N., Lott, B.D. (1982). Effect of atmospheric ammonia on laying hens performance. Poult. Sci., 61 (9): 1815-1817. http://dx.doi.org/10.3382/ps.0611815 PMid:7134135

13. Thiele, H. H., Pottgüter, R. (2008). Management recommendations for laying hens in deep litter, perchery and free range systems. Lohmman Information 43, 53-63.

14. Sterling, K.G., Bell, D.D., Pesti, G.M., Aggrey, S.E. (2003). Relationships among strain, performance, and environmental temperature in commercial laying hens. J App Poult Res. 12, 85-91. http://dx.doi.org/10.1093/japr/12.1.85

15. Xin, H., De Shazer, J.A., Beck, M. M. (1987). Post-effect of ammonia on energetics of laying hens at high temperatures. Transactions of the ASAE. 30 (4): 1121-1125. http://dx.doi.org/10.13031/2013.30530

16. Czarick, M., Farichild, B. (2012). Relative humidity... The best measure of overall poultry house air quality. Poultry Housing Tips [Internet] [cited 2015 November 5]; 24 (2). Available from: https://www.poultryventilation.com/tips/vol24/n2

17. Oarad, Z., Marder, J., Soller, M. (1981). Effect of gradual acclimatization to temperature up to 44°C on productive performance of the desert Bedouin fowl, the commercial white Leghorn and the two crossbreds. Br Poult Sci. 22, 511-520. http://dx.doi.org/10.1080/00071688108447918

18. Talukder, S., Islam, T., Sarker S., Islam, M.M. (2010). Effects of environment on layer performance. J Bangladesh Agril Univ. 8 (2): 253-258.

19. Appleby, M.C., Hughes, B.O., Elson, H.A. (1992). Poultry production systems: Behaviour, management and welfare. CAB International, Wallingford, United Kingdom.

20. Carlile, F.S. (1984). Ammonia in poultry houses: a literature review. World's Poult Sci J. 40 (2): 99-113. http://dx.doi.org/10.1079/WPS19840008

21. Ning, X. (2008). Feeding, defecation and gaseous emission dynamics of W-36 laying hens. Graduate Theses and Dissertations. Paper 11575. Iowa State University. [cited 2015 May 18] http://lib.dr.iastate.edu/etd/11575

22. Reece, F.N., Lott, B.D. (1983). The effects of temperature and the age on body weight and feed efficiency of broiler chickens. Poult Sci. 62 (9): 1906-1914. http://dx.doi.org/10.3382/ps.0621906 PMid:6634619

23. Li, H. (2006). Ammonia emissions from manure belt laying hen houses and manure storage. Retrospective Theses and Dissertations. Paper 1273 Iowa State University. http://lib.dr.iastate.edu/rtd/1273

13

DIAGNOSTIC CHARACTERISTICS OF CIRCOVIRUS INFECTION IN PIGS

Ivica Gjurovski, Branko Angelovski, Toni Dovenski, Dine Mitrov, Trpe Ristoski

*Faculty of Veterinary Medicine, "Ss Cyril and Methodius" University in Skopje
Lazar Pop Trajkov 5-7, 1000 Skopje, Republic of Macedonia*

ABSTRACT

The aim of this study is to compare the results from the histopathology and the immunohistochemical method in the diagnostic of Porcine circovirus type 2 (PCV2) infection in pigs. The circovirus infection is a pig disease that is caused by a small, spherical, nonenveloped virus with a single stranded DNA genome which is spread throughout the pig industry worldwide. The circovirus is the etiological agent of a several pig diseases which today are thought to be the cause of the greatest economical loses in pig production. The most important of these diseases is the PMWS (post-weaning multisystemic wasting syndrome). In this article we have performed an investigation of four farms on which there had been a previous clinical diagnosis of the Post-weaning multisystemic wasting syndrome. The examination was performed on thirty pigs from these farms, from two to five months old, which had the most severe symptoms of the disease. Necropsy, histopathology and immunohistochemical diagnostic methods were performed. The most significant necropsy findings were the enlarged lymph nodes (especially the inguinal, mediasinal and the mesenteric lymph nodes). The main histopathological changes were located in the lymphatic organs presented by B and T lymphocyte depletion and increase in the number of the macrophages. PCV2 antigen and nucleic acid were detected in almost all of the examined tissues. The examination showed that the histopathological and immunohistochemical methods provide complementary results in diagnosing PCV2 in pigs.

Key words: histopathology, immunohistochemistry, porcine circovirus type 2, post-weaning multisystemic wasting syndrome

INTRODUCTION

The circovirosis presents one of the most significant virus diseases in pig production in the world. The etiological agent of this disease is a small, nonenveloped, spherical virus with a single stranded DNA genome which belongs to the Circoviridae family (1, 4, 5).

The virus was first isolated on a PK-15 cell culture and was considered non-pathogenic (25). Later, a virus was isolated from pigs with PMWS with a different genotype than the virus present on the PK-15 cell culture (11, 19). The virus present in the pigs with PMWS was marked as Porcine

---

Corresponding author. Assist. Prof. Trpe Ristoski, PhD
E-mail address: tristoski@fvm.ukim.edu.mk
Present address: Department of Pathology and Forensic Medicine
Faculty of Veterinary Medicine-Skopje
"Ss. Cyril and Methodius" University in Skopje
Lazar Pop Trajkov 5-7, 1000 Skopje, Republic of Macedonia

circoviruse type 2 (PCV2), and the virus present on the PK15 cell culture was marked as Porcine circovirus type 1 (PCV1) (17, 19).

PCV2 is the causal agent of several pig diseases which are collectively known as Porcine circovirus diseases - PCVD in Europe, or porcine circovirus-associated diseases (PCVAD) in North America (9). Most significant among them is the Post-weaning multisystemic wasting syndrome (PMWS); and the other diseases in this group are: Porcine dermatitis and nephropathy syndrome (PDNS); porcine respiratory disease complex (PRDC); proliferative and necrotizing pneumonia (PNP); enteritis; as well as some reproductive diseases (4, 8, 9, 12, 23).

It is noted that the PCVD, especially the PMWS, have the greatest impact on pig production. In the European Union alone it is estimated that the annual loss caused by the PCVD is more than 600 million Euros. PMWS affects pigs between the age of 7 and 20 weeks, mainly older pigs and in the early fattening period, but the diseases has also been described in pigs between the age of 1 and 6 months (1, 10).

The most characteristic damages of the PMWS develop in the immunological system of the pigs expressed by depletion of the lymphocytes in the lymphoid tissues, changes of the cell subpopulation in the peripheral blood and change in the cytokines expression in the diseased pigs (1, 3, 7).

The diagnosis for the porcine circovirosis is based on three criteria. The first criterion is the clinical picture which is consisted of loss of body weight, skin pallor, respiratory disorders and occasionally jaundice (14, 15, 21). The second criteria is the finding of characteristic histopathological lesions in the tissues, and the third criteria is the finding of PCV2 (antigen and/or nucleic acid) in the microscopic lesions (6, 7, 22).

Lately the PCR method gets more attention in the diagnosis of the porcine circovirosis (2, 13, 16, 20, 24). This method is based on the isolation of DNA (from viruses, bacteria, other microorganisms etc.) from the tissue samples and its amplification for easier demonstration of the existence of the causal agent in the examined sample. There are several types of the PCR method out of which the most used are the quantitative (qPCR) and the nested (nPCR). The advantage of the PCR method compared to the other previously mentioned is the short time necessary for establishing the diagnosis and quantification of the amount of the virus present in the examined material.

The "golden standard" in the PCV2 diagnosis is the method that includes finding of tissue changes and in the same time detection of the PCV2, which makes the in situ hybridization and immunohistochemical method the most often used method (18, 22).

MATERIAL AND METHODS

Animals

In this article, we have reviewed the investigation of four farms from different regions in the Republic of Macedonia, where a clinical diagnosis for PMWS has been previously set. All farms were farrow to finishing units (the common way of breeding in Macedonia). The first farm had 400 sows in the herd and a total of 8000 finishing pigs produced per year. The second farm has produced 20000 finishing pigs per year and had 1000 sows. The third and fourth farm have produced 14000 finishing pigs per year per farm and had 650 sows in each of the farms. The examination was performed *post mortem* on thirty pigs from these farms, age from two to five months old, which had the most severe symptoms of the disease. The materials were taken not later than twelve hours after the animals' death. A complete

necropsy was performed on all of the pigs and samples were collected from the following tissues: lymph nodes (mesenteric, superficial inguinal, mediastinal and submandibular), lungs, liver, spleen, kidneys, tonsils, jejunum, ileum and colon. The samples for histopathology and immunohistochemistry were fixed in a 10% formalin solution. Samples from all the previously listed tissues were frozen at -80°C for further PCR investigation.

Histopathology and immunohistochemistry

Tissue samples from the lymph nodes (mesenteric, superficial inguinal, mediastinal and submandibular), lungs, liver, spleen, kidneys, tonsils, jejunum, ileum and colon were collected at the necropsy and were fixated in 10% formalin, dehydrated, embedded in paraffin wax, sectioned at 3-4 μm and stained with haematoxylin and eosin (HE). F217 2C6-H9-A2 monoclonal antibodies and En Vision Kit (Dako ChemMate, Denmark) were used for immunostaining of the tissue sections which allowed us to assess low, moderate or large amounts of PCV2 antigen.

RESULTS

Clinical symptoms

The most important clinical symptoms observed before death were: wasting, weight loss, decreased rate of weight gain, lymph node enlargement, respiratory distress, dyspnea, skin pallor and occasionally icterus were diagnosed.

Macroscopic findings

In some of the pigs the presence of red papules and macula was noted, as well as hemorrhagic and necrotizing skin lesions. In the necropsy, the most evident finding was the enlarged lymph nodes (especially the inguinal, mediasinal and the mesenteric lymph nodes). The lungs had the following findings: cranio ventral lung consolidation in ten pigs, lack of pulmonary collapse in almost all of the pigs, interstitial pneumonia and lung edema. The liver was atrophic and discolored; white spots on the kidneys and catarrhal to hemorrhagic enteritis in twenty pigs were predominantly found.

Histopathology

The microscopic lesions in the lymphatic organs (the lymph nodes, tonsils, spleen and the Payer's patches) in all of the pigs were mainly expressed in the form of lymphocyte depletion and necrosis in the cortex and the paracortex of the lymph nodes, as well as the presence of giant cells in the same areas (Fig. 1).

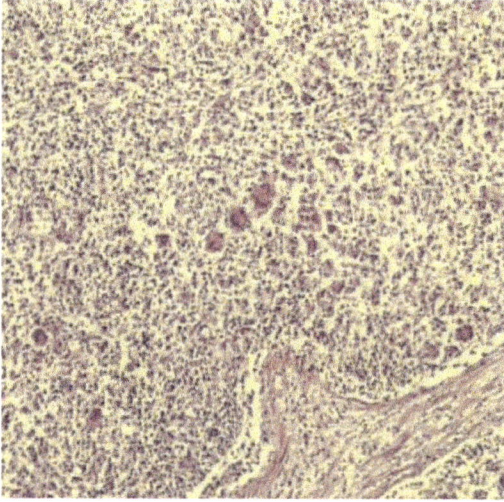
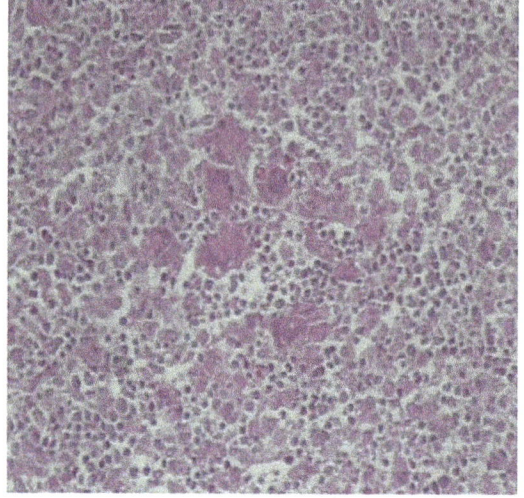

(a)   (b)

Figure 1. Giant (syncytial) cells in the lymph node of the infected pigs. H.E.x10 (a) and x 20 (b)

In the lymph follicles and the parafollicular areas lymphocyte depletion and infiltration with large histiocytic cells was found. Large multinucleated cells were found in the lymph nodes, Payer's patches and lamina propria of the intestinal villi.

In the lungs, a multifocal lymphohistiocytic to granoulomatous interstitial pneumonia with the presence of histiocytes and multinucleated giant cells in the interalveolar walls was found (Fig. 2). Five of the pigs had necrotizing pneumonia.

Changes in the liver consisted of lymphohistiocytic infiltration, disorganization of the hepatic lobules, and in few samples, a perilobular fibrosis.

Lymphohistiocytic infiltration was also found in the kidneys, the intestines and also in most of the other tissues. The finding in the kidneys consisted of tubulointerstitial lymphoplasmatic and granulomatous nephritis.

Immunohistochemistry

The immunohistochemical method revealed the presence of the PCV2 antigen in most of the examined pigs. The presence of the antigen is found in all the lymphoid tissues (specifically in the cells' cytoplasm), while in the non lymphoid tissues it was less present. The presence of the antigen in the tissues shows positive correlation with the presence

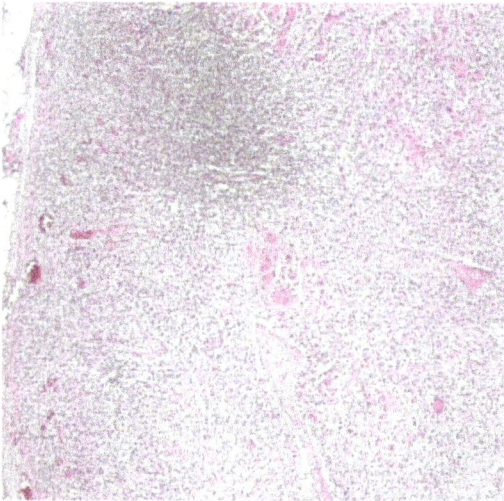
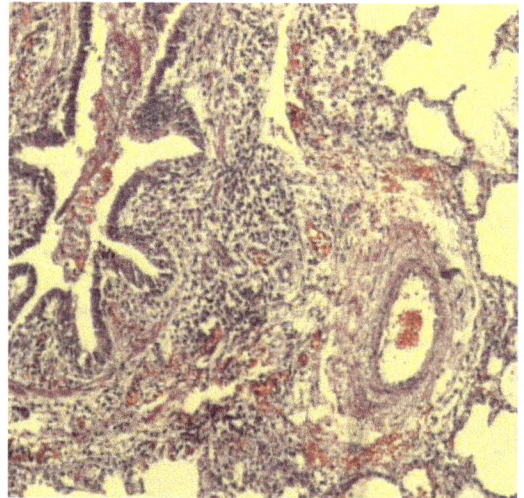

(a)   (b)

Figure 2. Lymphoid depletion in the tonsil (a) and lymphohistiocytic interstitial pneumonia in the lungs (b). H.E.x10 (a) and x 20 (b)

of the histopathological lesions in the same tissues. The antigen is mostly present in the necrotic areas of the lymph follicles and less present in the giant cells and the mononucleated phagocytes of the lymph follicles (Fig. 3).

circovirosis were found. Most significantly affected are the lymphoid tissues expressed by lymphocyte depletion, histiocytic infiltration and presence of a giant multinucleated cells. The findings suggest immunosuppression.

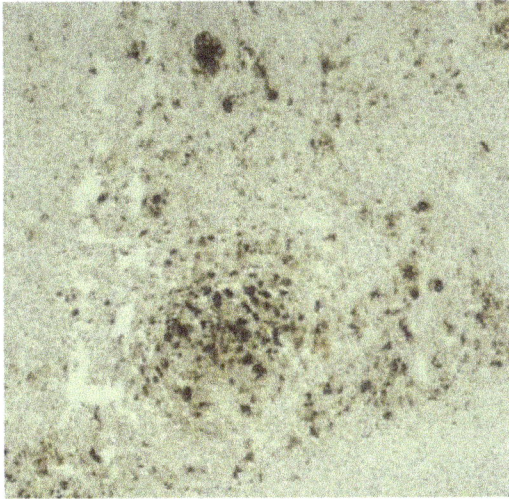

(a)

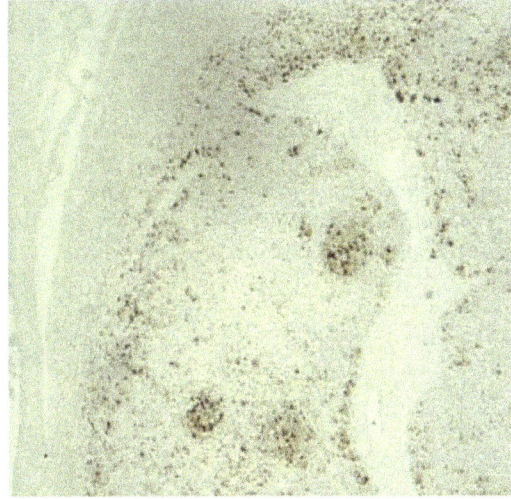

(b)

Figure 3. Abundant presence of porcine circovirus antigen in nuclei of lymphocytes and histiocytes of tonsil. IHC x 20 (a) and x10 (b)

In the lungs, the PCV2 antigen is found in the large cells in the hyperplastic bronchial lymph tissue (BALT), in the epithelial alveolar cells, interstitial mononucleated cells, as well as the inflammatory exudates of the bronchi, bronchiole and alveoli.

In the liver, the antigen is mostly present in the centroacinar areas, especially in the hepatocytes, the epithelial cells of the bile ducts and in the Kupffer cells.

In the kidneys, the PCV2 antigen is widely present not only in the inflammatory cells, but also in the epithelial cells, in the interstitial inflammatory infiltrate and in the tubular cells.

DISCUSSION

This article described the histopathological and immunohistochemical findings and also made a comparison of these findings in thirty pigs from four farms in the Republic of Macedonia. All the pigs have PMWS symptoms. From the presented histopathological and immunohistochemical diagnoses it is evident that there is a close correlation between the finding of the PCV2 antigen, and the degree of the tissue lesions. The examinations included the parenchymatous organs of the animals and changes which are characteristic for the porcine

The use of the immunohistochemical method helped to determine the presence and the distribution of the PCV2 antigen in the tissues. The previously presented histopathological and immunohistochemical findings can confirm that the virus has a tropism towards the lymphoid tissue as it has been previously concluded by the other articles (1, 4, 7). It has been confirmed that both methods give satisfying results in the diagnosis of the porcine circovirosis. The "golden standard" in the diagnosis of porcine circovirosis consists of three parts: clinical symptoms (weight lose, pallor, respiratory distress, jaundice), histopathological findings (lymphocyte depletion and the presence of multinucleated giant cells) and confirmation of the presence of the virus DNA in the tissues using immunohistochemistry and in-situ hybridization.

In recent time, the PCR (polymerase chain reaction) method is being widely used. This method consists of only several steps which makes the time necessary for diagnosis significantly shorter (with the conventional method, about 7-78 hours, and with the real time quantitative PCR method, only about 45 minutes). Most of the studies recommend the real time quantitative PCR (qPCR) method. However, there are differences in opinion on what amount (threshold) of the virus in the serum should be present in the diagnosis of PCV2: $10^{6.21}$, $10^{6.91}$, 10^7 and $10^{7.43}$ viral copies/ ml. It is important that the sensitivity and the specificity obtained with the qPCR tests (used separately or combined with serology) are not enough to replace the histopathology plus the detection of PCV2 in the tissues (8).

According to the proposal of some authors the diagnosing of a herd should be based on two elements: 1) significant increase in the mortality of post weaning pigs followed by clinical signs compatible with PCV2 compared to the histological data for the herd, and 2) individual diagnosing of PMWS in at least one in three to five necropsies of pigs combined with the mentioned increase in the mortality. At the same time, other reasons for increased mortality should be excluded.

CONCLUSION

The results gained in this examination showed that the histopathological and the immunohistochemical method combined with the clinical diagnostics are sufficient to confirm or deny the presence of PCV2 infection in the pig population.

In future investigation, in order to improve diagnostic accuracy, beside the histopathological and the immunohistochemical method, the PCR method has to be introduced in the diagnosis of the PCV2, as well as comparison of the results between these methods.

REFERENCES

1. Ristoski, T., Cvetkovik, I., Joaqim, S. (2009). Circovirus diseases in swine. Mac Vet Rev 32, 1, 5-11.

2. Gan-Nan, C., Jyi-Faa, H., Jing-Tsang, C., Hau-Yang, T., Jyh-Jye, W. (2010). Fast diagnosis and quantification for porcine circovirus type 2 (PCV-2) using real-time plymerase chain reaction. J Microbiol Immunol Infect 43(2): 85–92. http://dx.doi.org/10.1016/S1684-1182(10)60014-X

3. Grau-Roma, L., Lorenzo, F., Joaqim, S. (2010). Recent advances in the epidemiology, diagnosis and control of diseases caused by porcine circovirus type 2. The Veterinary Journal 187, 23–32. http://dx.doi.org/10.1016/j.tvjl.2010.01.018 PMid:20211570

4. Joaquim, S., Tuija, K., Martí, C. (2012). The natural history of porcine circovirus type 2: From an inoffensive virus to a devastating swine disease? Veterinary Microbiology 165, 13–20.

5. Nicolas, R., Tanja, O., Béatrice, G., André, J. (2011). Epidemiology and transmission of porcine circovirus type 2 (PCV2). Virus Research 164, 78– 89.

6. McNeilly, F., Kennedy, S., Moffett, D., Meehan, B.M., Foster, J.C., Clarke, E.G., Ellis, J.A., Haines, D.M., Adair, B.M., Allan, G.M. (1999). A comparison of in situ hybridization and immunohistochemistry for the detection of a new porcine circovirus in formalin-fixed tissues from pigs with post-weaning multisystemic wasting syndrome (PMWS). Journal of Virological Methods 80, 123–128. http://dx.doi.org/10.1016/S0166-0934(99)00043-9

7. Rosell, C., Segalés, J., Plana-Durán, J., Balasch, M., Rodríguez-Arrioja, G. M., Kennedy, S., Allan, G. M., McNeilly, F., Latimer, K. S., Domingo, M. (1999). Pathological, immunohistochemical, and in-situ hybridization studies of natural cases of postweaning multisystemic wasting syndrome (PMWS) in pigs. J. Comp. Path., 120, 59–78. http://dx.doi.org/10.1053/jcpa.1998.0258 PMid:10098016

8. Joaquim, S. (2012). Porcine circovirus type 2 (PCV2) infections: Clinical signs, pathology and laboratory diagnosis. Virus Research 164, 10– 19. http://dx.doi.org/10.1016/j.virusres.2011.10.007 PMid:22056845

9. Tanja, O., Xiang-Jin, M., Patrick, G. H. (2007). Porcine circovirus type 2–associated disease: Update on current terminology, clinical manifestations, pathogenesis, diagnosis, and intervention strategies. J Vet Diagn Invest 19, 591–615. http://dx.doi.org/10.1177/104063870701900601

10. Calsaming, M., Segales, J., Quintana, J., Rosell, C., Domingo, M. (2002). Detection of porcine circvirus tupes 1 and 2 in serum and tissue samples of pigs with and without postweaning pultisystemic wasting syndrome. Journal of Clinical Microbiology 40, 1848 - 1850. http://dx.doi.org/10.1128/JCM.40.5.1848-1850.2002 PMCid:PMC130924

11. Ellis J, Hassard L, Clark E, Harding J, Allan G, Willson P, Strokappe J, Martin K, McNeilly F, Meehan B, Tood, D., Haines, D. (1998). Isolation of circovirus from lesions of pigs with postweaning multisystemic wasting syndrome. Canadian Veterinary Journal 39, 44 – 51. PMid:9442952 PMCid:PMC1539838

12. Ellis, J., Clark, E., Haines, D., West, K., Kreakowka, S., Kennedy, S., Allan, G, M. (2003). Porcine circovirus-2 and concurrent infections in the field. Veterinary Microbiology 98, 159 – 163. http://dx.doi.org/10.1016/j.vetmic.2003.10.008

13. Hamel, A.L., Lin, L.L., Sachvie, C., Grudeski, E., Nayar, G.P. (2000). PCR detection and characterization of type - 2 porcine circovirus. Canadian Journal of Veterinary Research 64, 44 - 52. PMid:10680656 PMCid:PMC1189580

14. Harding, J.C.S., Clark, E.G. (1997). Recognizing and diagnosing postweaning multisystemic wasting syndrome (PMWS) . Swine Health and Production 5, 201 - 203.

15. Kim, J., Chung, H.K., Jung, T., Cho, W.S., Choi, C., Chae, C. (2002). Postweaning multisystemic wasting syndrome of pigs in korea: Prevalence, microscopic lesions and coexisting microorganisms. Journal of Veterinary Medical Science 64, 57 - 62. http://dx.doi.org/10.1292/jvms.64.57

16. Magar, R., Larochelle, R., Thibault, S., Lamontagne, L. (2000). Experimental transmission of porcine circovirus type 2 (PCV2) in weaning pigs: a sequental study. Journal of Comparative Pathology 123, 258 - 269. http://dx.doi.org/10.1053/jcpa.2000.0413 PMid:11041995

17. Mankertz, A., Mankertz, J., Wolf, K., Bunk, H.J. (1998). Identification of a protein essential for replication of porcine circovirus. Journal of General Virology 79, 381 - 384. PMid:9472624

18. McNeilly, F., Kennedy, S., Moffet, D., Meehan, B.M., Foster, J.C., Clarke, E.G., Ellis, J.A., Haines, D.M., Adair, B.M., Allan, G.M. (1999). A comparison of in situ hybridization and immunohistochemistry for the detection of a new porcine circovirus in formalin - fixed tissues from pigs with post - weaning multisystemic wasting syndrome (PMWS). Journal of Virological Methods 80, 123 - 128. http://dx.doi.org/10.1016/S0166-0934(99)00043-9

19. Meehan, B.M., McNeilly, F., Todd, D., Kennedy, S., Jewhurst, V.A., Ellis, J.A., Hassard, L.E., Clark, E.G., Haines, D.M., Allan, G.M. (1998). Characterization of novel circovirus DNAs associated with wasting syndromes in pigs. Journal of General Virology 79, 2171 - 2179. PMid:9747726

20. Nayar, G.P.S, Hamel, A., Lin, L. (1997). Detection and characterization of porcine circovirus associated with postweaning multisystemic wasting syndrome in pigs. Canadian Veterinary Journal 38, 385 - 386. PMid:9187809 PMCid:PMC1576874

21. Quintana, J., Segales, J., Rosell, C., Calsamiglia, M., Rodríguez – Arrioja, G.M., Chianini, F., Folch, J.M., Maldonado, .J, Canal, M., Plana – Durán, J., Domingo, M. (2001). Clinical and pathological observations of pigs with postweaning multisystemic wasting syndrome. Veterinary Record 149, 357 - 361. http://dx.doi.org/10.1136/vr.149.12.357 PMid:11594382

22. Rosell, C., Segales, J., Plana – Duran, J., Balasch, M., Rodriguez – Arrioja, G.M., Kennedy, S., Allan, G.M., McNeilly, F., Latimer, K.S., Domingo, M. (1999). Pathological, immunohistochemical and in situ hibridization studies of natural cases of postweaning multisystemic wasting syndrome (PMWS) in pigs. J. Comp. Path., 120, 59 - 78. http://dx.doi.org/10.1053/jcpa.1998.0258 PMid:10098016

23. Segales, J. (2002). Update on postweaning multisystemic wasting syndrome and porcine dermatitis and nephropathy syndrome diagnostic. Journal of Swine Health and Production 10 (6): 277 - 281.

24. Segales, J., Allan, G.M., Domingo, M. (2005). Porcine circovirus diseases. Animal Health Research Reviews 6 (2): 119 - 142. http://dx.doi.org/10.1079/AHR2005106 PMid:16583778

25. Tischer, I., Mields, W., Wolff, D., Vagt, M., Griem, W. (1986). Studies on the pathogenicity of porcine circovirus. Archives of Virology 91, 271 - 276. http://dx.doi.org/10.1007/BF01314286 PMid:3778212

14

THE EFFECT OF ACUTE INFLAMMATION ON TOTAL ALKALINE PHOSPHATASE ACTIVITY IN DOGS

Zapryanova Dimitrinka

*Department of Pharmacology, Animal Physiology and Physiological Chemistry,
Faculty of Veterinary Medicine, Trakia University, 6000, Stara Zagora, Bulgaria*

ABSTRACT

The main purpose of this study was to investigate the effect of acute inflammation on total alkaline phosphatase (ALP) activity in dogs. In this study total ALP activity was determined in dogs with experimentally induced acute inflammation in order to characterize their potential value in this condition. For that, ALP concentrations were defined in plasmas from 9 mongrel male dogs (in an experimental group) and 6 mongrel male dogs (in a control group) at the age of 2 years and body weight 12-15 kg. The inflammation was reproduced by inoculation of 2 ml turpentine oil subcutaneously in lumbar region and same quantity saline in control dogs. Blood samples were collected into heparinized tubes before inoculation, then at hours 6, 24, 48, 72 and on days 7, 14, 21. The total ALP concentrations were determined with commercial kits (Human-GmbH, Germany) on an automatic biochemical analyzer (BS-3000 P, Sinnowa, LTD Nanjing China). The statistical analysis of the data was performed using one way analysis of variance (ANOVA), Statistica v.6.1 (StatSoft Inc., 2002). Statistically significant difference was not found between the groups, as well as within them. In conclusion, we can say that the total activity of ALP was not significantly affected in dogs with experimentally induced acute inflammation.

Key words: alkaline phosphatase activity, acute inflammation, dogs

INTRODUCTION

Alkaline phosphatase is a non-specific metalloenzyme which hydrolyzes many types of phosphate esters at an alkaline pH in the presence of zinc and magnesium ions. The enzyme is associated with microsomal and cell membranes and is present in many tissues. It is an "ectoenzyme" functioning in the external environment of the cell and is anchored to cell membranes by glycophosphatidylinositol (GPI) proteins (1). Cleavage of these proteins by bile acids, phospholipase D and proteases releases ALP from membranes resulting in increased ALP levels in serum/plasma. There are 2 isoenzymes (products of different genes) and several isoforms (produced from posttranslational modification of isoenyzmes) of ALP. The isoenzymes are produced from intestinal and tissue non-specific ALP genes and differ in amino acid sequence. Isoforms differ in catalytic sites and activity, immunogenecity, and electrophoretic mobility. In domestic animals several variants in ALP are identified: the bones, intestines and liver, but only in dogs there is another isoenzyme - corticosteroid-induced alkaline phosphatase (2). Routine measurement of ALP gives total serum activity (all isoforms) without specificity as to the source. In healthy normal animals, liver-ALP is the predominant isoform in blood. Inflammation accompanied by local and general systematic signs-enhanced fever and increase heart, and respiratory rates, which are indicators for nonspecific response and signs of inflammation. It has been demonstrated in this study that subcutaneous turpentine administration can be used as a simple

Corresponding author: Zapryanova Dimitrinka
E-mail address: zaprianowa@abv.bg
Present address: Department of Pharmacology, Animal Physiology and Physiological Chemistry, Faculty of Veterinary Medicine Trakia University, 6000, Stara Zagora, Bulgaria

method, which causes a local inflammatory process. The aim of the experiment was to determine the changes in plasma total ALP activity in dogs at different time points in acute inflammation induced by turpentine injection.

MATERIALS AND METHODS

Experimental animals and protocol design

The experiment was approved by the Ethic Committee at the Faculty of Veterinary Medicine. The experimental animals were provided by the municipality of Stara Zagora. The study was performed on 9 mongrel dogs (experimental group) and 6 mongrel dogs (control group) at the age of 2 years and body weight 12-15 kg. The dogs were housed in metal cages. They were exposed to a 12h light-dark cycle at room temperature (20-22^{0}C). The dogs were fed of commercial extruded dry food (Jambo dog®, Gallisman S.A., Bulgaria), and content: extruded cereal products, vegetable proteins, fats, dehydrated poultry meat, amino acids, extracts of sweet chestnut, vitamins, minerals, antioxidants. This food was assigned for dogs of medium physical activity after finishing their growth period (3). The food was given to dogs as a dry in the amount 250 g/day/dog average with permanent access to the clean water. The dog feeding was once a day, always at the same time.

Prior to the experiment, the animals were in the adaptation period of one month. During this period they were vaccinated with vaccine Nobivac®, Intervet International B.V and treated per oral against internal parasites with Caniverm®, Bioveta, A. S. Czech Republic, 1 tablet/10 kg b.w., and external parasites with Bolfo® Puder, Bayer, Germany. The acute inflammation was reproduced by inoculation of 2 ml turpentine oil in the lumbar region subcutaneously (s. c.) in experimental animals, whereas the control dogs were injected with the same volume of saline solution.

Biochemical analyses

Blood samples were collected from the puncture of the *v. cephalica antebrachii* into heparinized tubes before inoculation (hour 0) then at hours 6, 24, 48, 72 and on days 7, 14, 21 after turpentine injections. At the same time, blood was taken from controls. Heparinised blood was centrifuged (1500g, 10 minutes, room temperature) within 30 min after collection. Plasma was immediately separated and stored at -20°C until analysis. Total ALP-activity was determined by a kit from Human Diagnostics (GmbH), Germany. Enzyme analysis of the alkaline phosphatase level was done using a spectrophotometer (SPEKOL 11-Carlzeiss Jena, Germany). The rate of formation of p-nitrophenol is measured as an increase in absorbance of 405 nm wavelength light which is proportional to the alkaline phosphatase activity in the sample.

Statistical analysis

The statistical analysis of the data was performed using one way analysis of variance (ANOVA). The results were processed with software Statistica v.6.1 (StatSoft Inc., 2002). All results are presented as mean and standard error of the mean (Mean ± Err). The statistical significance of parameters was determined in the LSD test at p < 0.05.

RESULTS

The changes in the ALP concentrations during acute inflammation induced by turpentine injection are shown in Table 1. In the experimental and control groups, total alkaline phosphatase activities were followed during a period of 21 days. They were slightly influenced by those local, aseptic inflammatory stimuli. In the experimental group, initial levels (before inoculation) were 81,8±4,85 U/L and 72 hours after this, ALP levels began to rise (87,2±5,22 U/L) and remained high including on day 7 (88,2±5,06 U/L) of the study compared to baselines. After this period, the activities showed consistent downward trend and on the 21st day the mean values were 81,7±4,84 U/L. This study indicated differences in comparison to the control group at the 72th hours. On day 7, ALP levels reached peak elevation compared to the controls, but it was not significantly higher and the concentrations remained in the reference ranges. Inflammation accompanied by local and general systematic signs-enhanced fever (6 hour after inoculation), increase heart and respiratory rates at the 24th h, which are indicators for non-specific response and signs of inflammation (Table 2, 3 and 4).

Table 1. Blood total alkaline phosphatase activities (U/L) in healthy dogs (n = 6) and in dogs (n = 9) with experimentally induced acute inflammation

Time after inoculation	Inoculated dogs (n=9) mean ± SEM	Non-inoculated dogs (n=6) mean ± SEM
0 hour	81,81±4,85	79,53±5,88
6 hour	81,45±4,77	79,40±5,83
24 hours	83,44±4,65	80,10±5,68
48 hours	84,38±5,07	79,53±6,15
72 hours	87,22±5,22	80,03±6,23
Day 7	88,21±5,06	79,45±6,42
Day 14	85,53±4,96	79,31±6,11
Day 21	81,76±4,84	80,30±6,06

Table 2. Dynamics of internal body temperature (IBT) (°C) in healthy dogs (n = 6) and in dogs (n = 9) with experimentally induced acute inflammation with turpentine. Results are expressed as means ± standard errors of the means (SEM)

Time after treatment	IBT - control dogs	IBT - inoculated dogs
0 hour	38,63±0,16	39,27±0,17
6 hours	38,80±0,18	39,92±0,20***c
24 hours	38,81±0,19	39,46±0,15**
48 hours	38,66±0,17	39,20±0,09*
72 hours	38,68±0,12	39,10±0,17*
Day 7	38,60±0,17	38,65±0,15
Day 14	38,76±0,18	38,46±0,25
Day 21	36,65±0,19	38,85±0,08

For a given biochemical parameter: *($p < 0.05$), **($p < 0.01$) and ***($p < 0.001$) indicate significant differences between turpentine inoculated and control dogs. Different superscripts c indicate significant difference ($p < 0.001$) according to time within the experimental group (turpentine inoculated dogs).

Table 3. Dynamics of respiratory rate (RR) in healthy dogs (n = 6) and in dogs (n = 9) with experimentally induced acute inflammation with turpentine. Results are expressed as means ± standard errors of the means (SEM)

Time after treatment	RR - control dogs	RR - inoculated dogs
0 hour	28,66±2,81	35,88±2,44
6 hours	35,00±2,35	41,22±3,10
24 hours	35,00±4,17	48,00±4,21*b
48 hours	38,66±2,90	37,11±4,37
72 hours	34,00±4,47	34,00±2,15
Day 7	34,33±3,87	38,44±2,88
Day 14	35,50±4,42	29,77±3,25
Day 21	28,66±1,33	35,00±3,73

For a given biochemical parameter: *($p < 0.05$) indicate significant differences between turpentine inoculated and control dogs. Different superscripts b indicate significant difference ($p < 0.01$) according to time within the experimental group (turpentine inoculated dogs).

Table 4. Dynamics of pulse rate (PR) in healthy dogs (n = 6) and in dogs (n = 9) with experimentally induced acute inflammation with turpentine. Results are expressed as means ± standard errors of the means (SEM)

Time after treatment	PR - control dogs	PR - inoculated dogs
0 hour	87,33±5,35	101,88±8,88
6 hours	86,33±5,14	103,33±4,28
24 hours	82,33±4,46	98,77±6,92
48 hours	85,33±3,78	100,66±15,15
72 hours	82,00±4,20	82,77±5,25
Day 7	81,16±3,22	104,44±7,43*
Day 14	78,50±5,25	94,55±7,60
Day 21	80,00±4,25	91,66±7,76

For a given biochemical parameter: *($p < 0.05$) indicate significant differences between turpentine inoculated and control dogs

DISCUSSION

Alkaline phosphatase is a membrane-bound enzyme present in many tissues. Three major isoenzymes in dogs contribute to total serum ALP: bone, liver, and corticosteroid isoenzymes. Bone ALP accounts for about one-third of the total serum ALP and is elevated with conditions associated with increased osteoblastic activity. Liver ALP present on biliary epithelial cells and hepatocytes and has a half-life about 70 hours. Increased ALP activity is one of the most common abnormalities detected on serum chemistry profiles in ill dogs. ALP activity measurement has a high sensitivity (80%) for hepatobiliary disease, but its specificity is low (51%).

Inflammation or trauma can induce local swelling, mild pain, local erythema and variable fevers which are common findings in soft tissue inflammation. It has been demonstrated that subcutaneous turpentine administration can be used as a simple method, which causes a local inflammatory process (4). The results of the study are present in Table 1 and Table 2. In this study, changes in blood alkaline phosphatise concentrations were observed in dogs in response to turpentine injection. In this connection, the activities were slightly affected by aseptic stimuli; the experimental acute inflammation has lead to insignificantly increases in ALP at the 72nd hour and on days 7. In this experiment total ALP activity began to increase at the 72nd h after injection and remained so high up to day 14,

although they were within the normal ranges. The referent ranges for total ALP in dogs are 10-150 U/L (4). Turpentine oil which is a very powerful pyrogen, induces significant fever, which peaked 11 h after injection and continues for more than 24 hours (6). In our experimental group, the fever starts to rise 6 hours after treatment (39,92±0,20 ºC) and continued to the 72nd. This period coincides with elevation in ALP activities as compared to the baselines (the levels reached 87,2 U/L at 72nd hour). Some authors (7, 8) reported that the subcutaneous injection of turpentine in mice model induced local tissue damage and the inflammatory reaction to the oil is characterized by local inflammation, abscess formation, fever, loss of body weight, anorexia, lethargy. The same symptoms were observed in our study, whereas loss of body weight and anorexia were insignificant. There are some studies (9) which investigated changes in the ALP concentrations during acute and chronic wounds processes in animal and human models. They suggested that ALP activity is an acute inflammation marker since the enzyme levels are increased in acute wounds, but not in chronic inflammation processes. In our study, the elevation in the ALP levels is not significant because they remained in reference ranges for this species. Although, there are signs of non-specific response and inflammation - enhanced fever 6 hour after inoculation and increased respiratory rates at the 24th h. The fever continued to the 72nd h and at that time slight, insignificant elevation in ALP activities was also observed which continued until the 7th day (88,21±5,06 U/L), but stayed in the normal ranges (10-150 U/L). The mode of action of this potent pyrogen (turpentine injection) involves the production of localized necrotic damage which results in the sequential induction of some interleukins (TNFα and IL-1β) at the site of injury (6). The locally increased levels of them, particularly IL-1β, induce IL-6 synthesis and release into the circulation. IL-6 increases dramatically following a systemic inflammatory challenge and correlates significantly with the fever response. No significant changes in total activities of ALP of experimental groups were observed and this lead up to possible slightly increased permeability of liver cells plasma membrane. We could observe slightly elevated enzyme levels, presumably due to cellular damage which is characterized with altered permeability. We can assume that there is no significant disability in the liver function. The magnitude of ALP elevation may be proportional to the number of hepatocytes affected, so the lack of high levels (they were in the reference ranges) leads to the conclusion that in dogs, the liver function is not significantly affected by turpentine injection.

CONCLUSION

In conclusion, these results indicated that the total alkaline phosphatase activity was not significantly affected in dogs with experimentally induced acute inflammation by turpentine injection. Throughout the experiment (21 days), the levels remained in the reference ranges for this species.

REFERENCES

1. Shahbazkia, H.R., Sharifi, S., Shareghi, B. (2010). Purification and kinetic study of bone and liver alkaline phosphatase isoenzymes in the dog. Comparative Clinical Pathology, 19, 81-84.

2. Shahbazkia,H.R.,Aminlari,M.,Mohamad,A.R. (2009). Determination of alkaline phosphatase izoenzymes and isoforms in the dog serum by a simple anion exchange chromatographic method. Comparative Clinical Pathology, 18, 427-432.

3. NRC (2006). Chapter 15: Nutrient requirements and dietary nutrient concentrations. In: Nutrient requirements of dogs and cats. (pp. 354-370). National Academies Press, Washington, DC, USA.

4. Muthny, T, Kovarik, M., Tilser, I., Holecek, M. (2008). Protein metabolism in slow- and fast-twitch skeletal muscle during turpentine-induced inflammation. Int J Exp Path., 89, 64-71.

5. Hines R. (2012). Normal Feline & Canine Blood Chemistry Values Blood, Temperature, Urine and Other Values for Your Dog and Cat. (www.2ndchance.info/ normaldogandcatbloodvalues.htm)

6. Agular-Valles, A., Poole, S., Mistry, Y., Williams, S., Luheshi, G. N. (2007). Attenuated fever in rats during late pregnancy is linked to suppressed interleukin-6 production after localized inflammation with turpentine. The Journal of Physiology, 583, 391-403.

7. Renckens, R. J., Roelofs, J.T.H., De Waard, V., Florquin, S., Lijnen, H.R., Carmeliet, P., Van der Poll, T. (2005). The role of plasminogen activator inhibitor type 1 in the inflammatory response to local tissue injure. Journal of Thrombosis and Haemostasis, 3, 1018-1025.

8. Leon, L.R, Conn, C. A., Glaccum, M., Kluger, M.J. (1996). IL-1 type I receptor mediates acute phase response to turpentine, but not lipopolysaccharide, in mice. Am J of Physiol. Regulatory Integrative Comp Physiol., 271(6): R1668-75.

9. Krötzsch, E., Salgado, R.M., Caba, D., Lichtinger, A., Padilla, L., Di Silvio, M. (2005). Alkaline phosphatase activity is related to acute inflammation and collagen turnover during acute and chronic wound healing. Wound Repair and Regeneration, 13(2): A28-A48.

15

CLASSICAL AND MOLECULAR CHARACTERIZATION OF PIGEON PARAMYXOVIRUS TYPE 1 (PPMV-1) ISOLATED FROM BACKYARD POULTRY – FIRST REPORT IN MACEDONIA

Dodovski Aleksandar[1], Krstevski Kiril[1], Naletoski Ivancho[2]

[1]*Veterinary Institute, Faculty of Veterinary Medicine,*
University "Ss. Cyril and Methodius" Skopje, Macedonia
[2]*Joint FAO/IAEA Division of Nuclear Techniques in Food and Agriculture, Vienna, Austria*

ABSTRACT

Aim of this study was to characterize pigeon variant of Newcastle disease virus (NDV) isolated from backyard poultry using classical and molecular methods. In standard hemagglutination inhibition (HI) test both polyclonal NDV antiserum and monoclonal antibodies 161/617 specific for pigeon variants of NDV showed inhibition of heamagglutination of the isolated virus. Intracerebral pathogenicity index (ICPI) has shown that the isolate is mesogenic virus (ICPI = 0.81). One-step RT-qPCR for detection of M gene was performed indicating a presence of NDV and RT-qPCR for discrimination between lentogenic and velogenic strains based on F gene was also performed indicating a presence of virulent NDV. A portion of the F gene was amplified and sequenced for determination of virulence and phylogenetic characterization. The F protein cleavage site sequence of the isolate had multiple basic amino acids at residues 112–116 and a phenyl alanine at residue 117 (112RRQKR*F117) which is typical for velogenic strains. The nucleotide sequence of 374 bp was aligned to begin at nt 47 and finish at 420 immediately after the cleavage site and compared with other reference strains from the region and worldwide. In the phylogenetic tree, the isolate clustered into genotype VIb, typical for PPMV-1. This strain is phylogenetically very similar to other PPMV-1 isolated from pigeons in Macedonia. Poultry infected with PPMV-1 can spread the virus in the absence of clinical signs, thus PPMV-1's are constant threat to domestic poultry. This is the first report of evidenced spillover of PPMV-1 into poultry in Macedonia.

Key words: PPMV-1, backyard poultry, RT-qPCR, nucleotide sequencing

INTRODUCTION

Newcastle disease (ND) virus may be present in natural or experimental hosts in 241 species from 27 to 50 orders of birds and it is very likely that all birds are susceptible to infection, but the severity of the disease would depend on the type of the bird (19). The ND virus (NDV) belongs to order Mononegavirales, family Paramyxoviridae, subfamily Paramyxovirinae, genus *Avulavirus* (22). In this genus there are 11 serotypes of APMV, labeled APMV-1 to APMV-11 (9, 24). Newcastle disease virus is APMV-1, for which there are two different classifications based on genomic structure (2, 7, 12).

Since the first discovery of ND in 1926 (16) to date, four panzootics had occurred worldwide (3). The first isolation of virulent NDV responsible for the panzootics in pigeons is done by Kaleta et al. (18) in the sample from Iraq from 1978. In 1981 virus reaches Italy (8) and afterwards spreads globally to become panzootic by 1984/85 (5). Several authors consider that the reason for fast spread of the virus is developed international trade as well as races and exhibitions of pigeons (5). Pigeon strains most probably are a result of interspecies transmission of the virus which occurred several times in the past. Spread from pigeons to poultry must have happened earlier then 1980's because significant adaptation and evolution of these strains was present during the

---

Corresponding author: Ass. Dodovski Aleksandar, MsC

e-mail address: adodovski@fvm.ukim.edu.mk
Present address: Faculty for Veterinary Medicine Veterinary Institute, Lazar Pop Trajkov, 5-7, 1000 Skopje Macedonia

epizootics in pigeons (29). Virus is characterized as an antigenic variant of NDV with use of monoclonal antibodies (mAb's) (6). Because of the antigenic difference and for pragmatic purposes these viruses are termed pigeon paramyxovirus type 1 (PPMV-1) viruses beside the fact being able to infect poultry but with decreased virulence (23). These viruses are also able to infect wild pigeons, doves and ornamental birds (17, 20). The disease in pigeons has an enzootic character with occasional spread to wild pigeons and doves and represents a constant threat to poultry (4).

Amino acid sequence of cleavage site (CS) of fusion (F) protein is a major determinant of virulence (25, 26), although other proteins have a role in virulence depending on the strain of the virus (14). In order for the virus to be virulent a basic amino acid at residue 113, a pair of basic amino acid at residues 115 and 116 and phenylalanine at residue 117 of the F gene is required (10).

For proper diagnosis it is not enough only to detect NDV or prove infection with the virus, but it is also necessary to distinguish whether the virus is virulent or not by recommended classical and molecular methods (30). Nucleotide sequencing can determine virulence and can assess genetic makeup, genotype and phylogenetic characteristics of NDV (11, 21, 27). These techniques allow only 250 nucleotides to be sufficient for reliable phylogenetic analysis (2, 21, 27).

The role of pigeons in epizootiology of NDV in Macedonia has not been studied previously. The aim of this study was to characterize PPMV-1 isolated from backyard poultry by classical and molecular methods and to assess its phylogenetic relationship with other NDV isolates.

MATERIAL AND METHODS

Virus and virus isolation

Pool of internal organs obtained from dead chickens were homogenized in antibiotic medium using sterile sand, checked for sterility and inoculated in to the 9-11 days old embryonated chicken eggs (ECE). All dying embryos and remaining embryos after the incubation period of five days were checked for haemagglutination activity according to recommended protocols (29). Isolated virus was named as follows: serotype/host/

country of origin/laboratory identification number (reference number)/year of sampling.

GenBank accession numbers of the viruses used for construction of the phylogenetic tree are shown in parentheses in Fig. 2. Several sequences without accession numbers were obtained from colleagues from the region. Accession number of the Macedonian strain is given in the results section.

Strain under investigation was isolated from backyard chicken on 10.02.2010 from village Rankovce in the northeastern part of Macedonia (N 42o10'03. E 22o07'03.) Isolation was donefrom the pool of visceral organs. Strain was labeled as NDV/chicken/Macedonia/231/2010 according to serotype/host/location/laboratory number/sampling date.

Hemagglutination inhibition test (HI test)

The supernatant of allantoic fluid was collected and used in standard HI test using polyclonal NDV antiserum and monoclonal antibodies (mAb): U85 for detection of classical strains, 161/617 for detection of PPMV-1 strains and 7D4 for detection of F and La Sota vaccine strains.

In vivo pathogenicity test

The pathogenicity of PPMV-1 isolate was assessed by intracerebral pathogenecity index (ICPI) test. One-day-old specific pathogen free (SPF) chickens were inoculated intracerebrally with 0.1 ml of a 1:10 dilution of infective allantoic fluid. Chicks were monitored during an 8-day observation period and scored daily as normal (score 0), sick (score 1), and dead (score 2). Total scores were determined and the mean daily scores were calculated to obtain the ICPI.

Preparation of viral RNA, real-time reverse transcription-polymerase chain reaction (RT-qPCR) and reverse transcription-polymerase chain reaction (RT-PCR)

Viral RNA was extracted from allantoic fluid of ECE using Invisorb Spin Virus RNA Mini Kit (Invitek, Germany) following manufacturers protocol.

One step RT-qPCR for detection of matrix (M) gene was performed with iScript One-Step RT-PCR Kit for Probes (Bio-Rad) with primers and hydrolysis probe as described by Wise et al. (31): forward primer M+4100

5'-AGTGATGTGCTCGGACCTTC-3', reverse primer M-4220   5'-CCTGAGGAGAGGCATTTGCTA-3' and hydrolysis probe M+4169 5'- (FAM) TTCTCTAGCAGTGGGACAGCCTGC(TAMRA) - 3'. Thermal protocol was as follows: 50 ^{0}C 10 min, 95 ^{0}C 5 min and 40 cycles on 95 ^{0}C 10 seconds and 55 ^{0}C 30 seconds.

The procedure for detection of fusion (F) gene is the same as described above except for primers and hydrolysis probe used: forward primer F+4839 5'-TCCGGAGGATACAAGGGTCT-3', reverse primer F-4939 5'-AGCTGTTGCAACCCCAAG-3' and hydrolysis probe F+4894 (VFP-1) 5'-(FAM) AAGCGTTTCTGTCTCCTTCCTCCA(TAM RA)-3' and the temperature of annealing of primers which was 58 ^{0}C instead of 55 ^{0}C, according to Wise et al. (31).

Two-step RT-PCR for the F gene was performed according to methods described by Collins et al., (10) with primers according to Aldous et al., (2) where forward primer was used instead of random primers in the RT step. In the PCR step forward primer MSF1 5'-GACCGCTGACCACGAGGTTA-3' and reverse primer #2 5'-AGTCGGAGGATGTTGGCAGC-3' were used with the thermal protocol of 94 ^{0}C for 3 min, 42 cycles of 94 ^{0}C for 1 min, 50 ^{0}C for 1 min and 72 ^{0}C for 3 min, and final extension at 72^{0}C for10 min. The PCR product of 700 base pairs (bp) was synthesized, subjected to electrophoresis in 1.5% agarose gel and the DNA band was excised from the gel and purified using QIAquick Gel Extraction Kit (Qiagen, Valencia, CA). The purified PCR product was used for sequencing.

Nucleotide sequencing and analysis of sequence data

The sequence of the amplified 374 bp region of the F-gene was obtained using Big Dye Terminator v3.1 kit (Applied Biosystems, USA) and F-gene-specific primers, forward primer #7 5'-GACCGCTGACCACGAGGTTA-3' and reverse primer#2 5'-TTAGAAAAAACACGGGTAGAA-3' according to Aldous et al., (2). All sequencing reactions were performed with fluorescent dideoxynucleotide terminators in the ABI 310 automated sequencer (Applied Biosystems Inc., Foster City, CA) and sequencing product was purified with 50 µl of ethanol (96-100%), 2 µl of 3M sodium acetate and 2 µl of 125 mM EDTA. Sequence editing was performed with BioEdit Sequence Alignment Editor version 7.0.9.0 while alignment with Clustal V method was done in MEGA5 software (MEGA, version 5). The same region of the F-gene was used to construct phylogenetic trees and to classify PPMV-1 isolate among other class II genotype reference sequences. Phylogenetic analysis was performed using MEGA5 software (MEGA, version 5) (28). The evolutionary distances were inferred using un-rooted maximum-likelihood method with 1,000 bootstrap replicates to give credibility to the grouping and included the first, second, and third coding and noncoding positions.

RESULTS

Virus was isolated from a holding of 40 chickens, out of which five have died. Clinical signs involved inapetence, stretched wings and dispnoea. Gross lesions were located predominantly in the respiratory system and involved congestion and edema of the lungs. Haemagglutination activity of allantoic fluid was detected after the second passage in inoculated ECE. Infective allantoic fluid has demonstrated inhibition of haemagglutination with polyclonal NDV serum with titer of 8 log^2 while it was negative for H5N1 and H7N1 antisera. When tested with mAb's it demonstrated inhibition of haemagglutination with mAb 617/161 with titre of 5 log^2 while it was negative for mAb U85 and mAb 7D4. Value of ICPI was 0.81 classifying the virus as mesogenic strain regarding pathogenicity. On the basis of RT-qPCR for detection of the M and the F gene, the virus proved to be virulent strain of class II NDV with Ct values of 21.3 and 27.5, respectively. These results were confirmed with RT-PCR for the F gene with visible band on the gel with expected size of 700 bp.

GenBank accession number of the partial F gene nucleotide sequence is KC915211. Nucleotide sequencing of the CS of the F gene revealed amino acid motif characteristic for virulent strains of NDV 112RRQKR*FIG119 (Fig. 1). Based on the position in the phylogenetic tree it can be concluded that this strain belongs to genotype VI, subgenotype VIb. Results obtained from HI test and phylogenetic tree clearly indicate that this strain is PPMV-1 although isolated from chicken.

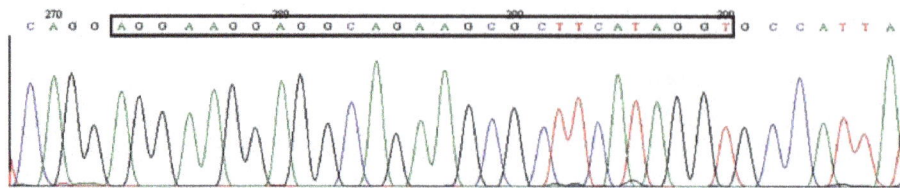

Figure 1. Electropherogram of part of the nucleotide sequence of the F gene of NDV/chicken/Macedonia/231/2010 encompassing the cleavage site (framed)

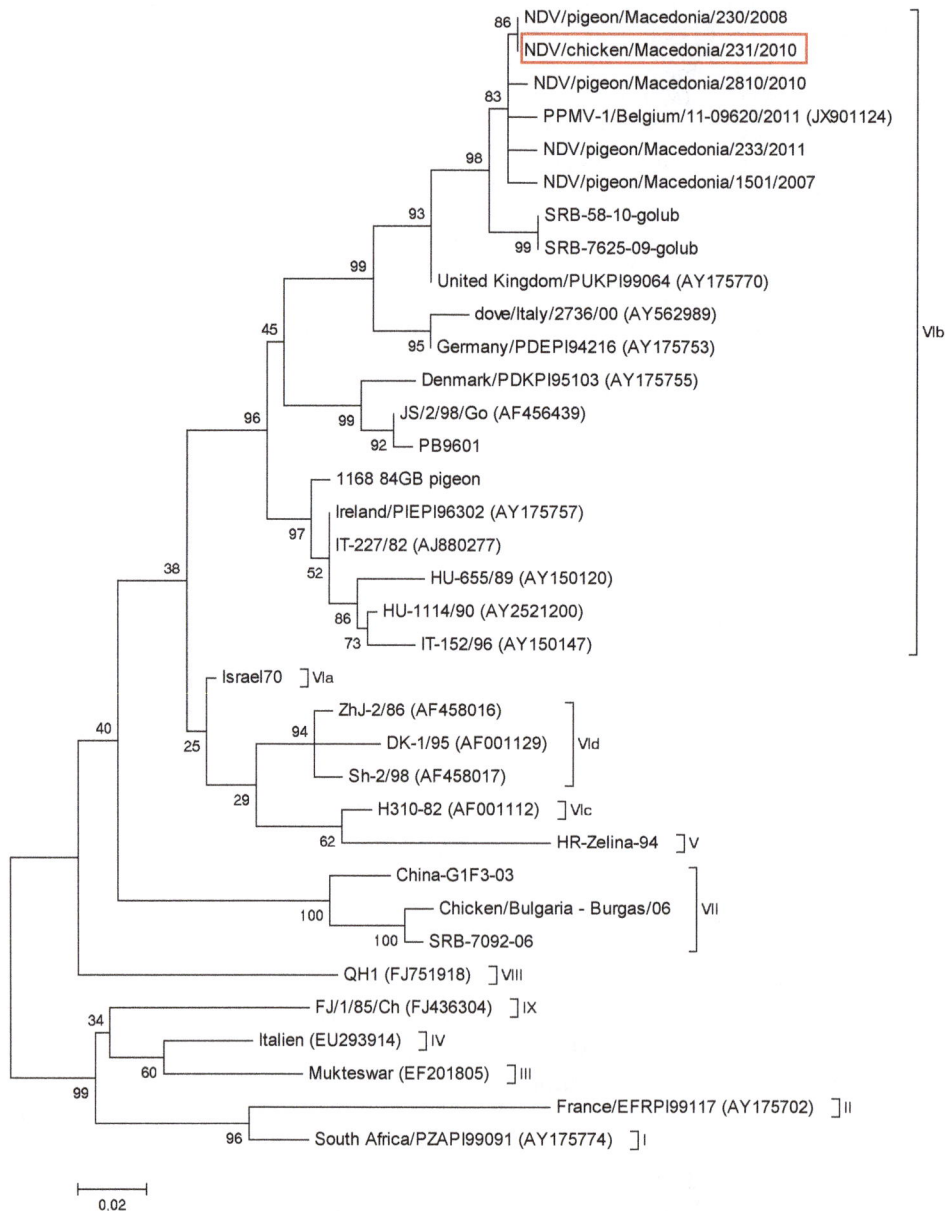

Figure 2. Phylogenetic tree based on the partial nucleotide sequence of the F gene (nt 47 – 420). Classification of the genotypes is marked on the right side of the tree. Tree is constructed with 'maximum-likelihood' method in MEGA 5.1. with "bootstrap" 1000 in order to give credibility to the grouping. Strain investigated in this study is framed. GenBank accession numbers where available are shown in parentheses.

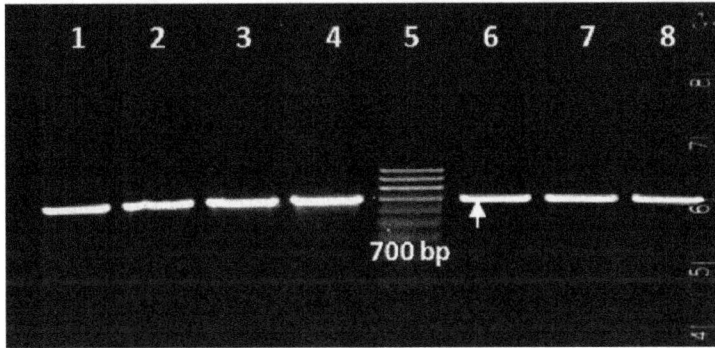

Figure 3. Results of PCR visualization of strain NDV/chicken/Macedonia/231/2010 using primers ' MSF1 и #2 (Aldous et al., 2003), Size 700 bp; (arrow)1-4, 7-8 Different PPMV-1 strains isolated in Macedonia; 5- Marker 100-1000 bp

DISCUSSION

Despite vaccination PPMV-1 is still enzootic in many countries, and birds other than domestic pigeons, such as doves and wild birds and birds in ZOOs, get infected (1, 23). Most PPMV-1 strains have reduced virulence for chickens, but because of the presence of virulent cleavage site motif of the F gene they belong to the group of virulent strains (1, 23, 29). Simultaneous presence of virulent CS of the F gene with lower ICPI values is not uncommon for PPMV-1 and it is previously reported (11, 23). This phenomenon is not associated with the F protein (13) but with replication complex consisting of nucleoprotein, phosphoprotein and polimerase protein (15). It is reported that PPMV-1 isolates from dead racing pigeons with nervous signs possessing amino acid motif of the CS of the F gene 112RRQKR*FIG119 have highly variable but low ICPI values (average 0,69) while PPMV-1 with 112GRQKR*FIG117 have high values of ICPI (average 1,44) (23). These results support recommendation that *in vivo* pathogenecity test should always be accompanied by sequencing (13).

Based on the partial nucleotide sequence of the F gene segment, strain NDV/chicken/Macedonia/231/2010 belongs to genotype VI, subgenotype VIb according to classification by Czegledi et al., (12). This subgenotype is further divided into two groups (28) and according to this classification Macedonian strain belongs to the group VIb/1 of recent European strains (EU/re). This group of strains (VIb/1) probably originated in North-East Africa (29). Strain NDV/chicken/Macedonia/231/2010 possess amino acid CS motif

of the F gene 112RRQKR*FIG119 that classifies it in virulent viruses (10) which is characteristic for PPMV-1 isolated from the 1990s onwards (23).

Pigeon variants are very contagious and can spread from infected pigeons to other pigeons or other poultry when inadequate biosecurity measures are present. Poultry infected with PPMV-1 can spread the virus in the absence of clinical signs. Thus they are a constant threat to domestic poultry. In the EU during the period 2000-2009, 14 outbreaks of NDV caused by PPMV-1 in poultry are reported with most of the outbreaks occurring in small backyard and ornamental flocks (4). Based on the nucleotide sequence, strain NDV/chicken/Macedonia/231/2010 even though isolated from chickens belongs to PPMV-1 . This strain is phylogenetically very similar to other PPMV-1 isolated from pigeons in Macedonia in 2007, 2008, 2010 and 2011. Most probably chickens contracted the virus from infected pigeons carrying the virus. It is possible that other introductions of the PPMV-1 into poultry have occurred but have gone unnoticed. If there is a large reservoir of PPMV-1 in domestic and wild pigeons including other wild birds there is a large possibility for spread of the virus to poultry (4).

The phylogenetic tree perceives no clear geographical demarcation between these strains globally. Thus, although geographically distant, PPMV-1 strains are phylogenetically close. This is primarily due to the specificities of this industry where there is intense mixing of pigeons from different geographic locations as a result of international and internal trade, exhibitions of live birds, racing pigeons, etc. This is the first evidenced spillover of PPMV-1 into poultry in Macedonia.

ACKNOWLEDGEMENT

We would like to acknowledge:

1. Dr. Vladimir Savić from the Croatian Veterinary Institute, Poultry Centre, Zagreb, Croatia for the initial training in techniques performed in this study.

2. Dr. Dejan Vidanović from the Specialized Veterinary Institute Kraljevo, Serbia for provision of Serbian sequences.

3. Dr. Christian Grund from the National Reference Laboratory for Newcastle Disease, FLI-Riems, Germany for his generous help in performing the ICPI test.

4. Dr. Ruth Manvell from the Animal Health and Veterinary Laboratories Agency, Weybridge UK for supplying monoclonal antibodies used in this study.

REFERENCES

1. Aldous, E.W., Fuller, C.M., Mynn, J.K., Alexander, D.J., (2004). A molecular epidemiological investigation of isolates of the variant avian paramyxovirus type 1 virus (PPMV-1) responsible for the 1978 to present panzootic in pigeons. Avian Pathol 33, 258–269.

2. Aldous, E.W., Mynn, J.K., Banks, J., Alexander, D.J., (2003). A molecular epidemiological study of avian paramyxovirus type 1 (Newcastle disease virus) isolates by phylogenetic analysis of a partial nucleotide sequence of the fusion protein gene. Avian Pathol 32, 239–257.

3. Alexander, D.J, (2001). Newcastle disease The Gordon Memorial Lecture. Br Poult Sci 42, 5-22.

4. Alexander, D.J., (2011). Newcastle disease in the European Union 2000 to 2009. Avian Pathol 40, 547-558.

5. Alexander, D.J., Manvell, R.J., Lowings, J.P., Frost, K.M., Collins, M.S., Russell, P.H. and Smith, J.E., (1997). Antigenic diversity and similarities detected in avian paramyxovirus type 1 (Newcastle disease virus) isolates using monoclonal antibodies. Avian Pathol 26, 399-418.

6. Alexander, D.J., Russell, P.H., Parsons, G., Abu Elzein, E.M.E., Ballough, A., Cernik, K.,

Engstrom, B., Fevereiro, M., Fleury, H.J.A., Guittet, M., Kaleta, E.F., Kihm, U., Kosters, J., Lomniczi, B., Meister, J., Meulemans, G., Nerome, K., Petek, M., Pokomunski, S., Polten, B., Prip, M., Richter, R., Saghy, E., Samberg, Y., Spanoghe, L., and Tumova, B, (1985). Antigenic and biological characterisation of avian paramyxovirus type 1 isolates from pigeons-an international collaborative study. Avian Pathol 14, 365-376.

7. Ballagi-Prodany, A., Wehmann, E., Herczeg, J., Belak, S., Lomniczi, B., (1996). Identification and grouping of Newcastle disease virus strains by restriction site analysis of a region from the F gene. Arch Virol 141, 243–261.

8. Biancifiori, F., and Fioroni, A., (1983). An occurrence of Newcastle disease in pigeons: virological and serological studies on the isolates. Comp Immunol Microbiol Infect Dis 6, 247–252.

9. Briand, F-X., Henry, A., Massin, P., and Jestin, V., (2012). Complete Genome Sequence of a Novel Avian Paramyxovirus. J Virol 86, 7710.

10. Collins, M.S., Bashiruddin, J.B., Alexander, D.J., (1993). Deduced amino acid sequences at the fusion protein cleavage site of Newcastle disease viruses showing variation in antigenicity and pathogenicity. Arch Virol 128, 363-70.

11. Collins, M.S., Franklin, S., Strong, I, Meulemans, G., and Alexander, D.J., (1998). Antigenic and phylogenetic studies on a variant Newcastle disease virus using antifusion protein monoclonal antibodies and partial sequencing of the fusion protein gene. Avian Pathol 27, 90-96.

12. Czegledi, A., Ujvari, D., Somogyi, E., Wehmann, E., Werner, O. and Lomniczi, B, (2006). Third genome size category of avian paramyxovirus serotype 1 (Newcastle disease virus) and evolutionary implications. Virus Research 120, 36-48.

13. Dortmans, J.C.F.M., Koch, G., Rottier, P.J.M., Peeters, B.P.H., (2009). Virulence of pigeon paramyxovirus type 1 does not always correlate with the cleavability of its fusion protein. J Gen Virol 90, 2746-2750.

14. Dortmans, J.C.F.M., Koch, G., Rottier, P.J.M., Peeters, B.P.H., (2011). Virulence of Newcastle disease virus: what is known so far? Vet Res 42, 122.

15. Dortmans, J.C.F.M., Rottier, P.J.M., Koch, G., Peeters, B.P.H., (2010). The viral replication complex is associated with the virulence of Newcastle disease virus. J Virol 84, 10113-10120.

16. Doyle, T.M., (1927). A hitherto unrecorded disease of fowls due to a filter-passing virus. Journal of Comparative Pathology and Therapeutics, 40, 144-169.

17. Kaleta, E.F., (1992). Paramyxoviruses in free-living and captive birds, a brief account. In: Kaleta, E.F., Heffels-Redmann, U. (Eds.), Workshop on Avian Paramyxoviruses, vol. 27-29. Rauischholzhausen, Germany, 262-271.

18. Kaleta, E.F., Alexander, D.J. and Russell, P.H., 1985. The first isolation of the avian PMV-1 virus responsible for the current panzootic in pigeons? Avian Pathol 14, 553–557.

19. Kaleta, E.F., and Baldauf, C., (1988). Newcastle disease in free-living and pet birds. In D.J. Alexander (Ed.). Newcastle Disease (pp. 197_246). Boston: Kluwer Academic Publishers.

20. Lister, S.A., Alexander, D.J., Hogg, R.A., (1986). Evidence for the presence of avian paramyxovirus type 1 in feral pigeons in England and Wales. Vet. Rec. 118, 476-479.

21. Lomniczi, B., Wehmann, E., Herczeg, J., Ballagi-Pordany, A., Kaleta, E.F., Werner, O., Meulemans, G., Jorgensen, P.H., Mante, A.P., Gielkens, A.L., et al., (1998). Newcastle disease outbreaks in recent years in western Europe were caused by an old (VI) and a novel genotype (VII). Arch Virol 143(1), 49-64.

22. Mayo, M.A., (2002). Virus Taxonomy - Houston 2002. Arch Virol 147, 1071–1076.

23. Meulemans, G., Van den Berg, T.P., Decaesstecker, M., Boschmans, M., (2002). Evolution of pigeon Newcastle disease virus strains. Avian Pathol 31, 515-519.

24. Miller, P.J., Afonso,C.L., Spackman, E., Scott, M.A., Pedersen, J.C., Senne, D.D., Brown, J.D., Fuller, C.M., Uhart, M.M., Karesh, W.B., Brown, I.H., Alexander, D.J., and Swayne, D.E., (2010a). Evidence for a new avian Paramyxovirus serotype 10 detected in Rockhopper Penguins from the Falkland Islands. J Virol 84, 11496–11504.

25. Nagai, Y., Klenk, H.D., Rott, R., (1976). Proteolytic cleavage of the viral glycoproteins and its significance for the virulence of Newcastle disease virus. Virology 72, 494-508.

26. Ogasawara, T., Gotoh, B., Suzuki, H., Asaka, J., Shimokata, K., Rott, R., Nagai, Y., (1992). Expression of factor X and its significance for the determination of paramyxovirus tropism in the chick embryo. EMBO J 11, 467-472.

27. Seal, B.S., King, D.J., and Bennett, J.D., (1995). Characterization of Newcastle disease virus isolates by reverse transcription PCR coupled to direct nucleotide sequencing and development of sequence database for pathotype prediction and molecular epidemiological analysis. J Clin Microbiol 33, 2624-2630.

28. Tamura, K, Dudley, J, Nei, M, Kumar, S., (2007). MEGA 4: Molecular Evolutionary Genetics Analysis (MEGA) software version 40. Mol Biol Evol 24, 1596 – 1599.

29. Ujvari, D., Wehmann, E., Kaleta, E.F., Werner, O., Savic, V., Nagy, E., Czifra, G., Lomniczi, B., (2003). Phylogenetic analysis reveals extensive evolution of avian paramyxovirus type 1 strains of pigeons (*Columba livia*) and suggests multiple species transmission. Virus Res 96, 63-73.

30. World Organization for Animal Health (OIE), (2012). Chapter 2.3.14 Newcastle Disease. In: Manual of diagnostic tests and vaccines for terrestrial animals, version adopted May 2012. OIE, Paris, France.

31. Wise, M.G., Suarez, D.L., Seal, B.S., Pedersen, J.C., Senne, D.A., King, D.J., Kapczynski, D.R., and Spackman E., (2004). Development of a real-time reverse-transcription PCR for detection of Newcastle disease virus RNA in clinical samples. J Clin Microbiol 42, 329–338.

EFFECT OF STORAGE ON RESIDUE LEVELS OF ENROFLOXACIN IN MUSCLE OF RAINBOW TROUT (*ONCORHYNCHUS MYKISS*) AND COMMON CARP (*CYPRINUS CARPIO*)

Ralica Kyuchukova[1], Anelia Milanova[2], Aleksandra Daskalova[1], Deyan Stratev[1], Lubomir Lashev[2], Alexander Pavlov[1]

*[1]Department of Hygiene and Technology of Foods,
Faculty of Veterinary Medicine, Trakia University, Bulgaria
[2]Department of Pharmacology, Physiology of Animals and Physiological Chemistry,
Faculty of Veterinary Medicine, Trakia University, Bulgaria*

ABSTRACT

Since fluoroquinolones are one of the most commonly used antibacterial drugs in aquaculture, there is a risk of their residues to be found in the treated fish. The objective of this study was to examine the changes in enrofloxacin and ciprofloxacin levels during storage of rainbow trout and common carp muscle at -18 °C. The trout and carp were treated orally with a single dose of 10 mg/kg of enrofloxacin. Tissue samples were collected 24 h after the treatment and stored at -18 °C for 270 days either as a whole fish or as precut muscle samples. Results for trout revealed that in the precut samples enrofloxacin concentration decreased significantly only after 9 months of storage, whereas a significant decline in the ciprofloxacin level was observed much earlier (after 3 months). After 9 months of storage, the trout stored without being sliced and eviscerated showed significantly higher levels of both quinolones as compared to the precut muscle samples. The enrofloxacin levels in the carp musculature decreased considerably after 3 months of storage and stayed almost unchanged up to the end of the study, whereas the ciprofloxacin concentration continued to drop even after this period and after 270 days constituted 1/6 of the initial values.

Key words: ciprofloxacin, common carp, enrofloxacin, rainbow trout, residues, storage

INTRODUCTION

Fluoroquinolones are a group of synthetic antimicrobial agents widely used in human and veterinary medicine for treatment and prevention of infections caused by Gram-negative and Gram-positive bacteria (1). They are among the most often prescribed antibiotics in fisheries (2), but their use in aquaculture presents a risk to fish products' consumers, because of potential risk of residues in the food. Tissue disposition of fluoroquinolones, including enrofloxacin and ciprofloxacin, in fish species depends on several factors such as ambient

Corresponding author: Assoc. Prof. Ralica Kyuchukova, PhD
E-mail address: ralitsa.kjuchukova@abv.bg
Present address: Department of Hygiene and Technology of Foods,
Faculty of Veterinary Medicine, Trakia University, Bulgaria

water temperature and salinity, lipid content and properties of the drug molecule (3, 4). These factors have significant impact on the withdrawal time and depletion of residues from muscles and can be a prerequisite for the presence of undesirable levels of drugs. Information about the behavior of residues of antibiotics during frozen storage is scarce. Alfredson and Ohlsson (5) found significant reduction of sulfamethazine residues in muscle kept for 3 months at a temperature of -20 °C. The average decrease was 35% in bovine and 55% in porcine muscle (5). Other data showed a significant decrease of ampicillin residues in pork meat during the first 3 months of storage at -20 °C (6). Residual concentrations of ampicillin were found in the pork muscles after 8 months of storage at the same temperature (6). In our previous studies major reduction of the residues of amoxicillin (7), kanamycin (8), tobramycin (9), and ampicillin (10) in poultry or rabbit meat during storage at -18 °C was found. No significant reduction of trimethoprim in poultry meat (8) and gentamicin in rabbit meat was registered (10). In all cases, microbiological methods were used which limited the ability for detection of metabolites. This data shows that stability of antibacterial substances in mammals' and chickens' muscles differs significantly, depending on the individual drug and animal species. Moreover, little is known of the stability of antimicrobial drugs in fish muscle after different storage times at usual commercial conditions.

Because of insufficient data concerning the changes of antimicrobial residues in meat during storage, the aim of the present study was to investigate concentration changes in enrofloxacin and its metabolite ciprofloxacin contents in trout and carp meat during frozen storage.

MATERIAL AND METHODS

Drugs

Enrofloxacin (Baytril 5%, Part. No KP076SM, Bayer Animal Health Gmbh, Leverkuzen, Germany) was used for oral (p.o.) treatment of fish as 1% solution. Analytical standards of enrofloxacin hydrochloride (Part No. 20020323) and ciprofloxacin hydrochloride (Part No. FPCPF 070483) were supplied by Biovet Pestera (Bulgaria) and Actavis (Bulgaria), respectively.

Animals

Two years old rainbow trouts (*Oncorhynchus mykiss,* n=20) with mean body weight of 450 g were included in the experiments. They were supplied by a fish farm, located in Enina (Bulgaria). The animals were placed in two aerated tanks. Water temperature was 15°C and pH was 7.5.

Market-sized carps (*Cyprinus carpio*, n=11) with a mean body weight of 1000 g were purchased from a commercial fish farm in Nikolaevo (Bulgaria). The fish were placed in 2 tanks, containing 800 l of tap water (water temperature 17°C; pH 7.2) with constant aeration.

Experimental procedure

The experimental design was approved by the Ethics and Animal Welfare Committee at Trakia University, Stara Zagora. Euthanasia was performed under the Directive 2010/63/EU on the protection of animals used for scientific purposes requirements.

Control groups of trouts (n=5) and carps (n=5) were not treated with enrofloxacin and were used for obtaining of muscle tissue samples for preparation of blank samples and fortified samples with standard dilutions for quantitative analysis of the drugs.

The other trouts (n=15) and carps (n=6) were treated orally with a single dose of enrofloxacin via a gavage tube (1% solution at dose rate of 10 mg/kg body weight). Tissue samples were obtained from each fish after euthanasia by a percussive (manual) blow on the cranium with a hammer. Muscle samples were taken from six fishes from each species 24 hours after the treatment with the antibacterial agent. Each muscle sample was divided into six portions and they were stored at -18 °C. These samples were analyzed at day 0 (immediately after obtaining the samples), 15, 30, 90, 180 and 270 of the storage. The remaining 9 trouts were euthanized and stored as whole fishes (with internal organs), without cleaning and muscle samples were analyzed 180 and 270 days after the storage. Aqueous solutions of enrofloxacin hydrochloride and ciprofloxacin hydrochloride (1 mg/mL) were stored at the same conditions as samples for depletion check of the pure standards. These solutions were analyzed together with the muscle samples at the same time intervals.

HPLC analysis of enrofloxacin and ciprofloxacin concentrations

The tissue samples from muscles (0.5 g) were homogenized in 0.5 mL of 0.1 M phosphate buffer pH 7.4 with a homogenizer at high speed up to 1 min. To this homogenate, 6 mL of dichloromethane were added, and the samples were mixed for 1 min and centrifuged for 6 min at 1000xg. The aqueous layer was removed. The organic phase was collected in 10 ml tubes. It was evaporated in a vacuum evaporator (CentriVap Vacuum Concentration System, Labconco, Kansas, MO, USA) at 40 °C to dryness. The residue was dissolved in 500 μL of demineralized water. Aliquots from 20 μL were injected into the HPLC system.

HPLC system was equipped with Hypersil Spherisorb ODS-2 (C18)-150 4.6 -mm 5 μM column, a Surveyor LC Pump Plus, a Surveyor fluorescence detector, and a Surveyor Autosampler Plus (Thermo Fisher Scientific Inc., USA). The column was used at room temperature. The mobile phase consisted of acetonitrile in aqueous solution (25:75, v/v) of potassium dihydrogen phosphate (0.05 M) in water. The pH of the mobile phase was adjusted to 3.5 with phosphoric acid (85%). The flow rate was 0.6 mL/min, isocratic conditions. Excitation and emission wavelengths were set at 277 nm and 418 nm, respectively for determination of enrofloxacin and ciprofloxacin. Peak area integrations were carried-out using ChromQuest Chromatography Data System (Thermo Fisher Scientific Inc., USA). Standard curves for both fluororquinolones were prepared with tissues from untreated animals. The concentrations of calibration standards for enrofloxacin and ciprofloxacin were 1000, 750,

Table 1. Residues of enrofloxacin and ciprofloxacin in muscle samples (Mean ± SD) from trout (*Oncorhinchus mykiss*) and carp (*Cyprinus carpio*) after storage at -18 °C

Day of storage	Enrofloxacin (µg/g)	Ciprofloxacin (µg/g)
	Oncorhinchus mykiss	
0	5.94±4.89	0.58±0.24
15	5.60±3.62	0.47±0.30
30	5.43±4.19	0.47±0.39
90	5.46±5.07	0.30±0.23*
180	5.71±6.26	0.31±0.15*
270	3.69±4.17	0.23±0.12*
	Cyprinus carpio	
0	1.27±1.76	0.36±0.45
15	1.20±0.64	0.36±0.48
30	1.10±0.64	0.34±0.12
90	0.41±0.30	0.10±0.02*
180	0.35±0.21	0.04±0.05*
270	0.31±0.35	0.06±0.07*

*Statistically significant differences in comparison to the concentrations at day of storage 0 at P<0.05

500, 250, 100, 50, and 10 ng/mL. Retention times for enrofloxacin and ciprofloxacin were 3.88 min and 4.57 min, respectively. Limit of detection and limit of quantification for both compounds were 10 and 50 ng/mL. The overall recovery rate in tissue samples exceeded >75%.

The analysis was performed in the Central Scientific Laboratory of Trakia University.

Statistical analysis

Descriptive statistics was performed with Statistica for Windows (Statistica 6.0.1, USA). Data were presented as mean ± SD. Statistical analysis was performed with Mann–Whitney test. – P level < 0.05 was considered as significant.

RESULTS

Rainbow trout (Oncorhynhus mykiss)

Enrofloxacin residues in the meat of rainbow trout showed insignificant decrease during frozen storage the first six months (Table 1). Considerable decrease was observed after storage during the last 3 months, after 270 days of storage. The levels reached 3.69 µg/g, or 62% of the initial values (Fig. 1).

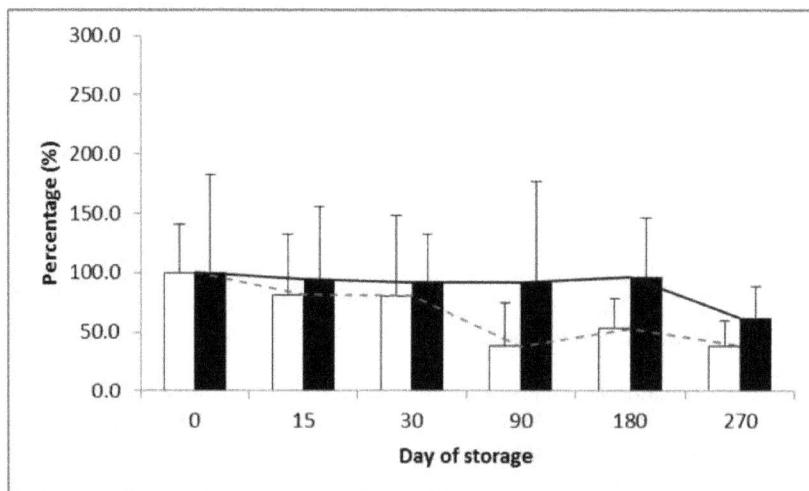

Figure 1. Levels of residues of enrofloxacin and ciprofloxacin, presented as percentage of the day 0 of storage, in muscle samples from trout (*Oncorhinchus mykiss*) after storage at -18 °C. ☐ and gray dashed line represent data for ciprofloxacin; ■ and black line represent data for enrofloxacin

Ciprofloxacin, which initial concentration (at 0 day) in the trout meat constituted about 10% of the enrofloxacin level, showed tendency for a gradual decrease. During the first 2 weeks of storage a decline of approximately 19% was observed (P>0.05) and subsequently after 9 months of storage, the ciprofloxacin concentration in the meat was less than 50% of the initial concentration (P<0.05). Significantly lower ciprofloxacin levels were measured after 3 months of storage (P<0.05).

The fish, stored without being sliced and eviscerated, showed different tissue levels of both fluoroquinolones as compared to the muscle samples which were cut into small pieces before storage. After 9 months of storage the enrofloxacin and ciprofloxacin residues were 8.24±3.99 μg/g and 0.56±0.47 μg/g, respectively. These values were higher than those obtained from the precut muscle samples (P > 0.05). Enrofloxacin concentrations were 38 % higher and the amount of ciprofloxacin was similar if compared to the initial concentrations of the drugs in the muscles.

Common carp (Cyprinus carpio)

Results obtained from the analyzed carp muscles showed that during the first month of storage there were no statistically significant changes in the tissue levels of both quinolones (Table 1). After 90 days of storage at -18 °C, enrofloxacin concentration decreased to 30% of the initial level and remained almost unchanged up to the end of the study

(Fig. 2). Ciprofloxacin level continued to drop even after 90 days of storage and at the end of the storage period its concentration constituted approximately 1/6th of the initial values. Its concentrations were statistically significantly lower after 3, 6 and 9 months of storage (P<0.05).

DISCUSSION

Rearing of fish species in farm conditions and international trade with aquaculture products have significantly developed during the last years. These tendencies determine extensive use of antibacterial drugs to control increased rates of diseases. Enrofloxacin is among the few drugs licensed for use in aquatic species with established Maximum Residual Limits of 100 μg/kg as the sum of the levels of enrofloxacin and ciprofloxacin in tissues (11). Literature data indicates variable withdrawal time in different fish species (12). Therefore depletion of drugs from edible tissues must be assessed in order to offer safe food on the market. In fish species, additional obstruction is the dependence of residues depletion time on the water temperature (4). Although they adopted strict criteria, there are cases of illegal use of drugs without following the required withdrawal time and Maximum Residual Limits which can be a reason for existence of residues in processed fish and requires information about the stability of enrofloxacin and its active metabolite under conditions of storage.

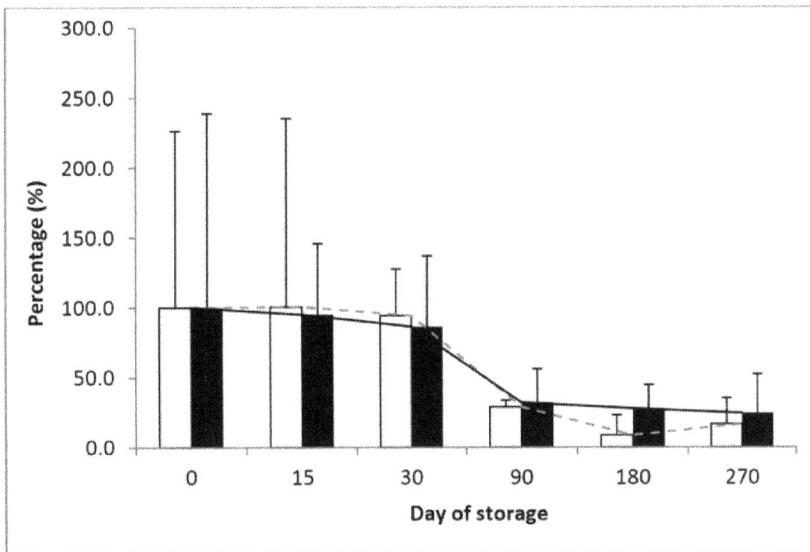

Figure 2. Levels of residues of enrofloxacin and ciprofloxacin in muscle samples from carp (*Cyprinus carpio*) after storage at -18 °C. Data are presented as percentage from the day 0 of storage. □ and dashed gray line represent data for ciprofloxacin; ■ and black line represent data for enrofloxacin

The data from our study show differences between trout and carp in the depletion time of fluoroquinolones after storage of muscle samples at -18 °C. Storage of trout meat for six months resulted in absence of significant changes ($P>0.05$) of enrofloxacin residues in meat and the highest decrease was observed after nine months. Insignificant changes were found in both enrofloxacin and ciprofloxacin levels in carp muscle during the first month of storage. Significant decrease of enrofloxacin levels was observed 90 days after freezing, which was earlier in carp samples if compared to trout. Similarly to these results, the concentrations of enrofloxacin in water samples frozen at -20°C for 28 days, were stored up to 90% in comparison to the samples, analyzed immediately (13). After 6 months of preservation of stock solutions of enrofloxacin at -20 °C the loss was less than 10% than in Rainbow trout fish meat, kept in the same freezer in the current study. After a longer period of storage, concentrations of fluoroquinolones in frozen water samples dropped off dramatically as in our experiment (14). Similar data were reported for tetracyclines, aminopenicillines and sulfonamides in frozen water in the EPA study (13) and in frozen meat samples. Verdon et al. (6) found 40% lower concentrations of ampicillin in pork meat kept at -20°C for 235 days and absence of changes at -70 °C. Trimetoprim degraded up to 50% in chicken meat after freezing at -18 °C for 30 to 90 days (8). Gentamicin was stable in rabbit's meat stored at same conditions for 45 days (10).

Enrofloxacin is dealkylated to pharmacologically active metabolite ciprofloxacin in several fish species, including trout and carp (15, 16, 17). Ciprofloxacin was found in the muscles of both investigated fish species and its depletion from this tissue differs from the data for the parent compound. Results showed that 15 days of storage lead to reduction of ciprofloxacin concentrations by 20% and by more than 50 % after the third month till the end of the experiment in trout muscles. The observed higher concentrations of enrofloxacin and ciprofloxacin in samples from whole trout, stored with internal organs, can be explained by additional penetration of fluoroquinolones to the muscles. Depletion pattern of ciprofloxacin concentrations in the carp muscles was similar to those in the samples from trout. Similarly, another fluoroquinolone compound such as gatifloxacin was stable in human plasma for 7 weeks at -20 °C (18).

CONCLUSION

Our data indicates that the samples from rainbow trout and their products can be stored frozen at temperature under -18 °C for a period of 6 months and to be analyzed within this term for determination of residues from enrofloxacin. For common carp meat, this period is 3 months. Administration of the drugs in modern aquaculture including antibiotics, requires knowledge for the withdrawal time of the drugs in each fish species. Freezing for months of whole and eviscerated fish results in different levels of fluoroquinolones in the muscles. Less residues are found in eviscerated fish during storage at -15, 16, 17 °C. A strong tendency toward enrofloxacin and ciprofloxacin decrease was observed in trout and carp muscles, although these drugs can be found in the samples after months of storage.

ACKNOWLEDGEMENTS

This research was financially supported by Faculty of Veterinary Medicine, Trakia University, Project 19/2011.

REFERENCES

1. Currie, D., Lynas, L., Kennedy, D.G., McCaughey, W.J. (1998). Evaluation of a modified EC Four Plate Method to detect antimicrobial drugs. Food Addit. Contam. 15, 651-660.
http://dx.doi.org/10.1080/02652039809374694
PMid:10209575

2. Samanidou, V.F., Evaggelopoulou, E.N. (2007). Analytical strategies to determine antibiotic residues in fish. J. Sep. Sci. 30, 2549-2569.
http://dx.doi.org/10.1002/jssc.200700252
PMid:17924582

3. Haritova, A., Fink-Gremmels, J. (2010). An in silico model for the prediction of muscle: plasma partition coefficients of feed contaminants. Book of Abstracts. 2nd Feed for Health Conference, p. 48. Tromso, Norway

4. Liang, J., Li, J., Zhao, F., Liu, P., Chang, Z. (2012). Pharmacokinetics and tissue behavior of enrofloxacin and its metabolite ciprofloxacin in turbot Scophthalmus maximus at two water temperatures. Chinese J. Oceanol. Limnol. 30, 644-653.
http://dx.doi.org/10.1007/s00343-012-1228-2

5. Alfredsson, G., Ohlsson, A. (1998). Stability of sulphonamide drugs in meat during storage. Food Addit. Contam. 15, 302-306.
http://dx.doi.org/10.1080/02652039809374645
PMid:9666889

6. Verdon, E., Fuselier, R., Hurtaud-Pessel, D., Couedor, P., Cadieu, N., Laurentie, M. (2000). Stability of penicillin antibiotic residues in meat during storage: ampicillin. J. Chromatogr. A. 882, 135-143.
http://dx.doi.org/10.1016/S0021-9673(00)00065-0

7. Pavlov, A., Vachin, I., Lashev, L. (1993a). Studies on amoxicillin residues in chicken meat and by-products during storage. Vet. Nauki 2, 94-98.

8. Dinkov, D., Pavlov, A., Lashev, L. (1998). Kinetics of the residue levels of kanamycin and trimethoprim in poultry meat at storage. Bulg. J. Vet. Med. 1, 105-112.

9. Pavlov, A., Lashev, L., Rusev, V. (2006). Studies on the residue levels of tobramycin in stored poultry products. Trakia J. Sci. 3, 20-22.

10. Pavlov, A., Vachin, I., Lashev, L., Tododrov, B. (1993b). Influence of the irradiation of rabbit meat on unbound ampicillin and gentamicin content. Soz. Ep-Hefte 16, 155-157.

11. EMEA/MRL/820/02-FINAL (2002). Enrofloxacin (Extension to all food producing species): Summary report (5) Committee for Veterinary Medicinal Products,
http://www.ema.europa.eu/ema/index.jsp?curl=pages/includes/document/document_detail.

12. Lucchetti, D., Fabrizi, L., Guandalini, E., Podesta, E., Marvasi, L., Zaghini, A., Coni, E. (2004). Long depletion time of enrofloxacin in rainbow trout (Oncorhynchus mykiss). Antimicrob. Agents Chemother. 48, 3912-3917.
http://dx.doi.org/10.1128/AAC.48.10.3912-3917.2004
PMid:15388452 PMCid:PMC521881

13. EPA (2010). Stability of Pharmaceuticals, Personal Care Products, Steroids, and Hormones in Aqueous Samples, POTW Effluents, and Biosolids. United States Office of Water Environmental Protection Agency (4303).

14. Okerman, L., Van Hende, J., De Zutter, L. (2007). Stability of frozen stock solutions of beta-lactam antibiotics, cephalosporins, tetracyclines and quinolones used in antibiotic residue screening and antibiotic susceptibility testing. Anal. Chim. Acta 586, 284-288.
http://dx.doi.org/10.1016/j.aca.2006.10.034
PMid:17386725

15. Xu, W., Zhu, X., Wang, X., Liping, D., Gan, Z. (2006). Residues of enrofloxacin, furazolidone and their metabolites in Nile tilapia (Oreochromis niloticus). Aquaculture 254, 1-8.
http://dx.doi.org/10.1016/j.aquaculture.2005.10.030

16. Fang, W., Zhou, S., Yu, H. (2007). Pharmacokinetics and tissue distribution of enrofloxacin and its metabolite ciprofloxacin in Scylla serrata following oral gavage at two salinities. Aquaculture 272, 180-187.
http://dx.doi.org/10.1016/j.aquaculture.2007.08.049

17. Xu, L., Wang, H., Yang, X., Lu, L. (2013). Integrated pharmacokinetics/pharmacodynamics parameters-based dosing guidelines of enrofloxacin in grass carp Ctenopharyngodon idella to minimize selection of drug resistance. BMC Vet. Res. 9, 126.
http://dx.doi.org/10.1186/1746-6148-9-126
PMid:23800340 PMCid:PMC3717066

18. Al-Dgither, S., Alvi, S.N., Hammami, M.M. (2006). Development and validation of an HPLC method for the determination of gatifloxacin stability in human plasma. J. Pharm. Biomed. Anal. 41, 251-255.
http://dx.doi.org/10.1016/j.jpba.2005.09.026
PMid:16311002

THE PARADOX OF HUMAN EQUIVALENT DOSE FORMULA: A CANONICAL CASE STUDY OF ABRUS PRECATORIUS AQUEOUS LEAF EXTRACT IN MONOGASTRIC ANIMALS

Saganuwan Alhaji Saganuwan, Patrick Azubuike Onyeyili

Department of Veterinary Physiology, Pharmacology and Biochemistry
College of Veterinary Medicine, University of Agriculture,
Makurdi, Benue State, Nigeria

ABSTRACT

There is abundant literature on the toxicity of *A. precatorius* seeds. However there is a need to define the toxicity limit of the *Abrus precatorius* leaf in monogastric animals. Human Equivalent Dose (HED) which is equal to animal dose multiplied by animal km (metabolism constant) divided by human km was used to project the LD_{50} of fifteen monogastric animals, where human km factor is body weight (kg) divided by body surface area (m²). Human Equivalent No-observable Adverse Effect Doses were determined by multiplying the animal no-observable adverse effect dose by animal weight (Wa) divided by human weight (Wh). The LD_{50} of the aqueous leaf extract of *Abrus precatorius* in mice was estimated to be between 2559.5 and 3123.3 mg/kg body weight. The LD_{50} extrapolated from mouse to rat (1349.3-1646.6 mg/kg), hamster (1855.3-2264.1 mg/kg), guinea pig (1279.5-1561.4 mg/kg), rabbit (618.4-754.7 mg/kg), monkey (593.7-724.5 mg/kg), cat (392.7-479.2 mg/kg), dog and baboon (371.1-452.8 mg/kg), child (297-362 mg/kg) and adult human (197.8-241.5 mg/kg) body weight respectively could be a reality. The therapeutic safe dose range for the animals was 1-12.5 mg/kg body weight for a period of 7 days, but at a dose ($\leq$ 200 mg/kg body weight) the leaf extract showed haematinic effect. However, at a higher dose (> 200 mg/kg), the extract showed haemolytic activity in rats, whereas at a dose ($\geq$25.0 mg/kg), the leaf extract might be organotoxic in hamster, guinea pig, rabbit, monkey, cat, dog, baboon, child and adult human if administered orally for a period of 7 days.

Key words: monogastric, toxicity, *Abrus precatorius*, mice, human

INTRODUCTION

Abrus precatorius is highly regarded as a universal panacea in a herbal medicine (49). The aqueous leaf extract of *Abrus precatorius* showed 99.4% clearance of *Plasmodium berghei* in mice within 11 days (47), significant antimicrobial activity against *Staphylococcus aureus, Streptococcus pyogenes, Klebsiella pneumoniae, Escherichia coli* and *Salmonella typhimurium* (4, 42, 43). The plant showed significant inhibition of human

metabolic breast cancer cell line (MDA-MB 231). The ethanolic extract of *Abrus precatorius* leaves may be used in the management of asthma (52). It also inhibited acetylcholine-induced contractions of both toad rectus abdominis and rat phrenic nerve-diaphragm muscle preparations and caused flaccid paralysis in the young chicks (56). Both natural and heat denatured forms of abrusagglutinin are potential immunomodulators (54).

The leaves are used to cure fever, stomatitis, bronchitis (29), epilepsy (6), neuronal damage (35) and diabetes (13). Two triterpernoid saponins isolated from aerial parts of *Abrus precatorius* exhibited activity against inflammation (5), gonorrhoea, diarrhea and dysentery (8). The ethanol acetate of the leaf extract showed anti-serotonergic activity in frog fundus strip (11). The leaves also have astringent, emetic, antihelmintic, alexeteric and diuretic properties in addition to being useful in cough (32), pharyngodynia, pectoralgia (28), strangury and vitiated condition of vata (25, 29). Isoflavanquinone, abruquinone B and abruquinone

Corresponding author: Dr. Saganuwan Alhaji Saganuwan, PhD
E-mail address: pharn_saga2006@yahoo.com
Present address: Department of Veterinary Physiology, Pharmacology and Biochemistry, College of Veterinary Medicine, University of Agriculture, P.M.B. 2373, Makurdi, Benue State, Nigeria

G isolated from aerial parts of the plant exhibited antitubercular, antiplasmodial, antiviral and cytotoxic activities (30). The leaves are sweet tasting due to the presence of glycyrrhizin component. The leaves are also used for the treatment of scratches, sores and wounds caused by dogs, cats and mice. Fresh leaves may be pressed on the gum for the treatment of stomatitis, skin cancer and nervousness (8), suppuration, acne, boils, abscesses, tetanus, rabies (58), colic, convulsion (27), cough, sore throat and insomnia (33). Aqueous extract of the plant has haematinic and plasma expander effects in mice (38).

The leaf components are made of choline, trigonellin (III) (22), flavonoids, total glycosides, saponin glycosides, saponins and tannins in higher concentration, but alkaloids, steroids and cardiac glycosides are present in moderate concentration. Calcium (10.2mg), magnesium (5.2mg), Sodium (6.8mg), Potassium (10.8mg), Phosphorous (2.4mg), nitrogen (30.5 mg) (45), triterpenoid saponin, 3-0-β-D-glucopyranosyl-(1→2)-β, D-glucopyranosyl subprogenin D together with six triterpenoids, subprogenin D, abrusgenic acid, triptotriterpenic acid B, abruslactone A, abrusogenin and abrusoside are also present (57). Other triterpenoids isolated are 20S, 220S)-β, 22-dihydroxycucubitacin, 24-diene-26, 29-dioc acid δ lactone, 3-0- (6'-methyl-β-D-glucurunopyranosyl)-3β, 22β-dihydroxylean-12-en-29-oic acid methyl ester, 3-0β-D-glucuronopyranosylsophoradiol methyl ester and sophoradiol (29). Abrusagglutinin, a low-toxicity protein present in every part of the plant is less lethal (LD_{50}=500µg/kg) than abrin A (LD_{50}=20µg/kg) (31).

The clinical features of *Abrus precatorius* leaf poisoning were pulmonary oedema and hypertension (16). The aqueous extract of *A. precatorius* leaf caused decreased levels of packed cell volume, haemoglobin concentration, red blood cell count, white blood cell count, mean corpuscular volume and mean corpuscular haemoglobin concentration in rats. The extract also resulted in increased levels of total serum protein, albumin, alanine amino transferase, aspartate amino transferase, alkaline phosphatase and total bilirubin. It also caused testicular degeneration characterized by decreased numbers of epithelial lining and reduction in sperm cells at dose range between 400 and 1600 mg/kg body weight (3). The foliage of *Abrus precatorius* contains abrin, which is among the most potent toxins. Clinical toxicosis was characterized by gastroenteritis, weakness and death (2, 10, 20). Abrin is present in the leaf and is known to cause hyperactivity of physiological system (8). The parenteral LD_{50} of abrin in mice is less than 0.1µg/kg (8). All parts of *Abrus precatorius* are toxic (9).

Acute toxicity study of aqueous extract of *Abrus precatorius* leaf in mice showed shallow respiration, sedation, weight loss, penile prolapsed and limbs paddling within 48 hours of extract administration. Haematological analysis revealed significant increased packed cell volume, red blood cell and white blood cell count (44). The biochemical analysis showed increased aspartate aminotransferase, alanine aminotransferase, alkaline phosphatase, creatinine, chloride ion, hypophospataemia, hyponatraemia, hypokalaemia and hypoglycaemia after 3 weeks of oral administration of the extract at dose range between 25.0 and 200 mg/kg body weight. At 12.5 mg/kg only the urea increased on the 7th day of the extract administration (46). *In vitro* cytotoxicity assay of *Abrus* leaf against rat myoblast (L_6) cell line showed that chloroform fraction was the most toxic with inhibitory concentration (IC_{50}) value of 43.7µg/ml followed by n-hexane fraction (44.3µg/ml). In vitro antiplasmodial assay against plasmodium chloroquiune-pyrimethanine resistant strain (K_1) showed that n-hexane fraction has the best activity with IC_{50} value of 12.1µg/ml followed by chloroform fraction (23.0µg/ml) (40). The LD_{50} of oral and intraperitoreal aqueous extract of *Abrus precatorius* leaf in mice were 2559.5 to 3123.2 mg/kg and 866 mg/kg body weight respectively (45). In view of the toxic potential of *Abrus precatorius* and also in line with the principle of replacement, reduction and refinement, the toxicity potential of the plant was extrapolated from mice to other fifteen species of monogastric animals.

MATERIAL AND METHODS

Literature on the medicinal uses, phytochemical components, toxicological effects, therapeutic and toxic doses of aqueous extract of *Abrus precatorius* leaf was searched. The toxicological doses and toxic effects of *Abrus precatorius* aqueous leaf extract in rats as reported by Adedapo et al. (2) were compared to toxicological doses and toxic effects of aqueous extract of *Abrus precatorius* leaf in mice as reported by Saganuwan (39), Saganuwan and Onyeyili (46) and Saganuwan et al. (44). Oral LD_{50}, (2559.5 – 3123.3 mg/kg) safe (12.5 mg/kg) and toxic (25 – 200 mg/kg) doses of aqueous extract of *Abrus precatorius* leaf were translated from mice to human, hamster, rat, guinea pig, rabbit, monkey, cat, dog, baboon, ferret, marmoset, squirrel monkey, micro-pig, mini-pig and child weighing 0.02, 60, 0.08, 0.15, 0.4, 1.8, 3, 7, 10, 12, 0.3, 0.35, 0.6, 20, 40, 20 kg body weight respectively (17, 37, 41, 48, 51, 55). The weights of the animals corresponded with the animal models used. The extract treatment doses

(400 – 1600 mg/kg) in rats were translated to human treatment doses. Saganuwan (39), Saganuwan and Onyeyili (46) and Saganuwan et al. (45) used 10% concentration of cold water extract of *A. precatorius* dry leaves. Adedapo *et al.* (2) used 50% cold water macerated extract of *Abrus precatorius* leaf for their study. Twenty (20) gramme and 150 g weighed mouse and rat between 5 – 7 weeks and 7 – 8 weeks respectively were used for the studies.

Animal-human and human-animal dose translations of LD_{50}, toxic and therapeutic doses of aqueous leaf extract of *Abrus precatorius* were determined using the human equivalent dose formula. Human Equivalent Dose (HED) is equal to animal dose multiplied by animal km factor divided by human K_m factor. The K_m factor is body weight (kg) divided by body surface area (m²). Human equivalent no-observable adverse effects dose is equal to animal no-observable adverse effect level (NOAEL) multiplied by animal weight (Wa) divided by human weight (Wh) to the power of 0.33 was used to confirm 12.5 mg/kg body weight of mice (relatively safe dose) translated to human and other animals' safe doses (4, 8, 9, 17, 34, 41, 51, 55).

A safety factor between 10th and 1000th was used to determine ideal safe therapeutic doses.

RESULTS

The range of LD_{50} estimated by Saganuwan (38, 39) was between 2559.5 and 3123.3 mg/kg body weight of mice. Adedapo et al. (3) did not conduct LD_{50} test on aqueous extract of *Abrus precatorius* leaf in rats. They investigated only haematological and biochemical effects of the extract on rats. The median lethal dose (2559.5-3123.3 mg/kg) of mice was translated to adult human LD_{50} (197.9-241.5 mg/kg), child (297-362.3 mg/kg), mini-pig (211.4-258 mg/kg), micro-pig (274.9-335.4 mg/kg), squirrel monkey (1107.6-1351.7 mg/kg), marmoset (1279.5-1561.4 mg/kg), ferret (1060.2-1293.8mg/kg), baboon and dog (371.1-452.8 mg/kg), cat (392.7-479.2 mg/kg), monkey (593.7-724.5 mg/kg), rabbit (618.4-754.7 mg/kg), guinea pig (1279.5-1561.4 mg/kg), rat (1349.3-1646.6 mg/kg) and hamster (1855.3-2264.1 mg/kg) respectively (Table 1).

Table 1. Mouse-human and human-other animals' extrapolated median lethal dose (LD_{50}) of aqueous leaf extract of *Abrus precatorius*

S/No.	Species	Body weight (kg)	BSA (m2)	K_m factor	LD_{50} (mg/kg)	Toxicity rating
1.	Mouse	0.02	0.007	2.9	2559.5-3123.3	Slightly toxic
2.	Hamster	0.08	0.02	4.0	1855.3-2264.1	,,
3.	Rat	0.15	0.025	6.0	1349.3-1646.6	,,
4.	Guinea pig	0.4	0.069	5.8	1279.5-1561.4	,,
5.	Rabbit	1.8	0.15	12.0	618.4-754.7	,,
6.	Monkey	3.0	0.24	12.5	593.9-724.5	,,
7.	Cat	7.0	0.37	18.9	392.7-479.2	Moderately toxic
8.	Dog	10	0.5	20.0	371.1-452.8	,,
9.	Baboon	12	0.6	20.0	371.1-452.8	,,
10.	Ferret	0.3	0.043	7.0	1060.2-1293.8	,,
11.	Marmoset	0.35	0.06	5.8	1279.5-1561.4	,,
12.	Squirrel monkey	0.6	0.09	6.7	1107.6-1351.7	,,
13.	Micro-pig	20	0.74	27.0	274.9-335.4	,,
14.	Mini-pig	40	1.14	35.1	211.4-258.0	,,
15.	Child	20	0.8	25.0	297-362.3	,,
16.	Adult human	60	1.6	37.5	197.9-241.5	,,

Note: Body weight and body surface area of animals and humans were taken from Reagan-Shaw et al. (7) and USEPA (55)

The therapeutic doses (12.5, 25, 50, 100 and 200 mg/kg) in mice translated to 1, 1.9, 3.9, 7.7 and 15.5 mg/kg body weight in human. On the other hand the therapeutic doses (400, 800 and 1600 mg/kg) in rats translated to 58.7, 117.3 and 234.7 mg/kg body weight in human (Table 2).

marmoset, squirrel, monkey, micro-pig, mini-pig, dog, baboon and mice to child translated doses are presented in Table 3.

At dose range between 400 and 1600 mg/kg body weight reported by Adedapo et al. (3), there was decreased RBC, PCV and Hb which were

Table 2. Mouse-human and rat-human equivalent therapeutic doses of aqueous leaf extract of *Abrus precatoirus*

Publications	Animal doses (mg/kg)	Human equivalent doses (mg/kg)
Saganuwan and Onyeyili (38, 46), Saganuwan (37), Saganuwan et al. (47)	12.5*	1.0*
	25	1.9
	50	3.9
	100	7.7
	200	15.5
Adedapo et al. (3)	400	58.7
	800	117.3
	1600	234.7

* = Safe dose for a period of 7 days

Human-animal equivalent therapeutic dose translation showed that 1 mg/kg body weight of adult human translated to 1.1 mg/kg in mini-pig and 9.1 mg/kg body weight in hamster respectively. But, 1.9 mg/kg body weight in human translated to 2.02 mg/kg in mini-pig and 18.1 mg/kg in hamster respectively. However, 15.5 mg/kg in human translated to 16.6 mg/kg in micro-pig and 145.0 mg/kg in hamster (Table 3). Human to hamster, rat, guinea-pig, rabbit, monkey, cat, baboon, ferret,

increased in mice (40, 44). White blood cells and lymphocytes were decreased in rat (3) (Table 4).

Alanine aminotransferase, aspartate aminotransferase, alkaline phosphatase, protein, albumin, globulin, albumin/globulin ratio were reported to have increased in rats and mice (3, 46). Total bilirubin, direct bilirubin and indirect bilirubin were reported to have increased in rat (3) but decreased in mice (46). Urea, creatinine, chloride ion, calcium ion and glucose increased as sodium ion

Table 4. Comparative haematological effects of aqueous extract of *Abrus precatorius* leaf

Parameters	Adedapo et al. (2)	Saganuwan (40)
Body weight	ND	↑
Red blood cells	↓	↑
Packed cell volume	↓	↑
Haemoglobin concentration	↓	NS
Mean Corpuscular Volume	↓	↑
Mean Corpuscular Haemoglobin	↑	↓
White Blood Cells Count	↓	↑
Neutrophils	↑	NS
Lymphocytes	↓	↑
Eosinophils	NS	↓
Monocytes	NS	↑
Basophils	ND	↓

Keys: ND=No data, NS=Not significant; ↑ =Increase; ↓ =Decrease

Table 3. Human-animal equivalent therapeutic doses of aqueous leaf extract of *Abrus precatorius*

Human	Hamster	Rat	Guinea pig	Rabbit	Monkey	Cat	Dog	Baboon	Ferret	Marmoset	Squirrel Monkey	Micro-pig	Mini-pig	child
								Animal-human translated doses (mg/kg)						
1.0	9.1*(1.0)	6.6*(0.9)	6.5*(1.2)	3.0*(0.9)	2.9*(0.9)	1.9*(0.9)	1.8*(1.0)	1.8*(1.1)	5.4*(0.9)	6.5*(1.2)	5.6*(1.2)	1.4*(1.0)	1.1*(1.0)	1.5*(1.0)
1.9	18.1	13.2	12.3	6.0	5.8	3.8	3.6	3.6	10.2	12.3	10.6	2.6	2.0	2.9
3.9	36.3	26.4	25.2	12.1	11.6	7.7	7.3	7.3	20.9	25.2	21.8	5.4	4.1	5.8
7.7	72.5	52.7	49.8	24.2	23.2	15.3	14.5	14.5	41.3	50.0	43.1	10.9	11.6	11.6
15.5	145.0	105.5	100.2	48.3	46.4	30.7	29.0	29.0	23.0	100.2	86.8	16.6	23.3	23.2

Note: * = Human-animal safe equivalent dose for a period of 7 days
The values in the brackets are the confirmed human equivalent safe doses approximated to 1 decimal place

Table 5. Comparative biochemical effects of aqueous extract of *Abrus precatorius* leaf

Parameters	Adedapo et al. (3)	Saganuwan and Onyeyili (37, 45)
Alanine aminotransferase	↑	↑
Aspartate aminotransferase	↑	↑
Alkaline phosphate	↑	↑
Cholesterol concentration	ND	NS
Protein	↑	↓
Albumin	↑	↑
Globulin	↑	↑
Albumin/globulin ratio	↑	↑
Urea	ND	↑
Creatinine	ND	↑
Total bilirubin	↑	↑
Direct bilirubin	↑	↓
Indirect bilirubin	↑	↓
Glucose	ND	↑
Sodium ion	ND	↓
Potassium ion	ND	↑
Calcium ion	ND	↓
Chloride ion	ND	↑
Biocarbonate ion	ND	NS
Phosphate ion	ND	↓

Keys: ND=No data, NS=Not significant; ↑ =Increase ↓ =Decrease

and phosphate ion decreased in mice (46). Adedapo et al. (3) didn't report the effect of aqueous extract of *Abrus precatorius* leaf on body weight, glucose, sodium ion, potassium ion, calcium ion, chloride ion, bicarbonate ion and phosphate ion (Table 5).

DISCUSSION

The mouse-human translated LD_{50} of 197.9-241.5 mg/kg body weight agrees with the report of Yamba et al. (58) indicating that the human translated LD_{50} should be between 10th and 100th of LD_{50} in mice. This shows that adult human is the most sensitive to acute poisoning of *Abrus precatorius* leaf followed by child, mini-pig, micro-pig, baboon, dog, cat, monkey, rabbit guinea pig, rat, hamster and mouse in that order (Table 1) invariably rating the extract as slightly to moderately toxic in monogastric animals (26, 40, 41). But the calculated higher LD_{50} of child (297 – 362.3 mg/kg) in comparison with the LD_{50} of adult human (197.9 – 241.5 mg/kg) may be caused by high body surface area of the child in comparison with that of the adult. Hence the child may require more amount of the extract than the adult. Generally the child weighing 20 kg should have developed

fully metabolic enzymes. High body surface area is given low km. Connotatively, fatty individuals may be less susceptible to *Abrus precatorius* poisoning than lean individuals. However 12.5 mg/kg body weight that translated to 1.0 mg/kg no observable adverse effect when administered for a period of 3 days to *Plasmodium berghei* infected mice, although the dose cleared 98.7% of the parasites in the blood within 9 days after the extract treatment (47). These findings agree with the report of Saganuwan (40) indicating that the Nupe ethnic group from Bida emirate has been using *Abrus precatorius* leaf for the treatment of both acute and chronic malarial symptoms. The use of Abrus leaf in the treatment of malaria among Nupes is sometimes either the last option after the conventional antimalarial drugs might have failed or due to poverty. The administration of 12.5 mg /kg body weight of the extract for 7 days did not cause any observable adverse effect on the treated mice but caused slight increase in the plasma urea level (37, 45). Therefore 1 mg/kg body weight translated dose for a period of 3 days may be safe in human, but when administered for a period of 7 days may likely cause slight increased plasma urea in human. Hence, one–tenth safety factor of mouse therapeutic dose can be adopted in human, whereas the 100th to 1000th safety factor of *Abrus precatorius* leaf extract may be adopted for doses between 10 and 100 mg/kg body weight of the extract. The least sensitive animal to *Abrus precatorius* aqueous leaf extract in this study may be mice, followed by hamster, rat and guinea pig respectively. However, doses higher than 1.5 mg/kg may be toxic to a child. Also doses higher than 9.1, 6.6, 6.5, 3.0, 2.9, 1.9, 1.8, 1.8, 5.4, 6.5, 5.6, 1.4 and 1.1 mg/kg body weight may be toxic to hamster, rat, guinea pig, rabbit, monkey, cat, dog, baboon, ferret, squirrel monkey, micro-pig and mini-pig respectively (Table 3). Animal human equivalent dose projections can be done in three ways; doses expressed in mg/kg body weight for the species where "the critical effect" leading to "the reference dose" are adjusted to mg/kg body weight$^{0.75}$ to reflect the dependence of pharmacokinetic elimination on metabolic rate-which may tend to scale with (body weight)$^{0.75}$ (1, 34, 53). Although when we scaled the body weight to 0.75 the estimated LD_{50s} were seriously higher in comparison with 0.67. A further adjustment factor may be applied to reflect the median human maximum tolerated dose (MTD) expected based on the identity and number of species that provided data that potentially could have been used as the basis for the reference dose (24). The expected geometric means of the ratios of human toxic potency ($\frac{1}{MTD}$) to the toxic potency estimated from the animal experiments ($\frac{1}{LD_{10}}$) or ($\frac{1}{TDL_0}$) are based on the ratios available for each species or combination of species shown (15). Looking from the single-species analyses to the cases for which data for increasing numbers of species are available for choice of "the most sensitive", it can be seen that the geometric mean ratios of the observed human potency to the human potency projected from the animal potency per (body weight)$^{0.75}$ tend to decline. This is the natural result of the fact that the lowest toxic dose inferred for data for more species will tend to make a more "conservative" prediction of human potency than when data are only available for a single animal species. Finally, the uncertainty in each type of animal-to-human toxic potency projection is inferred from variability of the ratios of the observed human potencies to the animal-projected potencies for different compounds. These variabilities are modelled as lognormal distributions with the standard deviations of the logarithms of the observed human to animal-projected potency ratios (24).

Increased RBC, PCV and haematocrit at dose range between 25-200 mg/kg body weight showed that the plant aqueous leaf extract, have haematinic effect at lower dose levels (44). But at higher dose levels (400-1600 mg/kg), it caused haemolysis with resultant hyperbilirubinaemia (3). However, at both lower doses (25-200 mg/kg) and higher doses (400-1600 mg/kg) the plant leaf extract caused increase in biochemical parameters with resultant deleterious effect on kidney, heart, intestine, lung, spleen and liver. But Adedapo et al. (3) should have conducted acute toxicity study on rats to serve as a guide for their selection of therapeutic doses instead of using predetermined doses. More so, their histopathological studies were restricted to testes, kidney and liver bearing in mind the fact that the plant is organotoxic. When Saganuwan and Onyeyili (40) treated mice with 25-200 mg/kg body weight of Abrus leaf extract for 21 days, the extract caused death of some mice, most especially at higher doses (25 – 200 mg/kg). But, it looked strange that Adedapo et al. (3) didn't report death in their experimental animals with serious kidney and liver damage. The plant has been reported to contain toxalbumin (phytoprotein), abrin, which may be responsible for the observed toxicity effects (21). Abrin consists of abrus agglutinin, and toxic lectins [a] to [d], the five toxic glycoproteins found in the plant. Abrus agglutinin is non-toxic to animal cells but a potent haemaglutinator (7). The toxic portion of abrin is heat-stable to incubation at 60 °C for 30 minutes, but at 80 °C most of the toxicity is lost in 30 minutes (36). Although the plant, particularly the seed is known to be highly poisonous due to presence of abrin (7, 12, 14, 21, 36), the leaf in the present study was observed to be slightly toxic. The incubation of the abrus leaf extract at 60 °C for several hours must have reduced the toxicity of the leaf (46). Although the extract was administered orally, abrin is very stable in the gastrointestinal tract, from where it is slowly absorbed and thereby making it less toxic (19). Abrins's toxic effect is due to its direct action on the membrane of parenchymal cells (e.g. liver, kidney cells and erythrocytes) (23) via the B chain (haptomere) that binds to galactosyl-terminated receptors on the cell membrane, which is a prerequisite for the entry of the other subunit, the A chain (effectomere). This inactivates the ribosomes, arrests protein synthesis, and causes cell death (50). The A-chain attacks the 60s subunits of the ribosomes and by cutting out elongation EF_2 stops synthesis of protein (18). So the extraction and concentration of aqueous extract of *Abrus precatorius* leaf at 60 °C (46) and unknown temperature (3) must have reduced toxic effects of the leaf extract in mice and rats respectively.

CONCLUSION

The translated mouse-human LD_{50} is 197.9-241.5 mg/kg body weight, showing high level of sensitivity of humans to *Abrus precatorius* leaf poisoning. The safe human therapeutic dose for a period of 3 days may be 1.0 mg/kg body weight. But the safe therapeutic doses for other animals are; hamster (9.1 mg/kg), rat (6.6 mg/kg), guinea pig (6.5 mg/kg), rabbit (3.0 mg/kg), monkey (2.9 mg/kg), cat (1.9 mg/kg), dog and baboon (1.8 mg/kg) and child (1.5 mg/kg) respectively. However, the administration of the safe doses for a period of 7 days may cause slight increase in the plasma urea.

REFERENCES

1. Ad Hoc Working Group (AHWG) (1992). Federal Coordinating Council for science, engineering and technology (FCCSET) Draft Report: A cross-section scaling factor for carcinogen risk assessment based on equivalence of mg/kg3 /day. Federal Register 57: 24152 – 24173.

2. Adedapo, A.A. (2002). Toxicological effects of some plants in the family euphorbiaceae in rats. PhD Thesis, University of Ibadan, Nigeria.

3. Adedapo, A.A., Omoloye, O.A., Ohore, O.G. (2007). Studies on the toxicity of an aqueous extract of the leaves of Abrus precatorius in rats. Onderstepport J Vet Res. 74, 31 36.
http://dx.doi.org/10.4102/ojvr.v74i1.137

4. Adelowotan, O., Aibinu, I., Adenipekun, E., Odugbemi, T. (2008). The in vitro antimicrobial activity of Abrus precatorius (L) Fabaceae extract on some clinical pathogens. Niger Postgrad Med. J. 15 (1): 32-37.
PMid:18408781

5. Anam, E.M. (2011). Anti-inflammatory activity of compounds isolated from the aerial parts of Abrus precatorius (Fabaceae). Phytomedicine 8(1): 24-27.
http://dx.doi.org/10.1078/0944-7113-00001
PMid:11292235

6. Anand, R.S., Kishire, V.O., Rajkumar, V. (2010). Abrus prectorius. A phytopharmacological review. J. Pharm. Res. 3(11): 2585-2587.

7. Budavari, S. (1989). The Merak Index: An Encyclopedia of Chemicals, Drugs and Biologicals, 10th ed., Rahway, New Jersey, Merck and Co. Inc
PMid:2666071

8. Burkill, H.M. (1997). The useful plant of West Tropical Africa, Vol 11, Royal Botanical Gardens, Kew.

9. Cheecke, P.R. (1998). Natural toxicants in feed, forage and poisonous plants. Interstate Publishers, Denville.

10. Cheecke, P.R., Shull, L.R. (1985). Natural toxicants in feeds and poisonous plants. The Connecticut: AVI Publishing Company.

11. Choudhari, A.B., Sayyed, N., Khairnar, A.S. (2011). Evaluation of antiserotonergic activity of ethyl acetate extract of Abrus precatorius leaves. J. Plant Res. 4(3): 570-572.

12. Davis, J.H. (1978). Abrus precatorius (Rosary pea). The most common lethal plant poison. J. Florida Med Assoc. 65, 189-191.

13. Dhawan, B.N., Patnaik, G.K., Singh, K.K., Tandon, J.S., Rastogi RP. (1977). Screening of Indian plants for biological activity. Indian J Exp Biol. 15, 208-219.
PMid:914326

14. Dreisbach, R.H., Robinson, W.O. (1987). Handbook of poisoning: prevention, diagnosis and treatment. Los Altos, Appleton and Lange, California 497.

15. Faustman, E.M., Allen, B.C., Karlock, R.J., Kimmel, C.A. (1994). Dose-response assessment for developmental toxicity. 1. Characterization of database and determination of no observed adverse effect levels. Fundamental Appl. Toxicol. 23, 478-486.
http://dx.doi.org/10.1006/faat.1994.1132

16. Fernando, C. (2011). Poisoning due to Abrus precatorius (Jequirity bean). Anaesthesia 56 (12): 1178-1180.

17. Freireich, E.J., Gehan, E.A., Rall, D. (1966). Quantitative comparison of toxicity of anticancer agents in mouse, rat, hamster, dog, monkey and man. Cancer Chemother. Rep. 50, 219-244.
PMid:4957125

18. Frohne, D., Pfander, H.J. (1983). A colour atlas of poisonous plants. Germany Wolfe Publishing Ltd., 291.
PMid:6683299

19. Galey, F.D. (1996). Plants and other natural toxicants. In: (Smith BP. Ed), Large Animals Internal Medicine, 2nd ed., Boston: Mushby Publishers.

20. Garg, S.K. (2005). Veterinary toxicology. New Delhi CBS publishers and Distributors, p321.

21. Ghosal, S., Dutta, S.K. (1971). Alkaloids of Abrus precatorius. Phytochemistry 10(1): 195-198.
http://dx.doi.org/10.1016/S0031-9422(00)90270-X

22. Hart, M. (1963). Jecquirity bean poisoning. N. Engl. J. Med. 268, 885-886.
http://dx.doi.org/10.1056/NEJM196304182681608

23. Hatts, D.S., S. Goble, R. (2002). A straw-man proposal for a quantitative definition of the reference dose. DOD conference on Toxicology risk assessment, Dayton, Ohio, 25, 2001, p 1-48.

24. Hemadari, K., Rao, S.S. (1983). Leucorrhoea and menorrhalgia, tribal medicine, Ancient Sci. Life 3, 40-41.

25. Hodge, H.C., Sterner, J.H. (1949). Toxicity rating. Am. Ind. Hyg. Assoc. Q. 10(4): 93. PMid:24536943

26. Iwu, M.M. (1993). Handbook of African medicinal plants. London: CRC Press Boca Raton Ann Arbot.

27. Kim, N.C., Kim, D.S., Kinghorn, A.D. (2002). New triterpenoids from the leaves of Abrus precatorius. Nat. Prod.Let.16 (4): 261-266. http://dx.doi.org/10.1080/10575630290020596 PMid:12168762

28. Kirtikar, K.R., Basu, B.D. (1980). Indian medicinal plants. Vol. 1, Dehra Dun: International Book Distributors.

29. Klassen, C.D. (2011). Casarett and Doall's. Toxicology: The basic science of poisoning. 6th ed., New York: Mc Graw-Hill.

30. Limmatvapirat, C., Sirisopanapom, Kittakoop, P. (2004). Antitubercular and antiplasmodial constituents of Abrus precatorius. Planta Med. 70 (3): 276-278. http://dx.doi.org/10.1055/s-2004-818924 PMid:15114511

31. Liu, C.L., Tsai, C.C., Lin, S.C. Wang, L.I., Hsu, C.I., Hwang, M.J., Lin, J.Y. (2000). Primary structure and function analysis of Abrus precatorius agglutinin A by site-directed mutagenesis, Pro (199) and amphiphilic alpha-helix H impairs protein synthesis inhibitory activity. J. Biol. Chem. 275 (3): 1897-1901. http://dx.doi.org/10.1074/jbc.275.3.1897 PMid:10636890

32. Mann, A., Gbate, M., Nda, Umar, A. (2003). Medicinal and economic plants of Nupeland. Bida: Jube Evans Books and Publications, p.191.

33. Mordent, J. (1986). Man versus beast: pharmacokinetic scaling in mammals. J. pharmaceut. Sci. 75, 1028–1040. http://dx.doi.org/10.1002/jps.2600751104

34. Premanand, R., Ganesh, T. (2010). Neuroprotective effects of Abrus precatorius Linn. Aerial extract on hypoxic neurotoxicity induced rats. Intern. J. Chem. Pharmaceut. Sci. 1(1).

35. Rajaram, N., Janardhanan, K. (1992). The chemical composition and nutritional potential of the tribal pulse, Abrus precatorius L. plant. Foods Human Nutr. 42(94): 285-290. http://dx.doi.org/10.1007/BF02194088

36. Reagan-Shaw, S., Nihal, M., Amhad, N. (2007). Dose translation from animal to human studies revisited. The FASEBJ 22, 659-661. http://dx.doi.org/10.1096/fj.07-9574LSF PMid:17942826

37. Saganuwan, S.A., Onyeyili, P.A. (2012). Haematonic and plasma expander effects of aqueous leaf extract of Abrus precatorius in Mus musculus. Campar Clinical Pathol. 21(6): 1249-1255. http://dx.doi.org/10.1007/s00580-011-1274-8

38. Saganuwan, S.A. (2011). A modified arithmetical method of Reed and Muench for determination of a relatively ideal median lethal dose (LD50). Afr. J. Pharm. Pharmacol. 5(12): 1543-1546. http://dx.doi.org/10.5897/AJPP11.393

39. Saganuwan, S.A. (2012). Toxicological and antimalarial effect of aqueous leaf extract of Abrus precatorius (Jacqurity bean) in Swiss albino mice. PhD Thesis, Usmanu Danfodiyo University, Sokoto Nigeria.

40. Saganuwan, S.A. (2012b). Principles of pharmacological calculations. 1st ed., Zaira: Ahmadu Bello University Press Ltd.

41. Saganuwan, S.A., Gulumbe, M.L. (2005a). In vitro antimicrobial activities testing of Abrus precatorius cold water leaf extract on Salmonella typhimurium, Escherichia coli and Klebesiella pneumoniae. J. Sci. Technol. Res. 4(3): 70-73.

42. Saganuwan, S.A., Gulumbe, M.L. (2005b). In vitro antimicrobial activities testing of Abrus precatorius cold water leaf extract on Streptococcus pyogenes and Streptococcuspneumoniae. Proc 2nd Annu Conf Nigerian Soc. Indigen Knowl Dev., 9th-12th Nov., Cross River State Univ. Technol Obubra, 93-97.

43. Saganuwan, S.A., Onyeyili, P.A., Etuk, U.E. (2009). Acute toxicity and haematological studies of aqueous extract of Abrus precatorius leaf in Mus Musculus, African Education Initiative Conf. p65.

44. Saganuwan, S.A., Onyeyili, P.A., Suleiman, A.O. (2011). Comparative toxicological effects of orally and intraperitoneally administered aqueous extracts of Abrus precatoriusleaf in Mus musculis. Herba Polonica 57(3): 32-44.

45. Saganuwan, S.A., Onyeyili, P.A. (2010). Biochemical effects of aqueous leaf extract of Abrus precatorius (Jecurity bean) in Swiss albino mice. Herba Polonica 56(3): 63-80.

46. Saganuwan, S.A., Onyeyili, P.A., Ameh, I.G., Etuk, E.U. (2011). In vivo antiplasmodial activity by aqueous extract of Abrus precatorius in mice. Rev. Latinoamer. Quin. 39(1-2): 32-34.

47. Sawyer, N., Ratain, M.J. (2001). Body surface area as a determinant of pharmacokinetics and drug dosing. Invest New Drugs 19, 171-177. http://dx.doi.org/10.1023/A:1010639201787 PMid:11392451

48. Sofi, M.S., Sateesh, M.K., Bashir, M.,Harish, G., Lakshmeesha, T.R., Vedashree, S., Vedamurthy, A.B. (2012). Cytotoxic and pro-apoptotic effects of Abrus precatorius L. on human metastatic breast cancer cell line, NDA-NB-231. Cytotechnology

49. Stirpe, F., Barbieri, L. (1986). Symposium: Molecular mechanisms of toxicity, toxic lectins from plants. Human Toxicol. 5(2): 108-109.
http://dx.doi.org/10.1177/096032718600500208

50. Sylva, M. (1998). Interspecies allometric scaling in pharmacokinetics of drugs. Acts Pharm Hung. 68 (6): 350-354.

51. Taur, D.J., Patil, R.Y. (2011). Effect of Abrus precatorius Leaves on milk induced leukocytosis and eosinophilia in the management of asthma. Asian Pacific J. Tropical. 1(1): 40-42.
http://dx.doi.org/10.1016/S2221-1691(11)60119-6

52. Travis, D.C., White, R.K., Ward, R.C. (1990). Interspecies extrapolation of pharmacokinetics. J. Theoretical Biol. 142, 285 - 304.
http://dx.doi.org/10.1016/S0022-5193(05)80554-5

53. Tripathi, S., Maith, T.K. (2005). Immunomodulatory role of native and heat denatured agglutinin from Abrus precatorius. Int. J. Biochem. Cell Biol. 37(13): 451-462.
http://dx.doi.org/10.1016/j.biocel.2004.07.015
PMid:15474989

54. US Environmental Protection Agency (USEPA) (1986). Guideline for carcinogen risk assessment. Fed Regist 51: 3392-4003.

55. Wambebe, C., Amosun, S.L. (1984). Some neutromuscular effects of crude extracts of the leaves of Abrus precatorius. J. Ethnopharmacol. 11(1): 49-58.
http://dx.doi.org/10.1016/0378-8741(84)90095-3

56. Watt, J.M., Breyer-Brandiwijk, A. (1962). The medicinal poisoning plants of Southern and Eastern Africa, 2nd ed., London: Livingstone publishers.
PMCid:PMC1957435

57. Xiao, Z.H., Wang, F.Z., Sun, A.J. (2011). A new triterpenoid saponin from Abrus precatorius Linn. Molecules 17(1): 295-302.
http://dx.doi.org/10.3390/molecules17010295
PMid:22210168

58. Yamba, O., Innocent, P.G., Odille, G.N. (2007). Biological and toxicological study of aqueous root-extract from Mitragyna inermis (Wild Okt) Rubiacea. Int. J. Pharmacol. 3(1): 80-85.
http://dx.doi.org/10.3923/ijp.2007.80.85

IMMUNOHISTOCHEMICAL DETECTION OF ESTROGEN RECEPTORS IN CANINE MAMMARY TUMORS

Elena Atanaskova Petrov[1], Ivica Gjurovski[2], Trpe Ristoski[2], Goran Nikolovski[1],
Pandorce Trenkoska[3], Plamen Trojacanec[4], Ksenija Ilievska[4],
Toni Dovenski[5], Gordana Petrushevska[6]

*[1]Department of Internal Medicine of Small Animals,
Faculty of Veterinary Medicine, Ss. Cyril and Methodius University in Skopje, Macedonia
[2]Department of Pathology, Faculty of Veterinary Medicine,
Ss. Cyril and Methodius University in Skopje, Macedonia
[3]Veterinary Clinic D-r Naletoski, Str. 1244/3, Skopje, Macedonia
[4]Department of Surgery, Faculty of Veterinary Medicine,
Ss. Cyril and Methodius University in Skopje, Macedonia
[5]Department of Reproduction, Faculty of Veterinary Medicine,
Ss. Cyril and Methodius University, Skopje, Macedonia
[6]Department of Pathology, Medical Faculty,
Ss. Cyril and Methodius University in Skopje, Macedonia*

ABSTRACT

Mammary tumors are among the most common neoplasms in intact female dogs.They have a complex morphology, usually affecting middle age and older bitches. Almost 50% of the mammary tumors in dogs are malignant neoplasms. Prognosis is based on several factors: stage, age, tumor size, metastasis, histopathology, ovariectomy status and hormone-receptor activity. Immunohistochemical (IHC) measurement has become increasingly an important diagnostic and prognostic parameter, with the development of monoclonal antibodies against nuclear estrogen and progestin receptors. The aim of this study was to detect the presence of ER receptors in malignant canine mammary tumors and to identify their association with the clinical course of the tumor. Mammary tumor samples have been obtained by mastectomy from dogs presented at our clinic. Detailed clinical examination, CBC and basic serum biochemical profile were performed in all patients. Surgery was the only treatment. Histopathological examination and immunohistochemical detection of estrogen α receptors (ERα) was performed on 8 formalin-fixed, paraffin-embedded tissue samples, using the PT LINK immunoperoxidase technique. Histopathological examination of the mammary tumor samples (n=11) revealed tubular adenocarcinoma (n=6,54.5%) and ductal adenocarcinoma (n=3, 27.3%), one patient with benign adenoma and one with mastitis. Patients with positive ER tumors are alive, without remission, while 3 of the patients that were ER negative died due to lung metastases. According to our results, it can be concluded that the appearance and development of canine mammary tumors is highly connected with ovarian steroid hormones and that immunostaining of the tumors may be used as a good prognostic parameter in these patients.

Key words: dog, mammary tumor, histopathology, immunohistochemy, ERα receptors

INTRODUCTION

Canine mammary tumors are the most prevalent tumors in female dogs, representing around 42% of all tumors (1, 2). These neoplasms have a complex morphology - epithelial, mixed, and mesenchymal types (3).

Corresponding author: Prof. Toni Dovenski, PhD
E-mail address: dovenski@fvm.ukim.edu.mk
Present address: Faculty of Veterinary Medicine, Ss. Cyril and Methodius University in Skopje, Str. Lazar Pop Trajkov 5-7, Skopje, Macedonia

Most frequently mammary gland tumors are found in 5 years and older bitches (4). Mostly affected parts are the caudal abdominal and inguinal mammary glands. Fifty to almost 70% of dogs with mammary tumors have multiple tumours (2, 4, 5). When multiple tumors are present, different tumour types may be found in one patient. According to some studies 50% of the tumors are malignant; most of them are carcinomas (6).

Histologic diagnosis of cancer does not always imply a malignant clinical course. Reliable prognostic factors are necessary for evaluation of the individual risk for undesirable clinical result. There are some prognostic factors of malignant mammary tumors in dogs and these include: tumor size, lymph node status, histologic type, histologic malignancy grade, degree of nuclear differentiation and distant metastasis (7).

Although several studies have been carried out on the prognostic aspects of canine mammary neoplasms, some areas, especially the role of steroid hormone receptors, remain uncertain (8).

Estrogens and progesterone excreted from the ovary have an impact on mammary gland tissue and presents a risk factor associated with the development of mammary tumors. According to many studies preventive effect of sterilization has been reported. The relative risk for mammary neoplasms in female dogs spayed before the first estrous is 0.5%, after the first cycle 8%, after the second cycle 26%; with the protective effect being lost after about 4 cycles (9, 10). Beauvais et al. (11) analyzed these conclusions and they found that the data are limited with a risk of bias, so further investigations are necessary in order to confirm that statement.

When metastases are present, dogs may show nonspecific symptoms such as fatigue, lethargy, weight loss, dyspnoea, cough, lymphoedema or lameness. Clinical signs depend on the extent and location of the metastases which determines the occurrence and severity of the clinical signs (2, 5).

Prognosis depends on many factors (stage, age, tumor size, metastasis, histopathology, ovariectomy status and hormone-receptor activity). With the development of monoclonal antibodies against nuclear estrogen and progestin receptors, immunohistochemical (IHC) measurement has become increasingly important (12).

The occurrence and growth of most mammary gland carcinomas is estrogen dependent. Benign tumors and well-differentiated tumors are more likely to be ER-positive, whereas undifferentiated, anaplastic tumors are usually ER-negative (8). The level of progesterone receptors (PR) is used as marker for hormone responsiveness of the tumor and patient's prognosis. PR-negative neoplasms generally have worse prognosis than progesterone receptor-positive neoplasms (13).

The aim of the present study was to detect the presence of ER receptors in malignant canine mammary tumors and to identify its association with clinical course of the tumor.

MATERIAL AND METHODS

Thirteen mammary tumor samples have been obtained by mastectomy from female dogs (6-13 years old, none of them were spayed) presented at the University Veterinary Hospital at the Faculty of Veterinary Medicine-Skopje. Medical history analyses showed that the first appearance of the tumor masses was noticed in a period of 1 month to one year before admission to the hospital and none of the patients were spayed. Rigorous examination was performed: assessment of the general condition, temperature, pulse, respiration, lymph node palpation, CBC and basic serum biochemical profile.

Surgical removal of the masses was the only treatment, with additional ovariohisterectomy in 7 patients. Following surgical excision, tissue samples were fixed in 10% formaldehyde, dehydrated, embedded in paraffin, then cut into 4 μm sections, and stained with hematoxylin and eosin (Merck, Darmstrad, Germany). All of the tumours were histologically classified into these categories: malignant tumours, benign tumours, unclassified tumours, and mammary hyperplasia/dysplasia (14).

Immunohistochemical detection of ERα was performed on 8 formalin-fixed, paraffin-embedded tissue samples. The procedure was performed on paraffin sections using the PT LINK immunoperoxidase technique (DakoChemMate, Denmark). For determination of ERα receptor expression, we used monoclonal antibody anti-ER from DAKO.

Corresponding positive and negative control were used. Two human score systems were used: ERi24, 45 and ERp. The ERi score was calculated as $P_1 + (2 * P_2) + (3 * P_3)$ where P_1, P_2, and P_3 are the estimated percentages of positive nuclei with low (P_1), medium (P_2), and high (P_3) intensity of immunostaining. The ERp score considered only the percentage of positive cells independent of the grade of intensity.

RESULTS

Most of the patients (11 out of 13) with mammary tumors were 12 – 13 years old. From a reproductive aspect, nine of the patients with malignant mammary tumors (81.8%) never had a litter and were not treated with exogenous hormones. Only one patient had history of false pregnancies after every oestrus cycle. Multiple nodular tumors were found in 9 patients, and solitary tumor in 4 patients (Fig. 1).

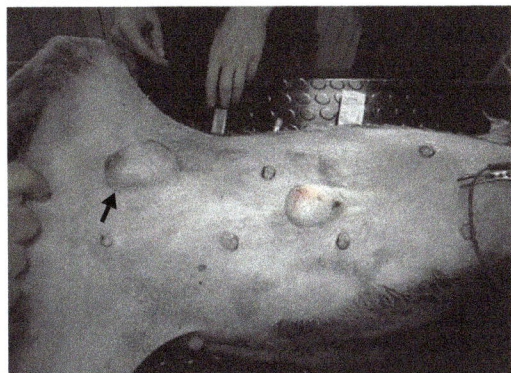

Figure 1. Solitary canine mammary tumor

Histopathology report made on 11 samples showed that six bitches had tubuloalveolar adenocarcinoma, three had ductal adenocarcinoma, there was one patient with benign adenoma and one with mastitis (Fig. 2). X-ray imaging was performed in 9 patients with diagnosed adenocarcinoma and 3 of them had lung metastases.

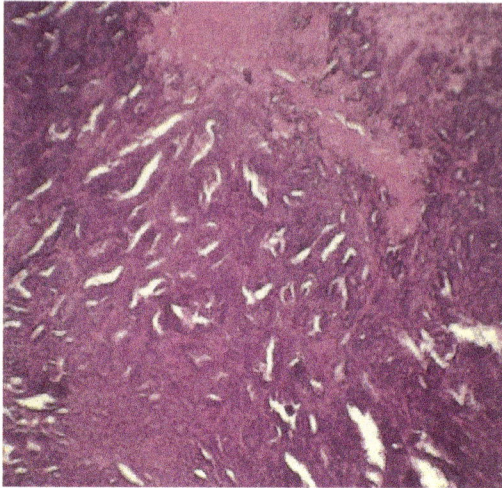

Table 1. Immunostaining percentage of ER and PR in different mammary tumors

Tumor type	ERα %
Adenocarcinoma- grade II-244	-
Adenocarcinoma- grade I- 241	20%
Adenocarcinoma - grade I-238	30%
Fibrosarcoma- grade III-237	-
Adenocarcinoma- grade III-233	-
Adenocarcinoma- grade I-223	30%
Ductal adenocarcinoma- grade II-193	2%
Adenocarcinoma - grade III194	-

Figure 2. Histopathology of mammary adenocarcinoma

In addition to the surgical removal of the tumors in seven patients, ovariohysterectomy was performed. Uterine enlargement characterized as Cystic Endometrial Hyperplasia (CEH) was noted in five patients with mammary tumors (Fig. 3), histopathology confirmed diagnosis of CEH.

Due to metastasis, two of the patient died two months after mastectomy (without ovariectomy) and one after one year. The others (n = 9) were controlled on a monthly basis. Six months after the treatment, these patients remained in good body condition, without any signs of health disorders. All of the patients with positive ER tumors are still alive, without remission. Three of the patients that were ER negative died due to lung metastases. Two of them (died 2 months after surgery) were presented in the Hospital with sings of dyspnoea due to lung metastases, anorexia, vomiting, decreased body temperature and lethargy. Third patient had remission six months after the surgical removal of the tumor and was euthanized six months later due to deterioration of the clinical condition.

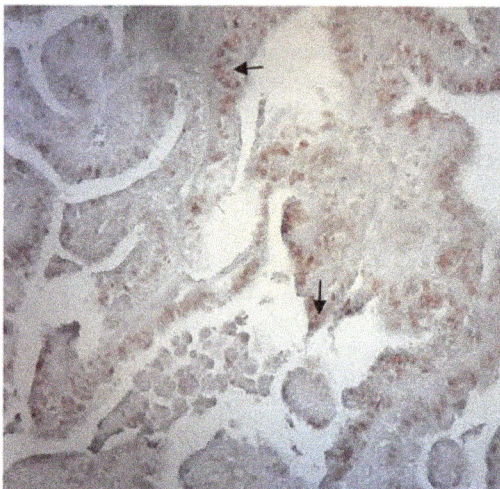

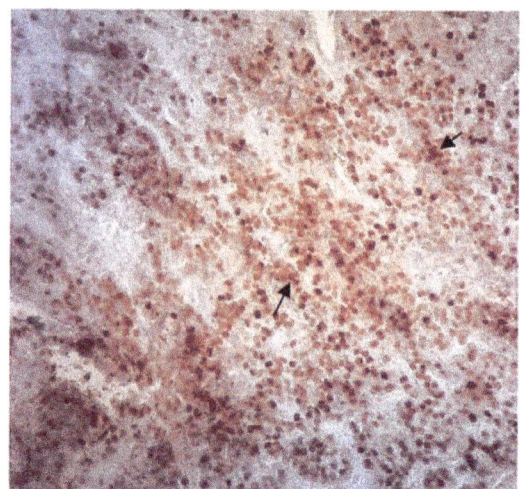

Eight malignant mammary tumors were immunohistochemically processed for ER analysis (Fig. 3). Four of the neoplasms (50%) were ER negative (Table 1).

Figure 3. Canine mammary adenocarcinoma showing expression of ERα in the nucleus of epithelial cells (IHC x40)

DISCUSSION

Ovarian steroids have proliferative effect on mammary epithelium that creates conditions for neoplastic proliferations. During the long luteal phase of the estrous cycle, mammary tissue is exposed to high concentrations of progesterone (10, 16). Mammary epithelial growth, proliferation and differentiation are regulated by the estrogen receptors (ER) and the complex cellular interactions that are mediated by a multitude of ligands, cofactors, and other stimuli. These receptors are also important for the physiological development and function of the mammary gland, but also play a role in the development and growth of mammary cancer (17). In our case 4 adenocarcinomas (50%) had positive ER immunostaining. Compared to the histopathology grade of the tumor, 3 (75%) were staged as grade I and one was grade II. Patients that had positive ER tumors are still alive and without remission, while 3 (75%) of the patients that were ER negative and histopathology grade III died within 20 days to one year after intervention due to metastases. Tumors which are positive for ER or PR or both, have a better prognosis than those that are negative for both receptors (18). Both ER and PR receptors were found in normal mammary tissues and benign tumors, but less common or absent in primary cancers and distant metastases. This is due to hormonal independency of the malignant mammary tumors (19, 20, 21).

The connection of uterine cystic glandular hyperplasia, pyometra and endocrine imbalance has been reported long time ago. Also the influence of progestogens on the development of canine mammary tumors and other nodular mammary changes has been reported (13). In our study, 5 patients with mammary tumors had cystic endometritis. Repeated progesterone influence during each metoestrus in cycling bitches leads to the gradual development of CEH, fluid accumulation and/or bacterial infection, with the most severe end stage being pyometra. Progesterone, especially after previous oestrogen influence, contributes to the development of disease because the influence of this hormone renders the uterus susceptible to bacterial infection and pyometra (22, 23). There are contradictory results regarding the benefit of ovariectomy performed together with mastectomy as well as the connection of abnormal oestrous cycle, false pregnancy, pregnancy, number of litters etc. to development of canine mammary tumors (12, 15, 24). Nine of our patient with mammary tumors had never whelped, one had one litter and one was with unknown history. False pregnancies were noted only in one patient with mammary tumors.

CONCLUSION

According to our study, with regard to other researches we can conclude that the appearance and development of mammary tumors in dogs is highly connected with ovarian steroid hormones and that positive immunohistochemical expression of the ER-s in tumors may be used as a good prognostic parameter in patients with mammary tumors.

REFERENCES

1. Moulton, J.E. (1990). Tumors of the mammary gland. In: Moulton J.E. (Ed.), Tumours in domestic animals (pp. 518–552). Berkeley: University of California Press.

2. Sorenmo, K. (2003). Canine mammary gland tumors. Vet Clin North Am Small Anim Pract. 33, 573–596. http://dx.doi.org/10.1016/S0195-5616(03)00020-2

3. Hellmen, E. (2005). Complex mammary tumours in the female dog: a review. Journal of Dairy Research 72, 90–97. http://dx.doi.org/10.1017/S002202990500124X PMid:16180726

4. Sorenmo, K.U., Kristiansen, V.M., Cofone, M.A., Shofer, F.S., Breen, A.M., Langeland, M., Mongil, C.M., Grondahl, A.M., Teige, J., Goldschmidt, M.H. (2009). Canine mammary gland tumours: a histological continuum from benign to malignant, clinical and histopathological evidence. Vet Comp Oncol. 7, 162–172. http://dx.doi.org/10.1111/j.1476-5829.2009.00184.x PMid:19691645

5. Misdorp, W. (2002). Tumors of the mammary gland. In: Meuten D.J. (Ed.), Tumors in domestic animals (pp. 575–606). Ames: Iowa State Press. http://dx.doi.org/10.1002/9780470376928.ch12

6. MacEwen, E.G., Withrow, S. (1996). Tumors of the mammary gland. Small Animal Oncology (pp. 356–372). Philadelphia: Saunders Company.

7. De Las Mulas, J. M., Millán, Y., Dios, R. (2005). A prospective analysis of immunohistochemically determined estrogen receptor α and progesterone receptor expression and host and tumor factors as predictors of disease-free period in mammary tumors of the dog. Veterinary Pathology Online 42 (2): 200-212. http://dx.doi.org/10.1354/vp.42-2-200 PMid:15753474

8. Nieto, A., Pena, L., Pérez-Alenza, M. D., Sanchez, M. A., Flores, J.M., Castano, M. (2000). Immunohistologic detection of estrogen receptor alpha in canine mammary tumors: clinical and pathologic associations and prognostic significance. Vet Pathol. 37 (3): 239–247. http://dx.doi.org/10.1354/vp.37-3-239 PMid:10810988

9. Lana, S.E., Rutteman, G.R., Withrow, S.J. (2007). Tumors of the mammary gland. In: Withrow S.J & MacEwen B.R. (Ed.), Small animal clinical oncology (pp. 455-477). Philadelphia: Saunders Company. http://dx.doi.org/10.1016/B978-072160558-6.50029-0

10. Murphy, S. (2008). Mammary tumours in dogs and cats. Inpractice 6, 334–339. http://dx.doi.org/10.1136/inpract.30.6.334

11. Beauvais,W., Cardwell, J. M., Brodbelt, D. C. (2012). The effect of neutering on the risk of mammary tumours in dogs – a systematic review. J Small Anim Pract. 53, 314–322. http://dx.doi.org/10.1111/j.1748-5827.2011.01220.x PMid:22647210

12. Las Mulas, J.M., Millan, Y., Dios R. (2005). A prospective analysis of immunohistochemically determined estrogen receptor alpha and progesterone receptor expression and host and tumor factors as predictors of disease-free period in mammary tumors of the dog. Vet Pathol. 42, 200-212. http://dx.doi.org/10.1354/vp.42-2-200 PMid:15753474

13. Cork, D. M. W., Lennard, T. W. J., Tyson-Capper, A. J. (2008). Alternative splicing and the progesterone receptor in breast cancer. Breast Cancer Res. 10 (3): 207. http://dx.doi.org/10.1186/bcr2097 PMid:18557990 PMCid:PMC2481493

14. Misdorp, W., Hellmen, E., Else, R.W. (1999). Mammary tumours and dysplasia in dogs and cats. Histologic classification of tumours of domestic animals. Second series (pp. 3-6). Washington DC: Armed Forces Institute of Pathology.

15. Sorenmo, K.U., Shoferm, F.S., Goldschmidt, M.H. (2000). Effect of spaying and timing of spaying on survival of dogs with mammary carcinoma. J Vet Intern Med. 14, 266–270. http://dx.doi.org/10.1111/j.1939-1676.2000.tb01165.x PMid:10830539

16. Thuroczy, J., Reisvaag, G. J. K., Perge, E., Tibold, A., Szilagyi, J., Balogh, L. (2007). Immunohistochemical detection of progesterone and cellular proliferation in canine mammary tumours. J Comp Pathol. 137 (2-3): 122–129. http://dx.doi.org/10.1016/j.jcpa.2007.05.005 PMid:17645888

17. Diaz, L. K., Sneige, N. (2005). Estrogen receptor analysis for breast cancer: current issues and keys to increasing testing accuracy. Adv Anat Pathol. 12 (1): 10–19. http://dx.doi.org/10.1097/00125480-200501000-00003 PMid:15614160

18. Port Louis, L.R., Varshney, K.C., Nair, M.G. (2012). An immunohistochemical study on the expression of sex steroid receptors in canine mammary tumors. ISRN VetSci. 1-7. http://dx.doi.org/10.5402/2012/378607 PMid:23738123 PMCid:PMC3658582

19. Rutteman, G.R., Misdorpl, W., Blankenstein, M.A., Van den Brom, W.E. (1988). Oestrogen (ER) and progestin receptors (PR) in mammary tissue of the female dog: Different receptor profile in non-malignant and malignant states. Br J Cancer. 58, 594-599. http://dx.doi.org/10.1038/bjc.1988.266 PMid:3219269 PMCid:PMC2246835

20. Mariotti, F., Giacomo, R., Subeide, M. (2013). Immunohistochemical evaluation of ovarian hormonal receptors in canine mammary tumors. Open J Vet Med. 3, 104-110. http://dx.doi.org/10.4236/ojvm.2013.32017

21. Spoerri, M., Guscetti, F., Hartnack, S., Boos, A., Oei, C., Balogh, O., Nowaczyk, R. M., Michel, E., Reichler, I. M., Kowalewski, M. P. (2015). Endocrine control of canine mammary neoplasms: serum reproductive hormone levels and tissue expression of steroid hormone, prolactin and growth hormone receptors. BMC Vet Res. 11, 235. http://dx.doi.org/10.1186/s12917-015-0546-y PMid:26370564 PMCid:PMC4570623

22. Chen, Y.M., Lee, C.S., Wright, P.J. (2006). The roles of progestagen and uterine irritant in the maintenance of cystic endometrial hyperplasia in the canine uterus. Theriogenology 66, 1537–1544. http://dx.doi.org/10.1016/j.theriogenology.2006.01.019 PMid:16472854

23. Hagman, R. (2014). Diagnostic and prognostic markers for uterine diseases in dogs. Reprod Dom Anim. 49 (2): 16–20. http://dx.doi.org/10.1111/rda.12331 PMid:24947856

24. Queiroga, F.L., Perez- Alenza, M.D., Silvan, G., Pena, L., Lopes, C., Illera, J.C. (2005). Role of steroid hormones and prolactin in canine mammary cancer. J Steroid Biochem Mol Biol. 94, 181–187. http://dx.doi.org/10.1016/j.jsbmb.2004.12.014 PMid:15862964

19

COMPARATIVE CLINICAL AND HAEMATOLOGICAL INVESTIGATIONS IN LACTATING COWS WITH SUBCLINICAL AND CLINICAL KETOSIS

Vania Marutsova[1], Rumen Binev[1], Plamen Marutsov[2]

*[1]Department of Internal Diseases, Faculty of Veterinary Medicine,
Trakia University, Students' Campus, 6000 Stara Zagora, Bulgaria
[2]Department of Veterinary Microbiology, Infectious and Parasitic Diseases,
Faculty of Veterinary Medicine, Trakia University, Students' Campus,
6000 Stara Zagora, Bulgaria*

ABSTRACT

Ketosis of lactating cows is among the most common metabolic diseases in modern dairy farms. The economic importance of the disease is caused by the reduced milk yield and body weight loss, poor feed conversion, lower conception rates, culling and increased mortality of affected animals. In the present study, a total of 47 high-yielding dairy cows up to 45 days in milk (DIM) are included. All animals were submitted to physical examination wich included checking the rectal body temperature, heart rate, respiratory and rumen contraction rates, and inspection of visible mucous coats. The body condition was scored, and blood β-hydroxybutyrate (BHBA) concentrations were assayed. The cows were divided into 3 groups: first group (control) (n=24) with blood β-hydroxybutyrate level <1.2 mmol/l, second group (n=15) with blood β-hydroxybutyrate between 1.2-2.6 mmol/l (subclinical ketosis) and third group (n=8) with blood β-hydroxybutyrate >2.6 mmol/l (clinical ketosis). Whole blood samples were obtained and analyzed for Red Blood Cell (RBC, 10^{12}/l), Hemoglobin (HGB, g/l), Hematocrit (HCT, %), Mean Corpuscular Volume (MCV, fl), Mean Corpuscular Hemoglobin (MCH, pg), Mean Corpuscular Hemoglobin Concentration (MCHC, g/l), White Blood Cell (WBC, 10^9/l), Lymphocytes (LYM, 10^9/l), Monocytes (MON, 10^9/l), Granulocytes (GRA, 10^9/l), Red Blood Distribution Width (RDW, %), Red Blood Cell Distribution Width Absolute (RDWa, fl), Platelets (PLT, 10^9/l) and Mean Platelet Volume (MPV, fl). In this study, deviations in the clinical parameters in the control group and in those with subclinical ketosis were not identified. The cows from the third group (clinical ketosis) exhibited hypotonia, anorexia and body weight loss vs. control group. Hematological analysis showed leukocytosis and lymphocytosis in cows with subclinical ketosis vs. control group. In cows with clinical ketosis WBC counts decreased (leukopenia), while hemoglobin content and hematocrit values are higher vs. control group. Blood BHBA values are higher in both groups of ketotic cows vs. the control group. The other analyzed parameters (RBC, MCH, MCHC, MCV, RDW, RDWa, MON, GRA, PLT and MPV) were close to control values.

Key words: ketosis, hematological parameters, β-hydroxybutyrate, dairy cows

INTRODUCTION

Metabolic disorders in ruminants are most frequently found in the transition period from late pregnancy to early lactation, as the animal's body suffers substantial changes. During the pregnancy,

Corresponding author: Dr. Rumen Binev, PhD
E-mail address: binew@abv.bg
Present address: Department of Internal Medicine and Clinical Toxicology, Faculty of Veterinary Medicine, Trakia University, Stara Zagora, Bulgaria

the metabolism of cows is adapted for the developing embryo (1), while during the early lactation the metabolism follows the increased production of milk.

Ketosis occurs most commonly after calving during the 2nd lactation (3-7 week postpartum) (2, 3) and considerably less afterwards (4). This period corresponds to an inadequate energy intake and increasing milk secretion, determining the occurrence of a negative energy balance (5).

Subclinical ketosis (SCK) is a pathological condition associated with an increased level of ketone bodies in the organism without symptoms for clinical ketosis (6). Health and economic consequences of subclinical ketosis are reduced milk yield (7, 31), reproductive disorders (8), low insemination index (9), prolonged service period, clinical and subclinical mastitis (10), abomasal dislocation (11), and/or clinical ketosis (12).

The periparturient period with metabolic and hormonal changes, stress factors has a significant impact on the health of dairy cows and decreases the resistance to various infections (13). The period of negative energy balance is of critical for appearance of clinical and subclinical ketosis. The increased blood concentrations of non-esterified fatty acids (NEFA) or β-hydroxybutyrate (BHBA) correlate positively with disturbances in dairy cows' health, reproduction and milk yield during the postpartum period (12, 14).

Marked hyperketonaemia is manifested clinically with reduced appetite, rapid weight loss and reduced milk yield. Sometimes, the animals exhibit nervous signs as pica, biting and licking unusual object, blindness (15). The faeces is usually hard, dry and scanty. Sometimes very high blood BHBA concentrations, clear clinical signs of ketosis could be absent (16).

Determination of the Body Condition Score (BCS) provides available information for the body reserves, for the determination of how dairy cows are prepared for the period of negative energy balance, full of stress and inappropriate diet (17). It can be used as an indicator for potential health problems in dairy cows, sheep and goats. The changes in BCS suggest the presence of inadequate energy supply and occurrence of postpartum metabolic disorders (18). Literature data about BCS before calving shows wide variety: $\leq$ 3.0 (19); 3.25 (20) and 3.00-3.50 (5). It is demonstrated that cows with BCS before calving which is > 3.5 has 2.5 times higher risk of developing type II ketosis (21).

Some hematological and biochemical parameters are indicators of physiological, nutritional, metabolic and clinical status of production animals, as an important part of health and welfare management (22). Several authors report that blood BHBA concentrations are a basic parameter for proper evaluation of ketosis, where BHBA is more stable than other ketone bodies (acetone and acetoacetate) (16, 23).

For diagnostic SCK in lactating cows, mainly 3 values of blood BHBA are noticed in the literature: more than 1.0 mmol/l (24, 25), more than 1.2 mmol/l 7, 26) and more than 1.4 mmol/l (12, 16, 27). If the blood BHBA is more than 1-1.4 mmol/l, there is 3 times greater risk for dislocation of the abomasum and/or development of ketosis (12, 16, 27). In our previous studies of goats with subclinical ketosis (28), blood BHBA concentrations between 0.8 and

1.9 mmol/l were established between the 10th and the 30th day of lactation. This data is comparable with type I subclinical ketosis in dairy cows. Subclinical ketosis and type I clinical ketosis (CK) occur usually between the postpartum days 14–21 and 5–50, respectively (16). Type II clinical ketosis is generally present during the first 14 days after calving, but could be encountered in cows up to the 30th day of lactation.

Blood BHBA values for clinical ketosis are: over 2.0 mmol/l (29), over 2.6 mmol/l (30) and over 3.0 mmol/l (2). Blood BHBA concentrations >3.0 mmol/l were established only in 20% of ketotic cows (14).

Considering the widespread occurrence of bovine ketosis at a global scale (31) and economic losses incurred by farmers, the early and accurate diagnosis is essential for prevention of this disease. On the other hand, it is known that circulating ketone bodies (acetone, acetoacetate and BHBA) have negative influence on all organs and physiological processes of the animal body. Alterations in blood biochemistry can be used for early diagnosis of metabolic diseases and taking preventive measures for herd health management and against economic losses in dairy production.

The aim of this study was to investigate changes in the clinical and hematological parameters in high-yielding cows suffering from subclinical and clinical ketosis.

MATERIAL AND METHODS

Animals

Studies were performed in dairy farms in the Republic of Bulgaria and Republic of Serbia between February and September 2014.

Experimental design

A total of 47 Holstein cows from 1st to 4th lactation were included in the study (n=29 from R. Bulgaria and n=18 from R. Serbia). Dairy cows were fed rations corresponding to the physiological state (lactation) of the studied groups. All cows were up to 45 days in milk (DIM). In this study, the blood BHBA threshold value for subclinical ketosis was set to $\geq$ 1.2 mmol/l, and for clinical ketosis – to $\geq$2.6 mmol/l. All cows were submitted to physical examination, body condition score evaluation and analysis of blood β-hydroxybutyrate concentrations.

Cows were divided into three groups:
- first group (n=24) with blood BHBA level <1.2 mmol/l – control cows;

- second group with blood BHBA between 1.2-2.6 mmol/l (n=15) – cows with subclinical ketosis;
- third group with blood BHBA >2.6 mmol/l (n=8) – cows with clinical ketosis.

Clinical investigations

All cows were submitted to examination of the rectal body temperature, heart rate, respiratory and rumen contraction rates, and visible mucous inspection using routine clinical diagnostic procedures.

Body condition scoring

Body condition scores were evaluated using a 5-point scale (1.0-5.0, at intervals of 0.25). The cows were scored visually by two investigators (32).

Blood samples and analyses

Blood samples were collected through puncture of the coccygeal vein using sterile 21G needles and vacutainers either anticoagulated with K_2EDTA - 3 ml or with gel and clot activator - 6 ml. (Biomed, Bulgaria). Samples were obtained in the morning before feeding.

Blood BHBA concentrations were determined immediately using a portable Xpress-I system (Nova Biomedical, UK). Samples for CBC analysis were transported and stored at 4^0C. Analysis was performed within 2 hours after sampling. The following parameters were determined: Red Blood Cell (RBC, $10^{12}/l$), Hemoglobin (HGB, g/l), Hematocrit (HCT, %), Mean Corpuscular Volume (MCV, fl), Mean Corpuscular Hemoglobin (MCH, pg), Mean Corpuscular Hemoglobin Concentration (MCHC, g/l), White Blood Cell (WBC, $10^9/l$), Lymphocytes (LYM, $10^9/l$), Monocytes (MON, $10^9/l$), Granulocytes (GRA, $10^9/l$), Red Blood Distribution Width (RDW, %), Red Blood Cell Distribution Width Absolute (RDWa, fl), Platelets (PLT, $10^9/l$) and Mean Platelet Volume (MPV, fl). Hematological investigations were analyzed on an automated analyser Exigo EOS Vet (Boule Medical AB, Sweden).

Statistical analysis

Statistical analysis was done with Statistica 6.0 (Windows) software, StatSoft, Inc. (USA, 1993) and ANOVA test. Results were presented as mean (x) $\pm$ standard deviation (SD). The level of statistically significance was $p < 0.05$.

RESULTS

Values of physical examination of cows with SCK showed no statistically significant changes vs. control group. Cows with CK, had a reduced average rumen contraction rate ($p<0.05$): 7.6±0.02 vs control values (11.4±0.02). Data from physical examinations (rectal temperature, heart rate, respiratory rate, rumen contraction rate) are presented in Table 1.

There were no changes in both groups of ketotic cows where inspection was performed of the color of visible mucosae, swelling, discharges and coat.

Reduced rumen contraction rate (hypotonia) was recorded, cows with clinical ketosis also exhibited anorexia and body weight loss.

The results of blood β-hydroxybutyrate concentrations and BCS in all cows included in experiment are presented in Table 2. Cows from group 2 (SCK) and group 3 (CK) BHBA levels were higher –1.57±0.55 mmol/l ($p<0.05$) and 4.75±1.36 mmol/l ($p<0.001$) respectively, compared to cows from the control group - 0.30±0.16 mmol/l.

Average BCS in control animals was 3.55±0.36, in SCK cows – 3.25±0.27 and in cows with clinical ketosis (group 3) – 2.51±0.31.

Table 1. Clinical parameters of cows from the control group (Group 1), with subclinical ketosis (SCK) (Group 2) and clinical ketosis (CK) (Group 3)

Parameters	Group 1 (control, n=24)	Group 2 (SCK, n=15)	Group 3 (CK, n=8)
Temperature (°C)	38.3±0.01	38.8±0.02	38.4±0.01
Heart rate (min⁻¹)	75.4±0.03	76.6±0.01	77.3±0.01
Respiratory rate (min⁻¹)	19.1±0.01	20.2±0.02	20.4±0.03
Rumen contractions (min⁻⁵)	11.4±0.02	9.7±0.01	7.6±0.02[1a]

Legend: [a]p<0.05; 1-vs control group; 2- vs group 2; 3-vs group 3

Table 2. Average blood concentrations of β-hydroxybutyrate (BHBA) and body condition scores (BCS) in cows from the control group (Group 1), with subclinical ketosis (SCK) (Group 2) and clinical ketosis (CK) (Group 3)

Parameters	Group 1 (control, n=24)	Group 2 (SCK, n=15)	Group 3 (CK, n=8)
BHBA (mmol/l)	0.30±0.16	1.57±0.55[1a]	4.75±1.36[1c]
BCS	3.55±0.36	3.25±0.27	2.51±0.31

Legend: $^a p<0.05$; $^e p<0.01$; $^c p<0.001$; 1-vs. control group1; 2- vs. group 2; 3-vs. group 3

Data reflecting changes in hematological parameters of both study groups are presented in Table 3. Cows with CK had higher HGB and HCT values - 109.37±12.11g/l and 29.86±4.32% respectively, vs. healthy cows (97.75±9.52 g/l and 26.72±3.00%; p<0.05). Total WBC values in cows with CK (group 3) were lower – 6.57±2.59 (10^9/l) (p<0.05) as compared with controls: 9.61±4.76 (10^9/l). Unexpectedly, higher WBC values were detected in cows with subclinical ketosis - 14.87±7.73 (10^9/l) (p<0.05), than in the control cows – 9.61±4.76 (10^9/l). In cows with SCK higher values were established of lymphocytes -

8.25±0.84 (10^9/l) (p<0.05) vs. control group - 4.89±0.77 (10^9/l).

The other hematology parameters (RBC, MCH, MCHC, MCV, RDW, RDWa, MON, GRA, PLT and MPV) were not significantly different than values in control animals.

DISCUSSION

This research confirmed that blood BHBA concentrations in cows with SCK is higher than 1.2 mmol/l and in cows with CK is higher than

Table 3. Hematological parameters in cows from the control group (Group 1), with subclinical ketosis (SCK) (Group 2) and clinical ketosis (CK) (Group 3)

Parameters	Group 1 (control, n=24)	Group 2 (SCK, n=15)	Group 3 (CK, n=8)
RBC (x10^{12}/l)	5.70±0.57	5.75±0.67	6.31±0.74
HGB (g/l)	97.75±9.52	99.73±8.17	109.37±12.11[1a]
HCT (%)	26.72±3.00	27.18±2.55	29.86±4.32[1a]
MCV (fl)	46.76±3.72	46.20±2.88	48.15±5.71
MCH (pg)	17.06±1.06	17.14±0.94	17.97±1.26
RDW (%)	21.79±2.54	20.82±4.13	21.45±1.85
RDWa (fl)	30.05±3.61	29.03±1.37	30.55±4.31
MCHC (g/l)	366.16±10.26	367.66±7.07	368.12±13.84
WBC (x10^9/l)	9.61±4.76	14.87±7.73[1a]	6.57±2.59[1a]
LYM (x10^9/l)	4.89±0.77	8.25±0.84[1a]	3.66±0.22
MON (x10^9/l)	0.82±0.10	1.14±0.11	0.57±0.02
GRA (x10^9/l)	3.80±0.77	5.13±0.77	2.44±0.15
PLT (x10^9/l)	354.62±98.45	365.53±139.38	397.87±126.19
MPV(fl)	6.44±0.93	6.01±0.65	6.40±0.85

Legend: $^a p<0.05$; $^e p<0.01$; $^c p<0.001$; 1-vs control group1; 2- vs group 2; 3-vs group 3

2.6 mmol/l, which are set as limited values for subclinical and clinical ketosis, respectively. Blood BHBA is an indicator of inappropriate oxidation of non-esterified fatty acids in the liver (33). It is used as early marker for detection of ketosis in ruminants (16, 23). Some researchers (24, 25) set a limit value >1.0 mmol/l, others (12, 16, 27) over 1.4 mmol/l, while in the present study value over 1.2 mmol/l is chosen as a limit of exhibited clinical sings (7, 26). Reduced blood glucose level and low insulin secretion are triggers for enhanced mobilization of lipids from the adipose tissue and deposition of triglycerides in the liver parenchyma and stimulation of ketogenesis (34).

Low values of BCS in cows with clinical ketosis correlated negatively with higher blood BHBA concentrations. Loss of appetite is a further reason for high blood ketone bodies concentrations. The weight loss until the 30th day of lactation has a considerable impact on the risk for development of ketosis, dislocation of the abomasum, milk yield reduction, disturbance of the reproductive performance and early embryonic death (35). Other authors (36) found that there was no relationship between the weight loss during the lactation and the incidence of metabolic diseases. Excessive fat deposition in the dry period correlates with increased occurrence of clinical ketosis in cows after calving (37). Literature and these results confirmed that the BCS is an important data for nutrition management of dairy herd.

The results from the complete blood count showed increased hemoglobin and hematocrit values only in cows with clinical ketosis. We suggest that these changes were due to higher erythrocyte counts in cows from group 3, although the differences were not statistically significant. Most authors (38) suggest that clinical and subclinical ketosis is not accompanied by changes in RBC, hemoglobin and hematocrit. There is literature data (39) for lower hemoglobin level and RBC counts in ketotic cows, as in these cases the erythropaenia was accompanied by anisocytosis and poikilocytosis.

Statistically significant increase of WBC is reported in this research in cows with SCK. It could be assumed that higher leukocyte counts were related to the wide spread of bovine enzootic leucosis in Bulgaria (40), and to the fact that 2 of cows (13.3%) presented signs of metritis. The leukocytosis in cows during the postpartum period is most commonly attributed to acute or chronic inflammations (mastitis, endometritis, metritis etc.) (22).

Reduction in WBC counts was shown in cows from group 3 (with clinical ketosis). Results in this investigation are in agreement with other reports (41, 42, 43). Lower WBC counts are reported in cows with enhanced catabolism in the periparturient period and increased blood BHBA levels (44). High levels of ketone bodies inhibit the cell proliferation in bone tissue (42), the *in vitro* chemotaxis of leukocytes (43) and respiratory activity of polymorphonuclear leukocytes (41).

In this study, we found statistically significant changes in lymphocyte counts (lymphocytosis) in cows suffering from SCK. This is consistent with the increased neutrophil and lymphocyte counts reported in lactating cows in consequence to the enhanced lipomobilisation, ketogenesis and hypoglycemia (45). On the other hand, high neutrophil and lymphocyte counts could result from stress and accompanying levels of glucocorticoids (cortisol) (46). The distinct immunosuppressive effects of high ketone bodies concentrations (BHBA and acetoacetate) (47) and oestrogens (48) are also acknowledged.

CONCLUSION

Clinical and subclinical ketosis among dairy cows in the first 45 days after delivery is quite prevalent. In practice, early detection is useful for treatment and assurance of good milk yields. The blood parameters, especially BCS and blood BHBA are excellent parameters for the nutritional status and health of dairy cows and could be utilized as markers for timely detection of metabolic disorders in cattle. Identification of problems at the herd is a signal for correction of the diet, preventive supplementation with rapid sources of energy etc., in order to reduce economic losses. Changes in hematology have a limited diagnostic value in clinical and subclinical ketosis, but our results provoke interest for further studies to clarify their meaning.

REFERENCES

1. Bell, A.W. (1995). Regulation of organic nutrient metabolism during transition from late pregnancy to early lactation. J. Anim. Sci. 73, 2804-2819. PMid:8582872

2. Oetzel, G.R. (2004). Monitoring and testing dairy herds for metabolic disease. Vet. Clin. North Am. Food Anim. Pract. 20, 651-674. http://dx.doi.org/10.1016/j.cvfa.2004.06.006 PMid:15471629

3. Kirovski, D., Šamanc, H., Cernescu, H., Jovanović, M., Vujanac, I. (2008). Fatty liver incidence on dairy cow farms in Serbia and Romania. International Symposium New Researches in Biotechnology", Romania, Buchurest, November 20th to 21st, Biotechnology, series F, special volume.

4. Radostis, O.M., Gay, C.C., Blood, D.C., Hinchcliff, K.W. (2000). Ketosis of ruminants. In: Radostits OM, DC Blood and CC Gay (Eds). Veterinary medicine: A textbook of the diseases of cattle, sheep, pigs, goats and horses. (pp. 1452-1462). 9th Edition. London: Sounders Company.

5. Nogalski, Z., Górak, E. (2008). Effects of the body condition of heifers at calving and at the first stage of lactation on milk performance. Med. Weter. 64, 322-326.

6. Duffield, T.F., Kelton, D.F., Leslie, K.E., Lissemore, K.D., Lumsden, J.H. (1997). Use of test day milk fat and milk protein to detect subclinical ketosis in dairy cattle in Ontario. Can. Vet. J. 38, 713-718. PMid:9360791 PMCid:PMC1576823

7. McArt, J.A., Nydam, D.V., Oetzel, G.R. (2013). Dry period and parturient predictors of early lactation hyperketonemia in dairy cattle. J. Dairy Sci. 96, 198–209.
    http://dx.doi.org/10.3168/jds.2012-5681
    PMid:23102961

8. Whitaker, D.A., Smith, E.J., da Rosa, G.O., Kelly, J.M. (1993). Some effects of nutrition and management on the fertility of dairy cattle. Vet. Rec. 133, 61-64.
    http://dx.doi.org/10.1136/vr.133.3.61
    PMid:8212484

9. Walsh, R., LeBlanc, S., Duffield, T., Leslie, K. (2004). Retrospective analysis of the association between subclinical ketosis and conception failure in Ontario dairy herds. Proc. World Buiatrics Congress / Med. Vet. Quebec, 34-152.

10. Suriyasathaporn, W., Heuer, C., Noordhuizen-Stassen, E.N., Schukken, Y.H. (2000). Hyperketonemia and udder defense: a review. Vet. Res. 31, 397-412.
    http://dx.doi.org/10.1051/vetres:2000128
    PMid:10958241

11. LeBlanc, S.J., Leslie, K.E., Duffield, T.F. (2005). Metabolic predictors of displaced abomasum in dairy cattle. J. Dairy Sci. 88, 159–170.
    http://dx.doi.org/10.3168/jds.S0022-0302(05)72674-6

12. Duffield, T.F., Lissemore, K.D., McBride, B.W., Leslie, K.E. (2009). Impact of hyperketonemia in early lactation dairy cows on health and production. J. Dairy Sci. 92, 571–580.
    http://dx.doi.org/10.3168/jds.2008-1507
    PMid:19164667

13. Meglia, G.E., Johannisson, A., Petersson, L., Persson Waller, K. (2001). Changes in some blood micronutritiens, leukocytes and neutrophil expression of adhesion molecules in periparturient dairy cows. Acta Vet. Scand. 42, 139-150.
    http://dx.doi.org/10.1186/1751-0147-42-139
    PMid:11455894 PMCid:PMC2202342

14. Ospina, P.A., Nydam, D.V., Stokol, T., Overton, T.R. (2010). Associations of elevated non-esterified fatty acids and β-hydroxybutyrate concentrations with early lactation reproductive performance and milk production in transition dairy cattle in the northeastern United States. J. Dairy Sci. 93, 1596–1603.
    http://dx.doi.org/10.3168/jds.2009-2852
    PMid:20338437

15. Hungerford, T.G. (1990). Diseases of cattle. In: Diseases of livestock, 9th Edition (pp. 34-347).

16. Oetzel, G.R. (2007). Herd-level ketosis – diagnosis and risk factors. Preconference seminar 7C: Dairy herd problem investigation strategies: transition cow troubleshooting American association of bovine practitioners, 40th Annual Conference, September 19, 2007 – Vancouver, BC, Canada

17. Waltner, S.S., McNamara, J.P., Hillers, J.K. (1993). Relationships of body condition score to production variables in high producing Holstein cows. J. Dairy Sci. 76, 3410-3419.
    http://dx.doi.org/10.3168/jds.S0022-0302(93)77679-1

18. Bewley, J.M., Schutz, M.M. (2008). Review: An interdisciplinary review of body condition scoring for dairy cattle. Professional Animal Scientist 24, 507-529.

19. Garnsworthy, P. (2008). Influences of body condition on fertility and milk yield. In: Proc dairy cattle reproduction council convention, 63-72.

20. Skidmore, A.L., Peeters, K.A.M., Sniffen, C.J., Brand, A. (2001). Monitoring dry period management. In: Brand, A., Noordhuizen, J. P. T. M., Schukken, Y. H. (Eds.), Herd Health and Production Management in Dairy Practice. (pp. 171–201). Wageningen Press

21. Gillund, P., Reksen, O., Grohn, Y.T., Karlberg, K. (2001). Body condition related to ketosis and reproductive performance in Norwegian dairy cows. J. Dairy Sci. 84, 1390–1396.
    http://dx.doi.org/10.3168/jds.S0022-0302(01)70170-1

22. Găvan, C., Retea, C., Motorga, V. (2010). Changes in the hematological profile of Holstein primiparous in periparturient period and in early to mid-lactation. Animal Sciences and Biotechnologies 43, 244-246.

23. Duffield, T.F. (2004). Monitoring strategies for metabolic disease in transition dairy cows. IVIS, 23rd WBC Congress, Québec, Canada.

24. Goldhawk, C., Chapinal, N., Veira, D.M., Weary, D.M., Keyserlingk, von M.A.G. (2009). Prepartum feeding behavior is an early indicator of subclinical ketosis. J. Dairy Sci. 92, 4971-4977.
    http://dx.doi.org/10.3168/jds.2009-2242
    PMid:19762814

25. Kinoshita, A., Wolf, C., Zeyner, A. (2010). Studies on the incidence of hyperketonemia with and without hyperbilirubinaemia in cows in Mecklenburg-Vorpommern (in Germany) in the course of the year. Tieraerztliche Praxis 38, 7-15.

26. Seifi, H.A., LeBlanc, S.J., Leslie, K.E., Duffield, T.F. (2011). Metabolic predictors of post-partum disease and culling risk in dairy cattle. Vet. J. 188, 216-220.
http://dx.doi.org/10.1016/j.tvjl.2010.04.007
PMid:20457532

27. Geishauser, T., Leslie, K., Tenhag, J., Bashiri, A. (2000). Evaluation of eight cowside ketone tests in milk for detection of subclinical ketosis in dairy cows. J. Dairy Sci. 83, 296-299.

28. Binev, R., Marutsova, V., Radev, V. (2014). Clinical and haematological studies on subclinical lactational ketosis in dairy goats. Agricultural Science and Technology 6, 427–430.

29. Andrews, A.H., Blowey, R.W., Boyd, H., Eddy, R.G. (2004). Bovine Medicine Diseases and Husbandry of Cattle. Second edition. USA: Blackwell Publishing Company.

30. González, F.D., Mui-o, R., Pereira, V., Campos, R., Benedito, J.L. (2011). Relationship among blood indicators of lipomobilization and hepatic function during early lactation in high-yielding dairy cows. J. Dairy Sci. 12, 251-255.
http://dx.doi.org/10.4142/jvs.2011.12.3.251

31. Suthar, V.S., Canelas-Raposo, J., Deniz, A., Heuwieser, W. (2013). Prevalence of subclinical ketosis and relationships with postpartum diseases in European dairy cows. J. Dairy Sci. 96, 2925–2938.
http://dx.doi.org/10.3168/jds.2012-6035
PMid:23497997

32. Edmonson, A.J., Lean, I.J., Weaver, L.D., Farver, T., Webster, G. (1989). A body condition chart for Holstein dairy cows. J. Dairy Sci. 72, 68–78.
http://dx.doi.org/10.3168/jds.S0022-0302(89)79081-0

33. LeBlanc, S. (2010). Monitoring metabolic health of dairy cattle in the transition period. J. Reprod. Dev. 56, 29–35.
http://dx.doi.org/10.1262/jrd.1056S29

34. Grummer, R.R. (1993). Etiology of lipid-related metabolic disorders in periparturient dairy cows. J. Dairy Sci. 76, 3882-3896.
http://dx.doi.org/10.3168/jds.S0022-0302(93)77729-2

35. López-Gatius, F., Santolaria, P., Yaniz, J., Rutllant, J., López-Béjar, M. (2002). Factors affecting pregnancy loss from gestation day 38 to 90 in lactating dairy cows from a single herd. Theriogenology 57, 1251-1261.
http://dx.doi.org/10.1016/S0093-691X(01)00715-4

36. Ruegg, P.L., Milton, R.L. (1995). Body condition scores of Holstein cows on Prince Edward Island, Canada: relationship with yield, reproductive performance, and disease. J. Dairy Sci. 78, 552–564.
http://dx.doi.org/10.3168/jds.S0022-0302(95)76666-8

37. Markusfeld, O., Galon, N., Ezra, E. (1997). Body condition score, health, yield and fertility in dairy cows. Vet. Rec. 141, 67–72.
http://dx.doi.org/10.1136/vr.141.3.67
PMid:9257435

38. Sahinduran, S., Sezer K., Buyukoglu T., Albay M.K., Karakurum M.C. (2010). Evaluation of some haematological and biochemical parameters before and after treatment in cows with ketosis and comparison of different treatment methods. J. Anim. Vet. Adv. 9, 266-271.
http://dx.doi.org/10.3923/javaa.2010.266.271

39. Belić, B., Cincović, M.R., Stojanović, D., Kovačević, Z., Vidović, B. (2010). Morphology of erythrocyte and ketosis in dairy cows with different body condition. Contemporary agriculture 59, 306-311.

40. Sandev, N., Ilieva, D., Sizov, I., Rusenova, N., Iliev, E. (2006). Prevalence of enzootic bovine leukosis in the Republic of Bulgaria in 1997-2004. Vet. Arhiv 76, 263-268.

41. Hoeben, D., Heyneman, R., Burvenich, C. (1997). Elevated levels of beta-hydroxybutyric acid in periparturient cows and in vitro effect on respiratory burst activity of bovine neutrophils. Vet. Immunol. Immunopathol. 58, 165-170.
http://dx.doi.org/10.1016/S0165-2427(97)00031-7

42. Hoeben, D., Burvenich, C., Massart-Leen, A.M., Lenjou, M., Nijs, G., Van Bockstaele, D. (1999). In vitro effect of ketone bodies, glucocorticosteroids and bovine pregnancy-associated glycoprotein on cultures of bone marrow progenitor cells of cows and calves. Vet. Immunol. Immunopathol. 68, 229-240.
http://dx.doi.org/10.1016/S0165-2427(99)00031-8

43. Suriyasathaporn, W., Daemen, A.J., Noordhuizen-Stassen, E.N., Dieleman, S.J., Nielen, M., Schukken, Y.H. (1999). Beta-hydroxybutyrate levels in peripheral blood and ketone bodies supplemented in culture media affect the in vitro chemotaxis of bovine leukocytes. Vet.Immunol. Immunopathol. 68, 177-186.
http://dx.doi.org/10.1016/S0165-2427(99)00017-3

44. Cincović, R.M., Belić, B., Radojičić, B., Hristov, S., Đoković, R. (2012). Influence of lipolysis and ketogenesis to metabolic and hematological parameters in dairy cows during periparturient period. Acta Vet. 62, 429-444.
http://dx.doi.org/10.2298/AVB1204429C

45. Belić, B., Cincović, M. R., Krčmar, Lj., Vidović, B. (2011). Reference values and frequency distribution of hematological parameters in cows during lactation and in pregnancy. Contemporary agriculture 60, 145-151.

46. Burton, J.L., Madsen, S.A., Chang, L.C., Weber, P.S., Buckham, K.R, Van Dorp, R., Hickey, M.C., Earley, B. (2005). Gene expression signatures in neutrophils exposed to glucocorticoids: A new paradigm to help explain "neutrophil dysfunction" in parturient dairy cows. Vet. Immunol. Immunopathol. 105, 197-219. http://dx.doi.org/10.1016/j.vetimm.2005.02.012 PMid:15808301

47. Hefnawy, A.E., Shousha, S., Youssef, S. (2011). Hematobiochemical profile of pregnant and experimentally pregnancy toxemic goats. J. Basic. Appl. Chem. 1, 65-69.

48. Wyle, F.A., Kent, J.R. (1977). Immunosuppression by sex steroid hormones. Clin. Exp. Immunol. 27, 407. PMid:862230 PMCid:PMC1540928

20

QUILL INJURY – CAUSE OF DEATH IN A CAPTIVE INDIAN CRESTED PORCUPINE (*HYSTRIX INDICA, KERR, 1792*)

Tanja Švara[1], Irena Zdovc[2], Mitja Gombač[1], Milan Pogačnik[1]

[1]*Institute of Pathology, Forensic and Administrative Veterinary Medicine*
[2]*Institute of Microbiology and Parasitology, Veterinary Faculty*
University of Ljubljana, Gerbičeva 60, 1000 Ljubljana, Slovenia

ABSTRACT

Indian crested porcupine (*Hystrix indica*) is a member of the family of Old World porcupines (*Hystricidae*). Its body is covered with multiple layers of quills, which serve for warning and attack if animal is threatened. However, the literature data on injuries caused by Indian crested porcupine are absent. We describe pathomorphological lesions in an Indian crested porcupine from the Ljubljana Zoo, which died after a fight with a younger male that caused a perforative quill injury of the thoracic wall, followed by septicaemia. Macroscopic, microscopic and bacteriological findings were detailed.

Key words: Indian crested porcupine (*Hystrix indica*), pathology, quill injury, pleuritis, septicaemia

INTRODUCTION

Indian crested porcupine (*Hystrix indica,* Kerr, 1792) is a member of the family of Old World porcupines (*Hystricidae*), which belong to the order *Rodentia* (1). These animals are large and heavy, with a total length of almost 1 m and a weight of 10-17 kg. The neck and shoulders are covered with multiple layers of quills, exploited in its defensive behavior. Indeed, when attacked, the Indian Crested porcupine uses the tactic of hind or caudal defense; it faces away from the adversary, raises its quills and rattles the hollow quills on its tail (3). If the predator persists past these threats, the porcupine launches a backwards assault, hoping to stab its attacker with its quills. It does this so effectively that most brushes between a porcupine and its predators end in the predator's death or severe injury (2). Quill injuries are more frequently attributed to the North American

porcupine (*Erethizon dorsatum*), a member of the New World porcupine family (*Erethizontidae*), with dogs, coyotes and wolves most commonly involved in such encounters. Severe pain, local tissue trauma, infection of deep tissues, quill migration into joints or vital organs and complications associated with penetration into thorax or abdomen are frequent consequences of those assaults (4-12).

We describe unusual pathomorphological lesions in an Indian crested porcupine from the Ljubljana Zoo, which died three weeks after perforative quill injury of the thoracic wall.

MATERIAL AND METHODS

An Indian crested porcupine was dissected at the Institute of Pathology, Forensic and Administrative Veterinary Medicine of the Veterinary Faculty in Ljubljana. Representative specimens of the thoracic wall, costal pleura, spleen, liver, small and large intestine, lungs and kidneys were fixed in 10% neutral buffered formalin for 24 hours, routinely embedded in paraffin, sectioned at 4 µm and stained with hematoxylin and eosin (HE).

Samples of the subcutaneous abscess, exudate from the thoracic cavity, spleen, liver, small intestine, lungs, heart and kidneys were taken for bacteriological culture. The samples were

Corresponding author: Assist. Prof. Tanja Švara, PhD
E-mail address: tanja.svara@vf.uni-lj.si
Present address: Institute of Pathology,
Forensic and Administrative Veterinary Medicine, Veterinary Faculty
University of Ljubljana, Gerbičeva 60, 1000 Ljubljana, Slovenia

inoculated on nutrient agar (Oxoid, Hampshire, UK) supplemented with 5% sheep blood, Drigalski agar and Sabouraud dextrose agar (Oxoid, Basingstoke, UK) with chloramphenicol (100 mg/l) and incubated at 37°C for 48 hours.

RESULTS

History

An adult, 10-year old alpha male Indian crested porcupine, weighing 14.5 kg from the Ljubljana Zoo suddenly died three weeks after a fight with a younger male from its own family. Immediately after the fight, the porcupine was treated with terramycin (oxytetracyclin) and supportive vitamin therapy.

Necropsy

At the necropsy, an oval subcutaneous abscess, measuring 7 cm x 4 cm x 2 cm, filled with white, creamy pus, was situated in the right costal region. Close to the abscess, a round-shaped perforation with purulent inflamed edges was observed in the intercostal muscles near the 6th right rib. An abscess, containing 0.5 litres of red-whitish, creamy pus and a large red clot, was formed in the thoracic cavity. A 13 cm long quill of an Indian crested porcupine was stuck in the right cranial lung lobe, which was diffusely necrotic (Fig. 1). The other lobes of the right lung were firm and the parenchyma contained purulent exudate, the left lungs were atelectatic and multifocally emphysematous. The pulmonary pleura was diffusely covered with a thick fibrin layer.

The parietal and the visceral layer of the pericardium were firmly adhered and an abscess measuring 2 cm x 1 cm x 0.5 cm was observed between the two layers. The right heart chambers were severely dilated. Numerous petechial hemorrhages, scattered throughout the kidney cortex, diffuse catarrhal enteritis and severe liver and spleen congestion were also observed.

Histopathology

Microscopically, the alveoli and bronchi of the right lung were diffusely infiltrated with numerous heterophils and some macrophages; small multifocal bacterial colonies were also observed. The parenchyma of the left lung was atelectatic and multifocally emphysematous. The pleura was multifocally covered with a thick fibrin layer, diffusely infiltrated by heterophils, few macrophages, erythrocytes and numerous bacteria. A thick band of parenchyma beneath the pleura was densely infiltrated with macrophages and heterophils (Fig. 2). The pericardium was thickened due to granulation tissue proliferation and diffusely adhered to the epicardium. Focally, there was an abscess filled with numerous degenerative heterophils and multifocal bacterial colonies.

Histopathological examination of other organs revealed several lesions consistent with septicemia, i.e. a multifocal purulent hepatitis and nephritis, marked lymphocyte depletion in the spleen and acute catarrhal desquamative enteritis.

Bacteriological culture

Bacteriological cultures of the spleen, lungs, heart and pus on blood agar yielded abundant growth of two types of haemolytic colonies, both

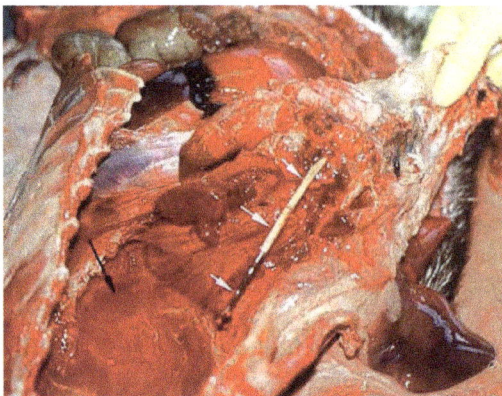

Figure 1. Thoracic cavity. Red-whitish, creamy pus filled the left pleural cavity (black arrow). A quill of an Indian crested porcupine is stuck in the right cranial lung lobe (white arrows)

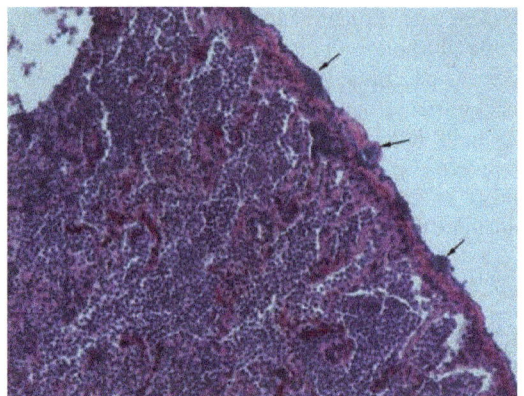

Figure 2. Lung. Pleura and a thick band of lung parenchyma beneath the pleura are densely infiltrated with heterophils, macrophages and numerous bacteria (arrows). HE staining, x 100

Gram-positive cocci. The predominant colonies were smooth, 2-3 mm in diameter, catalase and coagulase positive and were agglutinated with rapid test Monostaph plus (Bionor Laboratories AS, Klostergata, Norway). The biochemical characteristics were evaluated using the commercial kit API Staph (bioMerieux, Marcy I'Etoile, France) and the strain was determined as *Staphylococcus aureus*. The smaller (1-1.5 mm) colonies were catalase negative, Gram-positive cocci and therefore suspected to be streptococci.

The biochemical characteristics were evaluated using the commercial kit API Strep and the strain was determined as *Streptococcus agalactiae*. The culture was serologically typed according to the Lancefield classification system using the Streptococcal grouping kit (Oxoid, Basingstoke, UK) and classified in group B. Culture from the pus also yielded a few colonies of nonhaemolytic coryneform bacteria.

The samples from the kidney, liver and intestine were bacteriologically negative.

DISCUSSION

Despite a wide geographic range of the Indian crested porcupine (13), there is absence of literature data on injuries. All reported cases of porcupine quill injuries were related to a relative of the Indian crested porcupine, the North American porcupine (*Erethizon dorsatum*). In this species, the tip of its quill is covered with backward-pointing barbs and beyond them the shaft is smooth and hollow, which forces the quill, stuck in the tissue, to migrate into deeper layers (14). In injured dogs, porcupine quills are commonly seen in the external head and neck region, followed by the oral cavity, and are less often found in limbs and the truncal region. Inflammation or discharge and less often lameness and ocular signs occur in 10.8% of all injured dogs. Only in one case, a pneumothorax caused by quills in the cranial mediastinum and cranial lung lobe was reported (11).

Porcupine quills are not inert; they may harbor bacteria or act directly evoking septic or sterile foreign body reaction (8). *Staphylococcus aureus* (9, 10, 12) and *Staphylococcus intermedius* were isolated from ocular and orbital injuries (8), septic arthritis (10) and vertebral canal porcupine quill injury (12) in dogs and also septic tenosynovitis in the horse (9), all caused by a North American porcupine quill injury. A septic pleuritis, purulent bronchopneumonia with pyothorax, adhesive pericarditis and subsequent septicemia caused by *Staphylococcus aureus*, *Streptococcus agalactiae*

and *Corynebacterium sp.* were observed in our case. Liver, kidney and intestine were bacteriologically negative, most probably due to distribution of the lesions in these organs and less likely due to previous antibiotic treatment.

ACKNOWLEDGEMENTS

The authors wish to thank the ZOO Ljubljana for their cooperation and permission for the publication of data.

REFERENCES

1. Qumsiyeh, M.D. (1996). Mammals of the Holy Land (pp. 310–313). Lubbock: University Press.

2. Gupta, O. (2006). Encyclopedia of India, Pakistan and Bangladesh (p. 1014). Dehli: Isha Books.

3. Zherebtsova, O.V. (2000). Spiny cover and defense strategy of mammals. Transactions of the zoological institute RAS. 286, 169–174.

4. Milrod, S., Goel, D.P. (1958). Intraperitoneal foreign body granuloma caused by a porcupine quill. Med Serv J Can., 14, 504–507.
PMid:13577173

5. Mirakhur, K.K., Khanna, A.K. (1983). Removal of a porcupine quill from the temporal fossa of a dog. Canine Pract., 10, 38.

6. Daoust, P.Y. (1991). Porcupine quill in the brain of a dog. Vet Rec., 128, 436.
http://dx.doi.org/10.1136/vr.128.18.436-a
PMid:185354

7. Wobeser, G. (1992). Traumatic, degenerative, and developmental lesions in wolves and coyotes from Saskatchewan. J Wildl Dis., 28, 268–275.
http://dx.doi.org/10.7589/0090-3558-28.2.268
PMid:1602579

8. Grahn, B.H., Szentimrey, D., Pharr, J.W., Farrow, C.S., Fowler, D. (1995). Ocular and orbital porcupine quills in the dog: a review and case series. Can Vet J., 36, 488–493.
PMid:7585434; PMCid:PMC1687009

9. Magee, A.A., Ragle, C.A., Howlett, M.R. (1997). Use of tenoscopy for management of septic tenosynovitis caused by a penetrating porcupine quill in the synovial sheath surrounding the digital flexor tendons of a horse. J Am Vet Med Assoc., 210, 1768–1770.
PMid:9187727

10. Brisson, B.A., Bersenas, A., Etue, S.M. (2004). Ultrasonographic diagnosis of septic arthritis secondary to porcupine quill migration in a dog. J Am Vet Med Assoc., 224, 1467–1470.
http://dx.doi.org/10.2460/javma.2004.224.1467
PMid:15124888

11. Johnson, M.D., Magnusson, K.D., Shmon, C.L., Waldner, C. (2006). Porcupine quill injuries in dogs: a retrospective of 296 cases (1998-2002). Can Vet J., 47, 677–682.
PMid:16898110;   PMCid:PMC1482438

12. Schneider, A.R., Chen, A.V., Tucker, R.L. (2010). Imaging diagnosis - vertebral canal porcupine quill with presumptive secondary arachnoid diverticulum. Vet Radiol Ultrasound., 51, 152–154.
PMid:20402400

13. Gurung, K.K., Singh, R. (1996). Field guide to the Mammals of the Indian Subcontinent. Academic Press, San Diego
PMid:8862263

14. Banfield, A.W.F. (1987). The Mammals of Canada (pp. 233–235). Hong Kong: University of Toronto Press

21

HYPODERMOSIS IN NORTHERN SERBIA (VOJVODINA)

Zsolt Becskei[1], Tamara Ilić[2], Nataša Pavlićević[3], Ferenc Kiskároly[3], Tamaš Petrović[4], Sanda Dimitrijević[2]

[1]*University of Belgrade, Faculty of Veterinary Medicine,*
Department for Animal Breeding and Genetics, Belgrade, Serbia
[2]*University of Belgrade, Faculty of Veterinary Medicine,*
Department of Parasitology, Belgrade, Serbia
[3]*Veterinary Specialist Institute Subotica, Subotica, Serbia*
[4]*Scientific Veterinary Institute Novi Sad, Novi Sad, Serbia*

ABSTRACT

This paper describes the first documented case of cattle grub (hypodermosis) in Northern Serbia (Vojvodina). Subcutaneous warbles were determined in a six year old Simmental cow, at nine places along the spine. After the extirpation of larvae, based on the morphological characterisation, larvae of the third stage of *Hypoderma bovis* were diagnosed. The cow was administered therapeutic treatment, which had a favorable outcome, with no signs of recurrence. To the authors' best knowledge, the case described in this paper is the first documented case of hypodermosis in cattle in Northern Serbia (Vojvodina). As the climate changed in the past few decades, it is important to pursue detailed investigations of the prevalence of this parasitic myiasis, as there are few such literature data for the Southern region of Serbia. One should also not ignore the fact that species of the genus *Hypoderma* can cause myiasis in humans as well.

Key words: bovine, internal myiasis, oestridae, *Hypoderma bovis*, larval stage

INTRODUCTION

Hypodermosis is an ectoparasitic infestation, with impact both from the health and the economic aspect. The causes of this internal myiasis in cattle are larval forms of *Hypoderma bovis* and *H. lineatum*, and in deer, roe, and reindeer of *H. diana*, *H. actaeon* and *H. tarandi*. In addition to these 5 species, Zumpt reported two more species (*H. capreola* and *H. moschiferi*), whose names are used as synonyms for the species *H. diana* (1). An eighth species (*H. sinense*) was described by Pleske (2), and it was long believed that it was a synonym

Corresponding author: Dr. Zsolt Becskei, PhD
E-mail address: beckeizolt@gmail.com
Present address: University of Belgrade, Faculty of Veterinary Medicine
Department for Animal Breeding and Genetics
Str, Bulevar Oslobodjenja 18, 11000 Belgrade, Serbia

for the species *H. lineatum*. Otranto used molecular analyses to prove the presence of *H. sinense* as a separate species that is parasitizing in cattle in China (3).

The biology of the warble fly is complex, since *Hypoderma* passes through both the ecto- and endoparasitic stages of the life cycle. The parasitic phase in domestic and wild animals lasts around one year, but the adult female of the warble fly lives in an inactive form in the external environment for several days, and during that time (in flight or upon landing on skin), it lays eggs on the host's body (4). The model of animal breeding and favorable climatic conditions pose risk factors that favor the life cycle of the parasite (5).

The disease caused by the species *H. bovis* and *H. lineatum* mostly occurs between 25° and 60° latitude in the northern hemisphere, in more than 50 countries in North America, Europe, Africa and Asia (6). The accuratee prevalence of bovine infection with these *Oestridae* in Europe is not known. It varies from year to year, and is conditioned upon activities by ecological factors. It is known that the

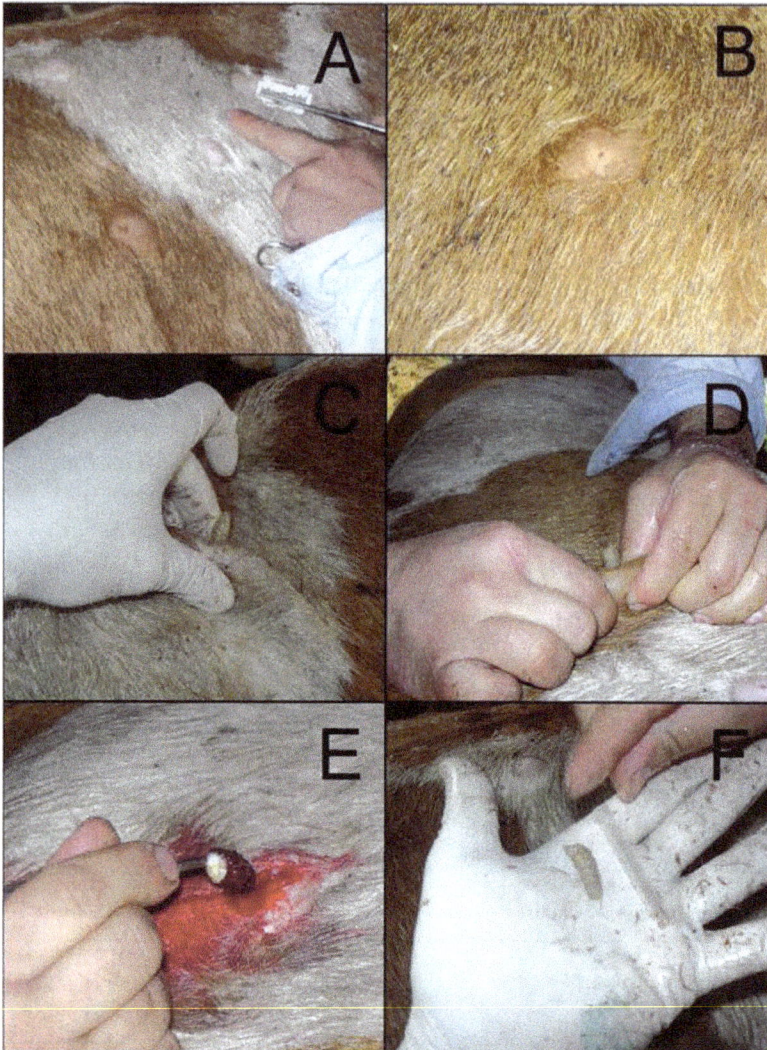

Figure 1. A. Localization of parasitic nodules along the hump; **B.** Cattle grub caused by *H. bovis;* **C.** and **D.** Manual extirpation of *H. bovis* larvae; **E.** Surgical extirpation of *H. bovis* larvae; **F.** Extirpated *H. bovis* larvae

lower temperatures in Eastern and Central Europe slow down the biological cycle of these parasites. Hypodermosis has a wide geographical distribution pattern in livestock as reported by Ahmed (7). In some cases, larvae can be found individually also in horses, donkeys, bison, sheep, and even in man (7, 8, 9).

CASE REPORT

This paper presents a case of hypodermosis diagnosed in May 2013 in a cow from the vicinity of Subotica (the settlement of Stari Žednik). The infested animal was 6 years old and originated from Southern Serbia where it was purchased in the cattle market. After being purchased, the cow was introduced to a homestead located in the epizootological territory of the North-Bačka District, where it was placed together with 10 dairy cows originating from this locality. The purchased cow was maintained in the barn, it was tethered, and it did not go out to pasture.

The owner contacted the local veterinarian when nodules were observed along the spine of the cow, and asked him to identify the cause of these changes.

Inspection and palpation established subcutaneously located nodular changes on the skin at nine points along the spine. The biggest number of established nodules was located along the hump, from the shoulder to the sacral part, and they were partly also distributed laterally to the left and to the right. Their dimensions ranged from 1.5 to 3.5 cm in diameter, and the hairs surrounding the opening of the warble were sticky with a dried secretion.

Following disinfection and removal of the hairs, the *Hypoderma* larvae were removed from the warbles. After removal of the larvae from the warbles, they were conserved in 70% alcohol. After the surgical procedures, the animal was treated with a combination of antibiotics (amoxicillin: Veyxyl LA 20%®), corticosteroids (Dexakel 0.2®, KELA, Belgium) and antihistaminic drugs (Ahistin 10%®, VETERINA, Croatia) in doses recommended by the manufacturer's prescription.

The analysis of morphological characteristics of larves served to identify third stage larves of the species *H. bovis*. The diagnosed larvae were light to dark brown in color, around 28 mm in length, their body exhibited funnel-shaped stigmatic plates, and it was established that they had no spines on the tenth (second-last) segment. A certain number of larvae were already in the stage when they begin to leave the animal through the opening formed previously by their mouth claws.

The antibiotic treatment of the cow was continued for next six days. The cow tolerated the intervention well and recovered rapidly. At the next physical checkups 7 and 30 days after intervention the cow was very active and in good condition and there were no sign of parasitical relapses.

DISCUSSION

Diphtheroid species of the genus *Hypoderma* have major significance due to the fact that they can cause myiasis in humans which can clinically manifest in different ways. They can cause so-called creeping disease (*myiasis linearis*, a migrating line), due to the *larva migrans* which occurs when the larvae penetrates into the skin through the openings of the hair follicle and sweat glands, and then migrates under the skin, forming a pruritic erythematous line (9).

Lagace-Wiens et al. (10) reported about the first two diagnosed cases of internal ophthalmomyiasis in humans in Canada, caused by the species *H. tarandi*. Infections of humans by the species *H. tarandi* are very rare and still not clarified to a sufficient degree. Both species (*H. bovis* and *H. Lineatum*) can cause infections in humans, and they are distributed in different areas of North America, Europe and Asia (3, 4, 7, 11). The third species that parasitizes in cattle and yaks in China

(*H. sinense*), can also be responsible for cases of infestation among the human population (10).

In the past century, the occurence of bovine hypodermosis in certain European countries indicates high prevalence: Slovakia (80%), Greece (49.2%), Italy (85%), Spain (52.3%), Great Britain (40%), and in Romania (32-42%) (12, 13). In southwestern Spain, the maximum annual temperatures are 20-21°C, the maximum summer temperatures are 29-30°C, which favors faster development and earlier appearance of the disease in the course of the year (7, 17).

Otranto et al. reported about the presence and spreading of hypodermosis in cattle in Albania, underscoring that this country poses a risk for the spreading of hypodermosis into other European countries (6). In the past 50 years, hypodermosis has been successfully eradicated in many countries of Northern Europe, such as Denmark, the Netherlands, the Czech Republic, Germany, France, and Switzerland (6).

France is one of the European countries that have introduced a programme for the eradication of hypodermosis, and in order for its effect to be satisfactory it is necessary that such programmes encompass larger epizootiological areas (13). Haine et al. presented data on the regional prevalence of hypodermosis in cattle in Belgium, which stood at 36-92% (15). Such a high prevalence of infection was conditioned by the size of the pastures and the effects of various relevant climatic factors (daily temperature, precipitation and relative humidity) (13, 14, 15, 16). The latest investigations conducted in Romania showed that, based on clinical examinations, the prevalence of hypodermosis was 16.21%, on parasitological section, 18.91%, while the seroprevalence was 27.27% (13).

This report of a diagnosed case is one of the few registered cases of hypodermosis in cattle in Serbia, but the first documented case in Vojvodina (Northern Serbia). The circulation of humans and goods, the transportation and acquiring of animals, create preconditions for the introduction of new sources of infection and the maintenance of this disease. The disease is mostly present in Central and Southern Serbia, in cattle that are kept in pasture during the summer and are outdoor rearing. Under such breeding conditions, cattle grub parasitize under the cattle's skin during the period from February to September. Since new infections can begin already in June, the same animal can become infected with two generations of larvae during the period from June to August (18). Since the animal in this case report is one that was purchased, it is clear that it had already been infected upon its introduction to the new herd.

Having in mind the geo-climatic characteristics of the region of Southern Serbia and the type of cattle breeding maintained in this locality, an even higher prevalence of cattle infection with cattle grub could be expected. The risk for the spread of this disease in Serbia is even further increased when one takes into consideration the close proximity of certain countries in this region (Greece, Albania, Romania, Turkey) in which hypodermosis in cattle is present (6, 13).

The clinical finding of *H. bovis* in a young ox from the territory of the Nišava District in 2006 and the finding in a parasitological section in a young ox from the territory of the Braničevo district in 2007 are individual cases recorded in Central and Southern Serbia by field veterinarians (18).

Due to its influence on meat, milk and leather production, hypodermosis results in major economic losses and it can also yield a negative effect on the general health condition and the immunological status of the diseased animals' organism (19). The implementation of efficient prophylactic measures against this disease is successfully controlled at national level in many European countries (4, 13, 14, 15).

There is no systematized data in Serbia on the prevalence of hypodermosis infection in cattle, either along the slaughter lines or in the records of the authorized services. There is also no statistical data available from the Serbian leather industry on damage and losses caused by cattle grub. The individual cases established through clinical examinations of cattle or at parasitological sections indicate the need for more detailed investigations and the keeping of records for each diagnosed case in order to establish the real incidence of hypodermosis in cattle in certain regions of Serbia. Such an approach is also of paramount epizootiological importance for the other countries of South-Eastern Europe surrounding Serbia (Croatia, Slovenia, Bosnia-Herzegovina, Romania, Bulgaria, Macedonia, Montenegro, and Albania).

ACKNOWLEDGEMENT

This paper was realized within the Project „Monitoring of game health and introduction of new biotechnological procedures in the detection of infectious and zoonotic agents – risk analysis regarding the health of humans, domestic and wild animals and environmental contamination" (Number TR31084) and Project „Implementation of EIIP/ISM bioinformatic platform in discovery of new therapeutic targets and potential therapeutic molecules" (Number 173001), financed by the Ministry of Education and Science of the Republic of Serbia.

REFERENCES

1. Zumpt, F. (1965). Myiasis in man and animals in the old world. Butter-worths. London, U.K., 217-229.

2. Plesek, T. (1926). Revue des especes palearctiques des Oestridae et catalogue raisonne de leur collection au Musee zoologique de l' academiedes Sciences. Annals Museum Zoology of Leningrad 24, 215.

3. Otranto, D., Traversa, D., Colwell, DD., Guan, G., Giangaspero, A., Boulard, C., Yin H. (2004). A third species of Hypoderma (Diptera: Oestridae) affecting cattle and yaks in China: molecular and morphological evidence. J Parasitol. 90, 958-965.
http://dx.doi.org/10.1645/GE-232R
PMid:15562593

4. Hassan, M., Khan, N.M., Abubakar, M., Waheed, H.M., Iqbal, Z., Hussain, M. (2010). Bovine hypodermosis - a global aspect. Trop Anim Health Prod. 42, 1615-1625.
http://dx.doi.org/10.1007/s11250-010-9634-y
PMid:20607401

5. Gorcea, C.F., Calescu, N., Gherman, M.C., Mihalca, D.A., Cozma, V. (2011). Diagnostic values of clinical, pathological and serologic findings in cattle hypodermosis in Peştişani, Gorj County Romania. Sci Parasitol. 12, 173-176.

6. Otranto, D., Zalla, P., Testini, G., Zanaj, S. (2005). Cattle grub infestation by Hypodema sp. in Albania and risk for European countries. Vet Parasitol. 28, 157-162.
http://dx.doi.org/10.1016/j.vetpar.2004.11.016
PMid:15725546

7. Ahmed, H., Khan, M. R., Panadero-fontan, R., Sandez, C. L., Farooq, M., Naqvi, SMS., Qayyum, M. (2012). Geographical distribution of hypodermosis (Hypoderma sp.) in Northern Punjab, Pakistan. Kafkas Univ. Vet. Fak. Derg. 18 (Suppl-A): A215-1219

8. Capinera, J.L. (2008). Encyclopedia of entomology. 2nd Edition. Vol. 1-4. Springer, Dordrecht, The Netherlands
http://dx.doi.org/10.1007/978-1-4020-6359-6

9. Van Hal, S.J.M., Hudson, B.J., Wong, D.A. (2004). Furuncular myiasis after contact with clothing (when washing clothes can be infectious). Clin Infect Dis. 39, 1552-1553.
http://dx.doi.org/10.1086/425505
PMid:15546103

10. Derraik, J.G.B., Hetah, A.C.G., Redemaker, M. (2010). Human myasis in New Zealand: imported and indiginously-acquired cases; the species of concern and clinical aspects. NZ Med J. 123, 1322.

11. Lagace-Wiens, P.R.S., Dookeran, R., Skinner, S., Leitch, R., Collwel, D.D., Galloway, D.T. (2008). Human ophthalmomyasis interna caused by Hypoderma tarandi, Northern Canada. Emerg Infect Dis. 14, 64-66.
http://dx.doi.org/10.3201/eid1401.070163
PMid:18258079 PMCid:PMC2600172

12. Anderson, J.R., (2006). Oestrid myiasis of humans. In: Colwell, D.D., Hall, M.J., Scholl, P.J. (Eds.) The oestrid flies biology, host-parasite relation'ships, impact and management (pp. 359). Oxford (UK): CABI Publishing.
http://dx.doi.org/10.1079/9780851996844.0201

13. O'Brien, D.J. (1998). Warble fy prevalence in Europe 1997 after COST 811. In: Boulard, C., Sol, J., Pithan, D., O'Brien, D.J., Webster, K., Sampimon, O.C. (Eds.), Improvements in the control methods for warble fy in livestock (pp. 20-23). European Commission. Brussels
PMid:9510819

14. Boulard, C., Avinerie, M., Argente, G., Languille, J., Pagept, L., Petit, E. (2008). A successful, sustainable and low cost control-programme for bovine hypodermosis in France. Vet Parasitol. 158, 1-10.
http://dx.doi.org/10.1016/j.vetpar.2008.07.026
PMid:18789582

15. Haine, D., Boelaert, F., Pfeiffer, D.U., Saegerman, C., Lonneux, J.F., Losson, B., Mintiens, K. (2004). Herdlevel seroprevalence and risk-mapping of bovine hypodermosis in Belgian cattle herds. Prev Vet Med. 65, 93-104.
http://dx.doi.org/10.1016/j.prevetmed.2004.06.005
PMid:15454329

16. Khan, M. R., Ahmed, H., Panadero-fontan, R., Sandez, C. L., Farooq, M., Naqvi, SMS., Qayyum, M. (2015). Risk mapping of bovine hypodermosis by using Geographical Information System (GIS) in cattle of subtropical region, Pakistan. Journal of Infection in Developing Countries 9 (8): 872-877.
http://dx.doi.org/10.3855/jidc.5387
PMid:26322880

17. Ahmed, H., Khan, M. R., Panadero-fontan, R., Mustafa, I., Sandez, C. L., Qayyum, M. (2013). Influence of epidemiological factors on the prevalence and intensity of Hypoderma sp. in cattle of Potowar Region, Pakistan. Pak. J. Zoo. 45 (6): 1495-1500.

18. Dimitrijević, S., Ilić, T. (eds) (2011). Clinical Parasithology. Faculty of Veterinary Medicine, University of Belgrade, Belgrade: Interprint D.O.O.

19. Khan, N.M., Iqbal, Z., Sajid, S.M., Anwar, M., Needham, R.G., Hassan, M. (2006). Bovine hypodermosis: Prevalence and economic significance in southern Punjab, Pakistan. Vet Parasitol. 141, 386-390.
http://dx.doi.org/10.1016/j.vetpar.2006.05.014
PMid:16787710

22

CARDIOTOXICITY STUDY OF THE AQUEOUS EXTRACT OF CORN SILK IN RATS

Adeolu Adedapo[1], Omotayo Babarinsa[1], Ademola Oyagbemi[1], Aduragbenro Adedapo[2], Temidayo Omobowale[3]

[1]*Department of Veterinary Physiology, Biochemistry and Pharmacology, University of Ibadan, Ibadan, Nigeria*
[2]*Department of Pharmacology and Therapeutics, University of Ibadan, Ibadan, Nigeria*
[3]*Department of Veterinary Medicine, University of Ibadan, Ibadan, Nigeria*

ABSTRACT

In the ear of corn there are silky strands which run its length and these strands are known as corn silks. Folk remedies show that the corn silks have been used as an oral antidiabetic agent in China for many years and as herbal tea in other world nations for the amelioration of urinary tract infection. The extract is being assessed for safety in this study using histopathological changes, as well as an electrocardiogram (ECG). Graded doses (200, 400 and 800 mg/kg) of aqueous CS extract were administered to rats for seven days. The fourth group which served as control received 3 ml/kg dose of distilled water. On the eighth day, ECG was evaluated in ketamine/xylazine-induced anaesthesia in rats to determine changes in the heart rate, P-wave duration, P-R interval, R-amplitude, QRS duration, QT interval and QTc. Hearts from the experimental animals were collected for histopathological changes. The results showed that there was a significant change in the heart rate (groups B and C), P-wave duration (group D), QT interval (groups B, C and D) and QTc (groups B, C and D) when compared to the control group. Histology also indicated that sections of the heart showed fatty infiltration of inflamed heart and areas of moderate inflammation of the atrium and ventricle. It could therefore be concluded from this study that though folklore indicated that corn silk (CS) is of high medicinal value, one must be careful in using this product as medicinal agent especially in patients with compromised heart conditions.

Key words: corn silks, ECG, histopathology, cardiotoxicity, rats

INTRODUCTION

Applications of complementary and alternative medicine have gained some prominent attention in recent times due to the fact that these form of medicine offer great opportunities in the discovery, development and production of potent, safe and inexpensive alternatives to existing synthetic chemotherapeutic agents (1, 2). Many of the plants with medicinal values have been used in different cultures of the world to treat many diseases and infections and drugs obtained from plant sources have been in use for a while now. In fact, rural dwellers used these herbs as therapeutic agents and medicament because they could procure them easily (3). It is on record that plants have provided a source of knowledge with respect to novel drug compounds because medicinal products obtained from plants have made tremendous contributions to human health and well being (4). One such plant-derived product is corn silk.

Corn silks look like strands of hair that are initially green in colour, then become red, and finally turn yellow. Corn silk threads may be steeped in boiling water to make tea. It has a variety of health benefits as it contains moderate amount of iron, potassium, zinc, phosphorus, magnesium and calcium. Corn silk tea may improve urinary tract infection and kidney stones (5). It is also known to be rich in proteins, vitamins, carbohydrates, fixed and volatile oils, steroids (such as sitsterol, stigma sterol, alkaloids, saponins, tannins) and flavonoid

Corresponding author: Dr. Adeolu Adedapo, PhD
E-mail address: aa.adedapo@ui.edu.ng
Present address: Department of Veterinary Physiology, Biochemistry and Pharmacology, Faculty of Veterinary Medicine, University of Ibadan, Nigeria

(6). Folk remedies show that corn silk has been used as an oral antidiabetic agent in China for decades, but the mechanism of its hypoglycaemic activity has not been elucidated (7). Corn silk has been used as tea for its diuretic properties, especially that it may help soothe irritation in the urinary system. Again, corn silk when used in conjunction with other herbs may help treat health conditions such as mumps or inflammation of urinary bladder or urethra (5). For those that suffer from high blood pressure, corn silk tea may be a gentle and natural way to help lower blood pressure. Because this tea is safe and gentle on the body, it makes it a preferred method for lowering high blood pressure as opposed to some over the counter medications which can come with some unexpected and unwanted side effects. Finally, it can keep blood pressure from dropping undesirably low as well, which makes this advantage useful for those that suffer from diabetes (6).

In this study, the aqueous extract of the corn silk was evaluated for safety or otherwise, especially because ethnomedicinal surveys have shown that its herbal tea is said to possess a lot of medicinal potential.

MATERIAL AND METHODS

Collection of fresh maize leaves and maize silk

Fresh corns with intact corn silk were collected from the Ayo farm in Abeokuta, Ogun State, Nigeria in June, 2014. After collection, the corn silks were dried for a few days and afterward pulverized in an electric blender into powdery form. It was the local maize variety that was used in this study.

Preparation of aqueous extract of maize silk

Each of the pulverized substances were soaked with 1000 ml of distilled water in a separate conical flask for 48 hours and then filtered. The filtrate was then concentrated using rotary evaporator and steam bath to obtain an aqueous extract. The extract was stored in refrigerator until its use for biological activities.

Experimental animals

Twenty healthy white strain albino female rats (100 – 140g) and thirty male mice (12 – 25g) used in this study were obtained from the Experimental Animal House of the Faculty of Veterinary Medicine, University of Ibadan, Nigeria. The animals were kept in cages within the animal house and allowed free access to water and standard livestock pellets. The animals were examined and found to be free of wounds, swellings and infections before the commencement of the experiment. All experimental protocols were conducted as directed by the National Institute of Health Guide for Care and Use of Laboratory Animals.

Chemicals and drugs

The chemicals and drugs which were used include the following: Normal saline, distilled water, Formalin, xylazine and Ketamine.

Acute toxicity of the aqueous extract of corn silk

The acute toxicity study of maize silk was conducted in line with the method of Sawadogo et al (8). Briefly, thirty male mice fasted for 16 hours were randomly divided into 6 groups of 5 animals each. Graded doses of the aqueous extract (200, 400, 800, 1,600 and 3,200 mg/kg) corresponding to groups B, C, D, E, F, and G respectively were separately administered to the mice in each test group using oral cannula. The control group or group A was administered with distilled water (3ml/kg) only. All animals were then given access to feed and water *ad libitum* and thereafter observed for a period of 48 hours for signs of acute toxicity, morbidity and mortality.

Sub acute toxicity of the aqueous extract of corn silk in rats

The sub acute toxicity study of maize silk was also carried out according to the method of Sawadogo et al (8). Twenty female rats were randomly divided into 4 groups of 5 animals each. Graded doses of the extract (200, 400 and 800mg/kg) representing groups B, C, and D respectively were separately administered to the rats in each test group using oral cannula. The control group or group A was administered with distilled water (3ml/kg) only. All animals were given feed and water *ad libitum* and thereafter observed for signs of toxicity, morbidity and mortality. The administration of the extract and distilled water was for 7 days only.

Electrocardiography (ECG) evaluation of rats administered with aqueous extract of corn silk

ECG of all the animals used for the evaluation of sub-acute toxicity was measured on the eight day i.e. 24 hours after the sub-acute toxicity was concluded. The rats were anaesthetized with 0.1 ml/100kg of ketamine/xylazine (v/v) to aid stabilization and the five electrodes of the ECG machine were placed at the appropriate position (both fore limbs, both hind limbs and chest). Hair was clipped to improve contact between the ECG pad and the skin. Electrode gel was used to improve contact between the patient and electrodes. The electrodes were connected to the ECG machine by colour-coded cables. The ECG was recorded in a calm and quiet environment. Standard lead II electrocardiogram was recorded in conscious rats using a 7-lead ECG machine (EDAN VE-1010, Shanghai, China). The machine was calibrated at 20mm/mV paper speed and 50mm/s paper speed. From the electrocardiogram, parameters such as heart rate, P-wave, QT, QTc etc were determined.

Histopathology

After the ECG measurement was concluded, all the animals used for the sub-acute toxicity study were sacrificed by over-dose of chloroform anaesthesia. The hearts from these animals were removed and placed in 10% formalin in normal saline for histological studies. These isolated organs were placed in an automatic tissue processor for 24 hrs and after these, the tissues were solidified in molten wax and sectioned using automatic tissue sectioner, fixed on slides with haematoxylin and eosin and thereafter stained slides were fixed with mountant, allowed to dry and viewed under the microscope (x400).

Statistics

All values were expressed as mean±S.D. The test of significance between two groups was estimated by Student's t test. "One-way ANOVA" with Dunnett's post-hoc test was also performed using GraphPad software version 4.00.

RESULTS

Acute toxicity study

In the acute toxicity test, no death was recorded in all the groups. All the mice appeared to be normal and none of them showed any visible signs of toxicity.

ECG

The electrocardiographs taken are represented in graph pads (Fig. 1-7) below. Group A – Control, Group B, Group C and Group D. There was significant change in heart rate (groups B and C), P-wave duration (group D), QT interval (groups B, C and D) and QTc (groups B, C and D) when compared to the control group.

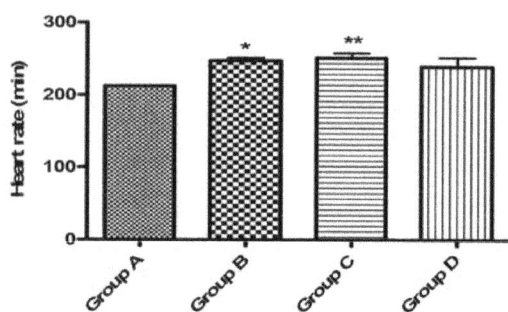

Figure 1. Heart rate (min). Asterisks (*) and (**) represented significant differences at $p<0.05$ and $p<0.01$ respectively when compared with the control (Group A)

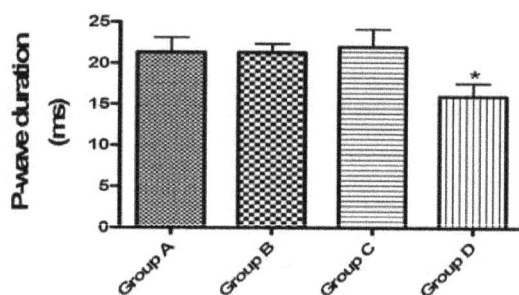

Figure 2. P-wave duration (ms). Asterisks (*) represented significant differences at $p<0.05$ when compared with Group A

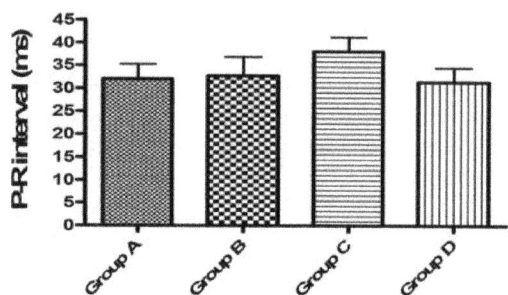

Figure 3. P-R interval (ms). No significant difference at $p<0.05$ was observed in this parameter when compared with Group A

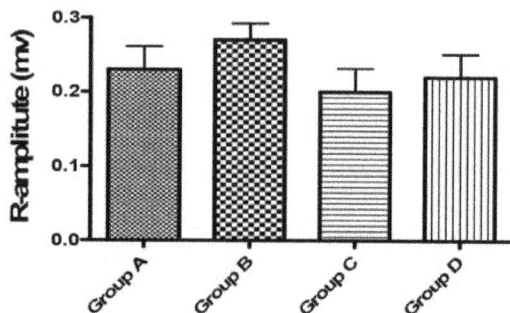

Figure 4. R-amplitude (mv). No significant difference at $p<0.05$ was shown in this parameter when compared with the control (Group A)

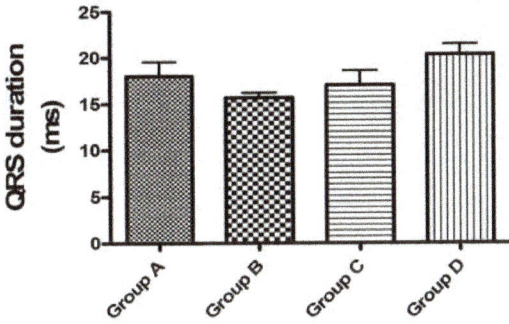

Figure 5. QRS duration (ms). No significant difference at p<0.05 was shown in this parameter when compared with the control (Group A)

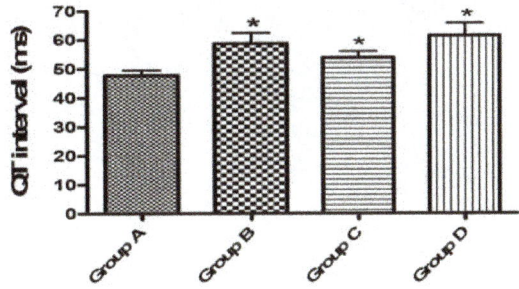

Figure 6. QT interval (ms). Asterisks (*) showed significant difference at p<0.05 when compared with the control (Group A)

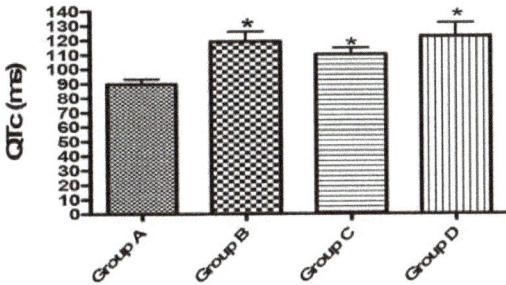

Figure 7. QTc (ms). Asterisks (*) indicates significant difference at p<0.05 when compared with the control (Group A)

Histopathology

Histological examination of the heart indicated that the extract caused pathological changes in this organ. For instance, the heart sections showed fatty infiltration of inflammed heart and areas of moderate inflammation of the atrium and ventricle. These observations are as depicted in the photomicrographs depicted below (Fig. 8a-d).

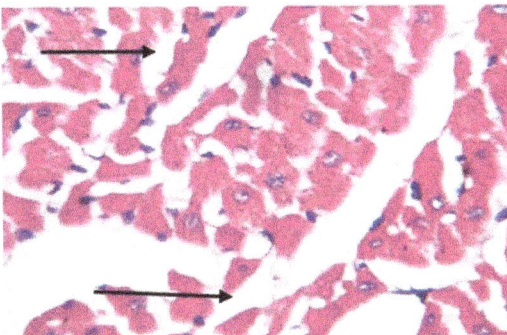

Figure 8a. Heart: Sections show fatty infiltration of inflammed heart of group B animal (X400)

DISCUSSION

Corn silk made from stigmas, is often a waste material from the cultivation of corn and is usually present in large quantities (9). In countries such as China, Turkey, United States and France, corn silk is used traditionally for the treatment of cystitis, edema, kidney stones, diuretic, prostate disorder, and urinary infections as well as bedwetting and obesity (10, 11, 12, 13, 14, 15). The mechanism of action may be related to the fact that it soothes and relaxes the lining of the bladder and urinary tubules, thereby reducing irritation and increasing urine secretion (16). The use of CS in traditional medicine has also showed that it has anti-fatigue, anti-depressant and kaliuretic activities (15, 17, 18). In addition to these properties, CS possesses excellent antioxidant activity (7, 19) and demonstrated radiation-protective as well as nephroprotective effects (20, 21). These excellent activities of CS prompted our need to evaluate it for safety in laboratory animals such as mice and rats.

The acute toxicity study showed that the aqueous extract of CS is safe for use medicinally because the 3200 mg/kg, the highest dose used in this study did not produce any lethal change in mice especially that the animals appeared normal and no mortality was recorded. This observation of safety in acute toxicity was similar to that of Ambike et al (22) who also observed that at 3.2 gm/kg, the aqueous extract of corn silk was safe for medicinal use. The lack of toxicity even up to 3200mg/dose of this extract guided our choice of doses in the sub acute toxicity study in which the extract was administered to rats for seven days and then examined for any toxic changes in the heart tissues using ECG and histopathology as indices of toxicosis.

In the ECG study, there was a significant change in heart rate (groups B and C), P-wave duration (group D), QT interval (groups B, C and D) and QTc

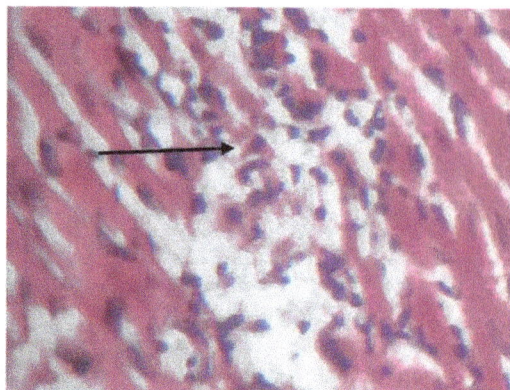

Figure 8b. Heart: Sections show focal area of inflammation (black arrow) in group C (X400)

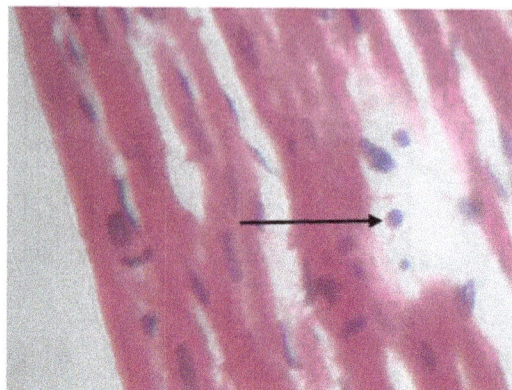

Figure 8c. Heart: Sections show area of infiltration by inflammatory cells (black arrow) in group C (X400)

(groups B, C and D) when compared to the control group. Administration of the extract to the rats for seven days thus led to increase in the heart rate for the animals in groups B and C, but not in group D (the highest dose - 800 mg/kg) in this study. The study thus showed that administration of the extract led to tachycardia in groups B and C animals. Tachycardia which is a fast heart rate (more than 100 beats per minute in humans) indicated that at these elevated rates, the heart is not able to efficiently pump oxygen-rich blood to the body. It also shows that at this condition of increased heart rate there may be increased work and oxygen demand by the heart, and as a result, there may be the development of rate related ischemia (23, 24, 25, 26, 27).

The P-wave represents depolarization of the atria and when it is of unusually long duration, it may be an evidence of atrial enlargement. In the present study, there was a shortening of P-wave duration (PWD) in group D animals. It was reported that shorter baseline PWD may be a pointer of a lower risk of persistent atrial fibrillation (AF) that may require cardioversion or AF-related hospitalization (28). It thus showed that the shortening of P-wave by the extract in this study is an indication of its having a cardiotonic effect on the heart. The QT interval is usually measured from the beginning of the QRS complex to the end of the T wave. When QTc interval is prolonged, it may become a risk factor for ventricular tachyarrhythmias and sudden death. This condition can arise as a genetic syndrome, or may be as a side effect of certain medications, but, an unusually short QTc can be seen in severe hypercalcemia (29, 30, 31, 32). In this study, all the tested doses brought about an increase in QT and QTc interval. It thus showed that the use of the extract for medicinal purposes is fraught with danger, hence cardiotoxicity. It must be noted that this is the first time that an ECG recording of the effect of corn silk extract in rats is being recorded.

Histological examination of the heart in this study corroborated the cardiotoxic changes brought

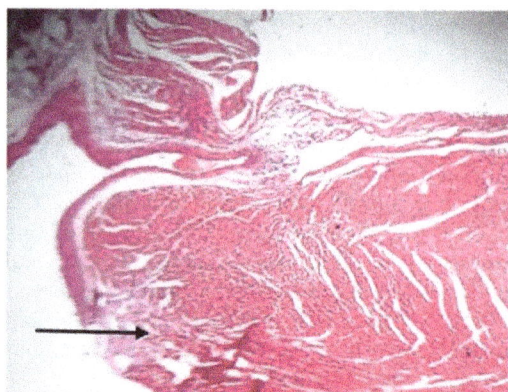

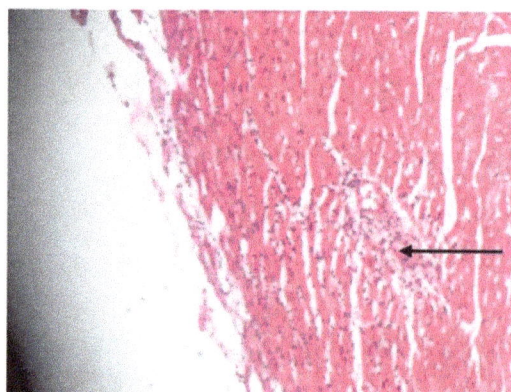

Figure 8d. Heart: Sections show focal areas of moderate inflammation of the atrium and ventricle (black arrows) in group D (X40; X100).

about with the use of this extract. Fatty infiltration of inflammed heart and areas of moderate inflammation of the atrium and ventricle were observed in this study in the tested groups. This histological change is similar to findings in arrhythmogenic right ventricular dysplasia/cardiomyopathy (33).

It could then be concluded from this study that lots of caution should be put in place when using this corn silk for medicinal purposes most especially in patient with compromised heart health condition.

ACKNOWLEDGEMENT

The study was carried out with the assistance of the University of Ibadan Senate Research grant (SRG/FVM/2010/10A) given to Dr. Adedapo.

REFERENCES

1. Rao, NK., Nammi, S. (2006). Antidiabetic and renoprotective effects of the chloroform extract of Terminalia chebula Retz. seeds in streptozotocin-induced diabetic rats. BMC Complement Altern Med. 6, 17.
http://dx.doi.org/10.1186/1472-6882-6-17
PMid:16677399 PMCid:PMC1540439

2. Aloulou, A., Hamden, K., Elloumi, D., Ali, MB., Hargafi, K., Jaouadi, B., Ayadi, F., Elfeki, A., Ammar, E. (2012). Hypoglycemic and antilipidemic properties of kombucha tea in alloxan-induced diabetic rats. BMC Complement Altern Med. 12, 63.
http://dx.doi.org/10.1186/1472-6882-12-63
PMid:22591682 PMCid:PMC3403982

3. Bhagwat, DA., Killedar, SG., Adnaik, RS. (2008). Anti-diabetic activity of leaf extract of Tridax procumbens. Intl J Green Pharm. 2, 126-128.
http://dx.doi.org/10.4103/0973-8258.41188

4. Saha, S., Verma, RJ. (2012). Efficacy study of Dolichos biflorus in the management of nephrotoxicity. Asian Pac J Trop Biomed. S1471-S1476.
http://dx.doi.org/10.1016/S2221-1691(12)60440-7

5. Guo, J., Liu, T., Han, L., Liu, Y. (2009). The effects of corn silk on glycaemic metabolism. Nutr Met. 6, 47.
http://dx.doi.org/10.1186/1743-7075-6-47
PMid:19930631 PMCid:PMC2785813

6. Hasanudin, K., Hashim, P., Mustafa, S. (2012). Corn silk (Stigma maydis) in healthcare: a phytochemical and pharmacological review. Molecules 17, 9697-9715.
http://dx.doi.org/10.3390/molecules17089697
PMid:22890173

7. Ebrahimzadeh, MA., Pourmorad, F., Hafezi, S. (2008). Antioxidant activities of Iranian corn silk. Turk J Biol. 32, 43-49.

8. Sawadogo, WR., Boly, M., Lompo, M., Some, N. (2006). Anti-inflammatory, analgesic and antipyretic activities of Dicliptera verticillata. Intl J Pharmacol. 2, 435-438.
http://dx.doi.org/10.3923/ijp.2006.435.438

9. Maksimović, Z., Malenčić, Đ., Kovačević, N. (2005). Polyphenol contents and antioxidant activity of Maydis stigma extracts. Bioresource Technol. 96, 873–877.
http://dx.doi.org/10.1016/j.biortech.2004.09.006
PMid:15627557

10. Bastien, JW. (1982). Pharmacopeia of qollahuayaandeans. J Ethnopharmacol. 8, 97–111.
http://dx.doi.org/10.1016/0378-8741(83)90091-0

11. Caceres, A., Giron, LM., Martinez, AM. (1987). Diuretic activity of plants used for the treatment of urinary ailments in Guatemala. J Ethnopharmacol. 19, 233–245.
http://dx.doi.org/10.1016/0378-8741(87)90001-8

12. Dat, DD., Ham, NN., Khac, DH., Lam, NT., Son, PT., Dau, NV., Grabe, M., Johansson, R., Lindgren, G., Stjernstrom, NE. (1992). Studies on the individual and combined diuretics effects of four Vietnamese traditional herbal remedies (Zea mays, Imperata cylindrica, Plantago major and Orthosiphon stamineus). J Ethnopharmacol. 36, 225–231.
http://dx.doi.org/10.1016/0378-8741(92)90048-V

13. Grases, F., March, JG., Ramis, M., Costa-Bauzá, A. (1993). The influence of Zea mays on urinary risk factors for kidney stones in rats. Phytother Res. 7, 146–149.
http://dx.doi.org/10.1002/ptr.2650070210

14. Yesilada, E., Honda, G., Sevik, E., Tabata, M., Fujita, T., Tanaka, T., Takeda, Y., Takaishi, Y. Traditional medicine in Turkey. V. (1995). Folk medicine in the inner Taurus Mountains. J Ethnopharmacol. 46, 133–152.
http://dx.doi.org/10.1016/0378-8741(95)01241-5

15. Hu, QL., Zhang, LJ., Li, YN., Ding, YJ., Li, FL. (2010). Purification and anti-fatigue activity of flavonoids from corn silk. Intl J Phys Sci. 5, 321–326.

16. Steenkamp, V. (2003). Phytomedicines for the prostate. Fitoterapia 74, 545–552.
http://dx.doi.org/10.1016/S0367-326X(03)00155-2

17. Velazquez, DVO., Xavier, HS., Batista, JEM., Castro-Chaves, CD. (2005). Zea mays L. extracts modify glomerular function and potassium urinary excretion in conscious rats. Phytomed. 12, 363–369.
http://dx.doi.org/10.1016/j.phymed.2003.12.010
PMid:15957371

18. Ebrahimzadeh, MA., Mahmoudi, M., Ahangar, N., Ehteshami, S., Ansaroudi, F., Nabavi, SF., Nabavi, SM. (2009). Antidepressant activity of corn silk. Pharmacologyonline 3, 647–652.

19. Maksimovic, ZA., Kovačević, N. (2003). Preliminary assay on the antioxidative activity of Maydis stigma extracts. Fitoterapia 74, 144–147. http://dx.doi.org/10.1016/S0367-326X(02)00311-8

20. Bai, H., Hai, C., Xi, M., Liang, X., Liu, R. (2010). Protective effect of maize silks (Maydis stigma). Ethanol extract on radiation-induced oxidative stress in mice. Plant Food Hum Nutr. 65, 271–276. http://dx.doi.org/10.1007/s11130-010-0172-6 PMid:20526679

21. Sepehri, G., Derakhshanfar, A., Zade, FY. (2011). Protective effects of corn silk extract administration on gentamicin-induced nephrotoxicity in rat. Comp Clin Pathol. 20, 89–94. http://dx.doi.org/10.1007/s00580-009-0943-3

22. Ambike, AA., Khandelwal, KR., Bodhankar, SL., Kadam, SS. (2000). Toxicity study and diuretic activity of corn silk, Zea mays L. Indian J Pharmacol. 32, 132-175.

23. Oosting, J., Struijker, BH., Janssen BJ. (1997). Autonomic control of ultradian and circadian rhythms of blood pressure, heart rate, and baroreflex sensitivity in spontaneously hypertensive rats. J Hypertens. 15, 401–410. http://dx.doi.org/10.1097/00004872-199715040-00011 PMid:9211175

24. Carvalho, MJ., van Den Meiracker, AH., Boomsma, F., Lima, M., Freitas, J., Veld, AJ., Falcao, DF. (2000). Diurnal blood pressure variation in progressive autonomic failure. Hypertens. 35, 892–897. http://dx.doi.org/10.1161/01.HYP.35.4.892

25. Custer, JW., Rau, RE. eds. (2008). Johns Hopkins: The Harriet Lane Handbook. 18th ed. Philadelphia, PA: Mosby Elsevier Inc.

26. Fauci, AS., Braunwald, E., Kasper, DL., Hauser, SL., Longo, DL., Jameson, JL., Loscalzo J. (2008). Harrison's Principles of Internal Medicine, 17th Edition. Amazon.com, Inc.

27. Moyer, VA. (2012). Screening for coronary heart disease with electrocardiography: U.S. Preventive Services Task Force recommendation statement. Annals Intern Med. 157 (7): 512–518. http://dx.doi.org/10.7326/0003-4819-157-7-201210020-00514

28. Padeletti, L., Santini, M., Boriani, G., Botto, G., Ricci, R., Spampinato, A. (2007). Duration of P-wave is associated with atrial fibrillation hospitalizations in patients with atrial fibrillation and paced for bradycardia. Pacing Clin Electrophysiol. 30, 961–969. http://dx.doi.org/10.1111/j.1540-8159.2007.00793.x PMid:17669078

29. Lodish, H., Berk, A., Kaiser, C., Krieger, M., Bretscher, A., Ploegh, H., Amon, A. (2000). Molecular Cell Biology (7th ed.). New York, NY: W. H. Freeman and Company. pp. 1021–1022, 1025, 1045.

30. Rang, HP. (2003). Pharmacology. Edinburgh: Churchill Livingstone. Page 149. ISBN 0-443-07145-4.

31. Callies, C., Fels, J., Liashkovich, I., Kliche, K., Jeggle, P., Kusche-Vihrog, K., Oberleithner, H. (2011). Membrane potential depolarization decreases the stiffness of vascular endothelial cells. J Cell Sci. 124, 1936-1942. http://dx.doi.org/10.1242/jcs.084657 PMid:21558418

32. Marieb, EN., Hoehn, K. (2014). Human anatomy and physiology. San Francisco, CA: Pearson Education Inc.

33. Gear, K., Marcus, F. (2003). Arrhythmogenic right ventricular dysplasia/cardiomyopathy. Circ. 107: e31-e33. http://dx.doi.org/10.1161/01.CIR.0000053943.38763.70 PMid:12569915

23

RETROSPECTIVE INVESTIGATION ON THE PREVALENCE OF PULMONARY HYPERTENSION IN DOGS WITH BRONCHIAL AND UPPER RESPIRATORY DISEASES

Chiara Locatelli, Daniela Montrasio, Ilaria Spalla, Giulia Riscazzi,
Matteo Gobbetti, Alice Savarese, Stefano Romussi, Paola G. Brambilla

*Department of Veterinary Sciences and Public Health (DIVET),
Università degli Studi di Milano, Via Celoria 10, 20133 Milan, Italy*

ABSTRACT

Bronchial and upper respiratory diseases have been associated with hypoxia and subsequent development of pulmonary arterial hypertension (PAH). However, there are no known studies assessing the prevalence of PAH in dogs with these conditions. The aim of this study was to assess the frequency of PAH in dogs with bronchial and upper respiratory diseases. Medical records of dogs with confirmed diagnosis (by endoscopic examination) of bronchial and/or upper respiratory diseases referred for cardiovascular investigation (January 2009 - May 2013) were retrospectively reviewed. Diagnosis of PAH was made by echocardiography (tricuspid regurgitation > 2.8 m/s and/or pulmonic regurgitation > 2.2 m/s); possible PAH was diagnosed when two or more specific echocardiographic findings were present. 52 dogs (30 with upper respiratory diseases, 17 with bronchial disease and 5 with both) were included. Diagnosis of PAH was performed in 3 dogs (5.7%). Two dogs were considered as probably affected by PAH; a total of 5 dogs (9.4%) resulted in being affected or probably affected by PAH. Our study shows that the prevalence of PAH in dogs with bronchial and/or upper respiratory diseases is low; PAH seems to occur mostly in older dogs and/or with very advanced disease: echocardiography may therefore be a useful tool in this category of patients.

Key words: dogs, pulmonary arterial hypertension, respiratory disease, tricuspid regurgitation

INTRODUCTION

In veterinary medicine, pulmonary arterial hypertension (PAH) is defined as pulmonary arterial systolic pressure greater than 25 mmHg (1). Right-heart catheterization is considered the "gold standard" in order to diagnose PAH (2, 3, 4). However it is rarely performed in veterinary medicine (1, 3, 4). In the absence of right ventricular (RV) outflow tract obstruction (e.g. pulmonary stenosis) or significant right-sided volume overload (e.g. tricuspid valve dysplasia), pulmonary arterial pressure can be inferred non-invasively with Doppler echocardiography, either by calculation of the maximal velocity of the regurgitant flow across the tricuspid (systolic pulmonary arterial pressure) or across the pulmonary valve (diastolic pulmonary arterial pressure) using the modified Bernoulli equation (4, 5, 6).

The severity of PAH is classified as mild, moderate, and severe based on the estimated pulmonary arterial pressure, with slight variations in cut off values among reports, in dogs affected by cardiovascular diseases (6, 7, 8).

PAH may occur through three mechanisms: increased left atrial pressure, increased pulmonary blood flow, and increased pulmonary vascular resistance. The pathophysiology of PAH is multifactorial and results from an imbalance of endogenous and exogenous pulmonary artery vasodilators and vasoconstrictors; this disequilibrium causes vasoconstriction, vascular smooth muscle cell proliferation and thrombosis, leading to an increased pulmonary vascular resistance in PAH (9, 10).

In people, chronic obstructive airway disease is one of the most common pulmonary causes of PAH (11). Chronic obstructive airway disease may

Corresponding author: Prof. Paola G. Brambilla, PhD
E-mail address: paola.brambilla@unimi.it
Present address: Department of Veterinary Sciences and Public Health (DIVET), Università degli Studi di Milano
Via Celoria 10, 20133 Milan, Italy

decrease the partial pressure of alveolar oxygen, which can result in hypoxia. In contrast to the systemic vasculature, which responds to hypoxia with vasodilatation to better perfuse hypoxic tissue, the pulmonary vasculature responds to hypoxia by pulmonic arterial vasoconstriction, which subsequently increases the pulmonary pressure (6). Few data is available on the PAH prevalence in dogs, except for selected conditions such as canine heartworm disease, left-sided heart failure and *Angiostrongylus vasorum* infection (12, 13, 14, 15, 16, 17).

Recently, some authors evidenced an association of pulmonary hypertension and increase serum CRP (C-reactive protein) concentrations in dogs affected by heartworm disease (12). Interestingly, the CRP concentration relates to the severity of endothelial arteritis, and not as a result of heartworm disease itself (12). The CRP concentration was still high even following adulticide treatment, and this underlined the possibility that CRP may be used as an early biomarker of pulmonary hypertension (12).

In veterinary medicine, lung disease, such as chronic pneumonia and lung fibrosis, chronic bronchitis, bronchiectasis, and upper respiratory disease such as tracheal collapse and laryngeal paralysis, have been associated with sustained or intermittent hypoxia and subsequent PAH development (10). PAH in dogs occurs mostly in patients with very advanced disease or those with predisposing conditions (9, 10). However, there are no known studies assessing the prevalence of PAH in dogs with bronchial and/or upper respiratory disease. The aim of this study was to assess the prevalence of PAH in dogs with bronchial and/or upper respiratory disease.

MATERIAL AND METHODS

The medical records of 1,063 dogs referred for cardiovascular investigation at the Cardiology Unit of the Department of Veterinary Science and Public Health between January 2009 and May 2013 were retrospectively reviewed. Only first visit cases were included in the study.

Inclusion criteria were: complete clinical records, radiographic, echocardiographic, a confirmed diagnosis by endoscopic examination of bronchial and/or upper respiratory disease and negative *Dirofilaria immitis* antigen test.

Exclusion criteria were: any cardiac and/or systemic disease that may cause PAH, except for mild mitral valve disease; diagnosis of *Angiostrongylus vasorum,* achieved using a Baermann faecal test performed at a veterinary diagnostic laboratory, or by detection of L1 larvae on a direct faecal smear or

bronchoalveolar lavage sample by a trained operator. The signalment, clinical history, and clinical signs (cough, dyspnoea, syncope, asthenia, weight loss, snoring, and reverse sneezing) were recorded.

Echocardiography was performed using an ultrasound system (MyLab 50, ESAOTE, Florence, Italy) equipped with a phased array transducer (7.5–10 MHz for small dogs, 5–7.5 MHz for medium dogs, and 2.5–3 MHz for large dogs and Doppler studies). Examinations were performed in awake dogs in left and right lateral recumbency, as recommended by the American Society of Echocardiography (18).

Echocardiographic and Doppler Examinations

The following echocardiographic parameters were evaluated:

B- and M- modes

1. Presence/absence of RV hypertrophy and/or dilation in the right parasternal long axis 4-chamber and short axis views at the level of the papillary muscle. The RV wall thickness was considered increased (RV hypertrophy) if it was greater than half the thickness of the left ventricular free wall (1). The RV chamber size was considered normal if it was smaller than or equal to one-half of the left ventricular thickness, mildly enlarged if greater than or equal to one-half the left ventricular thickness, or severely enlarged if greater than the left ventricle (5).

2. Presence/absence of flat or paradoxical interventricular septal motion in the right parasternal short axis and/or in M-mode at the level of the papillary muscle (10).

3. Presence/absence of main pulmonary artery enlargement based on the ratio between the diameters of the main pulmonary artery and the aorta (PA:AO ratio): a ratio greater than 0.98 was considered enlarged (1).

Doppler

1. Presence/absence of tricuspid regurgitation (TR): the TR systolic peak velocity (m/s) and peak systolic gradient (mmHg) were measured when present.

2. Presence/absence of pulmonic insufficiency (PI): the PI diastolic peak velocity (m/s) and peak diastolic gradient (mmHg) were measured when present. The presence and severity of PI were assessed through colour flow mapping, and the extension of the regurgitation jet and its width at the origin were evaluated (20).

3. Pulmonary artery systolic flow profiles: Type I (normal) was defined as a symmetric profile and

a rounded systolic peak; type II (mild and moderate PAH) as a peak velocity occurring during early systole and a long deceleration phase (asymmetric profile); and type III (severe PAH) was defined as having a notch in the deceleration phase (1).

4. Systolic time intervals: The acceleration time (AT), defined as the time to peak pulmonary artery flow velocity; RV ejection time (ET); and AT:ET ratio were assessed (21).

Doppler flow interrogations of the TR and PI jets were used to estimate the systolic and diastolic pulmonary arterial pressure respectively, allowing diagnosis and quantification of PAH (10). PAH was diagnosed when the TR systolic peak velocity (m/s) was greater than 2.8 m/s; the TR systolic peak velocity (m/s) and peak systolic gradient (mmHg) were used to classify the PAH severity (Table 1) (1, 4). The presence of PI with a velocity >2.2 m/s was considered suggestive of diastolic PAH (1, 4).

Statistical analysis

The Shapiro–Wilk test was used to verify normal distribution. Normally distributed data were expressed as the mean ± standard deviation. For data not normally distributed, the median and interquartile (IQR (25th to 75th percentile)) were calculated. Data were analyzed using statistical software (JMP version 7, JMP Headquarters, SAS Institute, Cary, NC, USA 27513).

RESULTS

Fifty-two clinical records fulfilled the inclusion criteria (35 males and 17 females), and represented 4.9 % of the total referral patients seen at the Cardiology Unit of the Department of Veterinary Science and Public Health between January 2009 and May 2013. Fourteen breeds were represented: 10 English Bulldogs (19%) resulted the prevalent,

Table 1. Classification of pulmonary hypertension based on TR (tricuspid regurgitation) peak systolic velocity and TR gradient [1]. (TR: tricuspid regurgitation)

	Mild	Moderate	Severe
TR peak systolic velocity (m/s)	> 2.8 to< 3.5	3.5 - 4.3	> 4.3
TR systolic gradient (mmHg)	> 31.4 a < 50	50 - 75	> 75

If TR/PI were absent, then PAH was considered possible when two or more of the following echocardiographic findings were recorded:

1. Presence of RV hypertrophy and/or dilation (5, 19)

2. Presence of main pulmonary artery enlargement (PA:AO ratio > 0.98) (1)

3. Presence of type II or III pulmonary artery systolic flow profile (1)

4. AT:ET < 0.31 and/or AT < 58 ms (21)

Endoscopic examination

Endoscopy was performed using either a rigid instrument equipped with a 18-cm optical length, 2.7-mm thickness (Karl Storz Hopkins II, Dr. Karl-Storz-Straße 34 Tuttlingen, Germany), 1-ccd camera (Wolf Endocam 551, Pforzheimer-Straße 32, 75438 Knittlingen, Germany),and xenon light source (Storz Xenon Nova 20131520, Dr. Karl-Storz-Straße 34 Tuttlingen, Germany) for examination of the nasal cavity, or a flexible video endoscope (4.9-mm diameter and 2-mm channel size, Fujinon Videobronchoscope EB-270 S7-3, Akasaka 9-chome, Minato-ku, Tokyo 107-0052, Japan) for examination of other respiratory airways.

7 males (70%) and 3 females (3%), followed by 8 crossbreeds dogs (15%), 5 males (62.5%) and 3 females (37.5%), 8 French Bulldogs (15%), 7 males (87.5%) and 1 female (12.5%) and 6 Yorkshire Terriers (11%), 2 males (33.3%) and 4 females (66.6%). The age ranged from 0.8 to 16 years (median 7 years; IQR: 3–12.25 years) and the weight from 2 to 40 kg (median 12 kg; IQR: 7.35–18 kg). All dogs showed at least one clinical sign: cough (50.1%), dyspnoea (50.1%), snoring (30.1%), exercise intolerance (15%), weight loss (9.4%), reverse sneeze (5.2%), and syncope (5.6%). Twenty-eight dogs (54%) showed more than one clinical sign simultaneously. The most common associations of symptoms were cough, dyspnoea and exercise intolerance (10.7%), cough and dyspnoea (21.4%), dyspnoea and snoring (10.7%).

Endoscopic examination

Seventeen dogs (33%; 8 females and 9 males) were diagnosed with bronchial disease (9 chronic bronchitis, 6 chronic bronchitis and bronchial collapse, 2 bronchial collapse). The prevalence on the total population referred was 1.6 %. Crossbreed dogs were the most represented (39%); the age

Table 2. Signalment, clinical signs, echocardiographic and Doppler data, PAH severity and endoscopic diagnosis of 5 dogs affected by PAH. (F: female; M: male; TR: tricuspid regurgitation)

	Breed	Sex	Age (years)	Clinical signs	TR peak velocity (m/s)	TR Gradient (mmHg)	Right ventricular hypertrophy/dilation	Pulmonary artery profiles	PAH	Bronchial Upper Respiratory Diseases	Endoscopic diagnosis
1	Poodle	M	11	Dyspnea	3.76	56.60	-	Normal	Moderate	Upper Respiratory Diseases	Laryngeal collapse and paralysis
2	Crossbreed	F	11	Cough and dyspnea	4.02	64.60	Mild	Normal	Moderate	Upper Respiratory Diseases	Tracheal collapse
3	French Bulldog	M	7	Weight loss	2.99	35.7	Mild	Normal	Mild	Upper Respiratory Diseases	Palatal disease
4	Yorkshire Terrier	F	5	Cough	-	-	Mild	Type II	Possible	Upper Respiratory Diseases	Tracheal collapse
5	Poodle	F	12	Cough	-	-	Mild	Type II	Possible	Bronchial Diseases	Chronic bronchitis

ranged from 1 to 15 years (median 12 years ; IQR: 11−13 years) and the weight from 3 to 16 kg (median 8 kg; IQR: 4−13.25 kg).

Thirty dogs (56.6%; 8 females and 22 males) were diagnosed with upper respiratory disease. Twenty-one of them resulted affected by brachycephalic airway obstructive syndrome (BAOS) (70 %; 5 female and 16 male), 3 by laryngeal paralysis, 2 by tracheal collapse, and 1 by laryngeal collapse; 3 dogs exhibited multiple upper respiratory disease simultaneously. The prevalence on the total population referred was 2.8 %. The most represented breeds were English and French Bulldogs (57%). The age ranged from 0.8 to 16 years (median 3.5 years; IQR: 3−10.25 years), and the weight ranged from 2 to 40 kg (median 13.85 kg; IQR: 10−21 kg). In the BAOS group specifically, the age ranged from 0.11 to 12 years (median 3 years; IQR: 2−4 years) and the weight from 8 to 26 kg (median 14 kg; IQR: 12−21 kg). Five dogs (9.5%; 1 female and 4 males), exhibited upper respiratory disease and bronchial disease simultaneously, 0.5 % the prevalence of this group on the total population referred to the Cardiology Unit during the study time.

Echocardiographic data

Mild RV enlargement was found in 4 dogs (7.5%) and mild RV hypertrophy in 2 dogs (3.8%).

One dog (1.9%) exhibited both RV hypertrophy and dilation simultaneously. No dog presented flat or paradoxical interventricular septal motion or main pulmonary artery enlargement.

TR was observed in 15 dogs (29%). The TR peak systolic velocity ranged from 1.51 m/s to 4.02 m/s (mean 2.62 ± 0.71 m/s), and the TR systolic gradient ranged from 9.10 mmHg to 64.60 mmHg (median 23.90 mmHg; IQR: 17.88−30.15 mmHg).

No dog showed pulmonary insufficiency. Type II pulmonary artery systolic flow profile was found in 2 dogs (3.8%) and was associated with mild RV hypertrophy in both. No dog presented an AT: ET ratio equal to or less than 0.31, and none exhibited an AT equal to or less than 58 ms. The mean AT: ET ratio was 0.48 ± 0.04, and the mean AT was 83.08±14.24 ms.

PAH was diagnosed in 3 dogs (5.7%) based on a TR peak systolic velocity >2.8 m/s. All three dogs were diagnosed with upper respiratory disease; therefore, the prevalence of PAH in this subgroup was 10%. Two dogs (one with bronchial disease and one with upper respiratory pathology) were considered likely to have PAH based on the presence of secondary specific echocardiographic findings. A total of 5 dogs (9.4%) had confirmed or probable PAH (Table 2), the prevalence in the overall referral population being 0.5 % and 1 % of dogs with valvular disease.

DISCUSSION

PAH is a well-recognized clinical condition in humans. Conversely, few data are available in dogs, except for PAH secondary to canine heartworm disease, mitral valve disease and *Angiostrongylus vasorum* infection (1, 6, 8, 9, 14, 15,16, 17, 22, 23, 24). The degree of hypoxia that can cause PAH likely exists in a large number of dogs with both upper and lower airway obstructive diseases (9). In particular, lung disease, such as chronic pneumonia, lung fibrosis, chronic bronchitis, bronchiectasis, and upper respiratory pathologies, such as tracheal collapse and laryngeal paralysis, have been associated with sustained or intermittent hypoxia and have been thought as theoretically causing PAH (5, 9, 10). Nevertheless, there are no known studies assessing the prevalence of PAH in dogs with respiratory disease, except for one study of West Highland White terriers, in which PAH occurred in more than 49% of dogs diagnosed with chronic interstitial pulmonary disease (19).

In humans, the prevalence of PAH in patients with at least one previous hospitalization for exacerbation of respiratory failure is 20%, and in patients with advanced respiratory disease, the prevalence is higher (>50%), although the severity is usually mild (2). In our population, the prevalence of PAH in dogs with bronchial and/ or upper respiratory diseases associated with potential hypoxia was low (5 dogs, 9.4%), even when both confirmed and possible PAH cases were considered, or very low (3 dogs, 5.7%) when only PAH diagnosed by TR velocity was considered. All 3 dogs with confirmed PAH were diagnosed with upper respiratory disease; therefore, the occurrence of PAH in this disease category was slightly high (3/30, 10%). Only mild and moderate PAH was identified.

In dogs with upper respiratory disease, PAH or possible PAH was diagnosed in 2 dogs with tracheal collapse, 1 dog with laryngeal collapse and paralysis, and 1 dog with BAOS (Table 2). Three of four dogs were older than the median age for the group (3.5 years); the only young dog showed echocardiographic signs of possible PAH and was diagnosed with very severe cervical tracheal collapse (Table 2). The occurrence of PAH in dogs with BAOS was also very low (1/21), though most of the dogs included in the study were young (median age 3 years). Interestingly, the only dog with BAOS (Table 2) diagnosed with PAH was older (7 years) than the rest of dogs with BAOS included in this study. Based on these results, we speculate that early surgical correction may be protective from PAH, but further studies are needed to confirm this hypothesis.

In our cases series, only one dog with bronchial disease presented echocardiographic signs suggesting possible PAH, and no dog with bronchial disease exhibited PAH. We found these data relatively surprising because chronic hypoxemia and increased airway resistance have been described as common findings in patients with advanced chronic bronchitis, and cor pulmonale is considered a possible consequence (25). The low occurrence of PAH in dogs with bronchial disease and in all dogs in our study may be due to the relatively poor vasoconstrictive response to hypoxia exhibited by dogs compared with other species (9, 10). Canine PAH seems to occur mostly during very advanced respiratory disease, as described in West Highland White terriers and suggested by several reports (9, 21).

Based on our results, we recommend an echocardiographic investigation only in older dogs with bronchial and/or upper respiratory disease or in dogs with advanced disease regardless of age. Echocardiographic and spectral Doppler assessments of tricuspid and pulmonic regurgitation are useful tool in this group of patients especially when utilized as a part of comprehensive assessment of PAH, and may supplement the methods traditionally used to investigate the respiratory system in canine patients (3, 26).

Diagnosis of PAH was based only on echocardiographic data: a TR systolic peak velocity greater than 2.8 m/s, a PI diastolic peak velocity greater than 2.2 m/s, the presence of a type II or III pulmonary artery systolic flow profile, and the presence of RV hypertrophy/dilation (4). Pulmonary hypertension was then classified as mild, moderate, and severe based on the tricuspid regurgitation peak systolic velocity and gradient. None of the dogs exhibited severe PAH; two dogs had moderate PAH, one mild, and two possible PAH. Potentially, some cases of PAH in our study population may have been undetectable using echocardiography (3). Cardiac catheterization is the "gold standard" to diagnose PAH, but in veterinary medicine, right heart catheterization is often considered unacceptably invasive by the clinician in a compromised patient, therefore the echocardiographic and spectral Doppler approach remains very common in clinical practice (3). When available however, catheterization enables measurement of multiple hemodynamic parameters that assist in the diagnosis and etiologic classification of PAH (1).

None of the dogs exhibited flat or paradoxic interventricular septal motion, main pulmonary artery enlargement, an AT: ET ≤ 0.31, or an AT ≤ 58 ms. These findings may be because very few dogs were diagnosed with PAH, and when present, PAH was mild or moderate, with no cases of severe PAH diagnosed. A median AT: ET of 0.48 and a median AT of 83 ms suggested a normal pulmonary pressure in the population and agree with previously reported values in healthy West Highland White terriers, which had a median AT:ET of 0.40 and a median AT of 73 ms (21).

None of the dogs with PAH presented syncope or exercise intolerance. The dogs with PAH included in our study only showed respiratory signs, with cough and dyspnoea as the most common clinical signs. These particular clinical signs likely reflect the underlying bronchial and/or upper respiratory disease causing PAH.

The epidemiological characteristics of our population agree with those previously reported, namely young English and French Bulldogs with BAOS, older large breed dogs (Labrador and Setter) with laryngeal paralysis, Yorkshire Terrier, typically middle-aged, with tracheal collapse, and older small breed dogs with chronic bronchitis (5, 27, 28, 29, 30).

This study has a number of limitations as a result of its retrospective nature. We only used non-invasive diagnostic approaches, and cardiac catheterization was not performed. PAH was diagnosed based only on certain echocardiographic and Doppler parameters (TR systolic peak velocity greater than 2.8 m/s, PI diastolic peak velocity greater than 2.2 m/s, presence of a type II or III pulmonary artery systolic flow profile, and presence of RV hypertrophy/dilation), and several parameters were not measured, including the TEI index and TAPSE (tricuspid annular plane systolic excursion). Moreover the lack of arterial blood-gas data could be an additional weakness in this study. Only cases with endoscopic diagnosis of bronchial and/or upper respiratory diseases were included; no parenchymal diseases, nor pleural diseases were included in our study.

Finally, most of the dogs diagnosed with BAOS were young and West Highland White terriers, a breed predisposed to PAH secondary to severe lung disease, was not included in the study (21). In conclusion, our study shows that the occurrence of PAH in dogs with bronchial and/or upper respiratory disease is low; PAH seems to occur mostly in older dogs or those with very advanced disease. The echocardiographic and spectral Doppler assessments of tricuspid and pulmonic regurgitation are useful tool in these classes of patients. Nevertheless, further prospective studies including different subsets of pathologies, clinical settings (acute vs chronic), disease severity (mild/moderate/severe) and the evaluation of clinical biomarkers (i.e. C-reactive protein) are needed to confirm these results.

Ethical approval

All applicable international, national, and institutional guidelines for the care and use of animals were followed. All procedures performed in studies involving animals were in accordance with the ethical standards of the institution or practice at which the studies were conducted. For this type of study, formal consent was not required.

REFERENCES

1. Kellihan, H.B., Stepien, R.L. (2010). Pulmonary hypertension in dogs: diagnosis and therapy. Vet Clin Small Anim. 40, 623-641.
   http://dx.doi.org/10.1016/j.cvsm.2010.03.011
   PMid:20610015

2. Galiè, N., Hoeper, M., Humbert, M. et al. (2009). Guidelines for the diagnosis and treatment of pulmonary hypertension. European Heart Journal 30, 2493-2537.
   http://dx.doi.org/10.1093/eurheartj/ehp297
   PMid:19713419

3. Soydan, L.C., Kellihan, H.B., Bates, L.B., Stepien, R.L., Consigny, D.W., Bellofiore, A., Francois, C.J., Chesler, N.C. (2015). Accuracy of doppler echocardiographic estimates of pulmonary artery pressures in a canine model of pulmonary hypertension. Journal of Veterinary Cardiology 17, 13 – 24.
   http://dx.doi.org/10.1016/j.jvc.2014.10.004
   PMid:25601540

4. Borgeat, K., Sudunagunta, S., Kaye, B., Stern, J., Luis Fuentes, V., Connolly, D. J. (2015). Retrospective evaluation of moderate-to-severe pulmonary hypertension in dogs naturally infected with angiostrongylus vasorum. Journal of Small Animal Practice 56, 196–202.
   http://dx.doi.org/10.1111/jsap.12309
   PMid:25483150

5. Johnson, L., Boon, J., Orton, E.C. (1999). Clinical characteristic of 53 dogs with Doppler - derived evidence of pulmonary hypertension 1992–1996. Journal of Veterinary Internal Medicine 13, 440–444.
   PMid:10499728

6. Kellihan, H.B., Stepien, R.L. (2012). Pulmonary hypertension in canine degenerative mitral valve disease. Journal of Veterinary Cardiology 14,149–164.
   http://dx.doi.org/10.1016/j.jvc.2012.01.001
   PMid:22364721

7. Pyle, R.L., Abbott, J., Maclean, H. (2004). Pulmonary hypertension and cardiovascular sequela in 54 dogs". International Journal of Applied Research in Veterinary Medicine 2, 99–109.

8. Serres, F.J., Chetboul, V., Tissier, R., Sampedrano, C.C., Gouni, V., Nicolle, A.P., Pouchelon, J.L. (2006). Doppler echocardiography-derived evidence of pulmonary arterial hypertension in dogs with degenerative mitral valve disease: 86 cases (2001–2005). Journal of the American Veterinary Medical Association 229, 1772–1778.
http://dx.doi.org/10.2460/javma.229.11.1772
PMid:17144824

9. Johnson, L.R., Hamlin, R.L. (1995). Recognition and treatment of pulmonary hypertension. In: Bonagura J.R.D. (Ed.), Kirk's Current Veterinary Therapy XII (pp 887 – 892). Philadelphia USA: WB Saunders.

10. Campbell, F.E. (2007). Cardiac effects of pulmonary disease. Veterinary Clinics North America Small Animal Practice 37. 949-962.
http://dx.doi.org/10.1016/j.cvsm.2007.05.006
PMid:17693208

11. Mc Laughlin. V.V., Rich. S. (2000). Corpulmonale. In: Braunwald E, Zipes DP, Libby P. (Ed.), Heartdisease: a textbook of cardiovascular medicine. 6th Edition. (pp 1936-1956). Philadelphia USA: WB Saunders.

12. Venco, L., Milhaylova, L., Boon, J.A. (2014). Right pulmonary artery distensibility index (RPAD index). A field study of an echocardiographic method to detect earl development of pulmonary hypertension and its severity even in the absence of regurgitant jets for Doppler evaluation in heartworm-infected dogs. Vet Parasitol. 206, 60-6.
http://dx.doi.org/10.1016/j.vetpar.2014.08.016
PMid:25218885

13. Swann, J., Sudunagunta, S., Covey, H.L., English, K., Hendricks, A., Connolly, D.J. (2014). Evaluation of red cell distribution width in dogs with pulmonary hypertension. Journal of Veterinary Cardiology 16, 227-235.
http://dx.doi.org/10.1016/j.jvc.2014.08.003
PMid:25465342

14. Sasaki, Y., Kitagawa, H., Hirano, Y. (1992). Relationship between pulmonary arterial pressure and lesionsin the pulmonary arteries and parenchyma, and cardiac valves in canine dirofilariasis. Journal of Veterinary Medical Science 54, 739–744.
http://dx.doi.org/10.1292/jvms.54.739

15. Nicolle, A.P., Chetboul, V., Tessier-Vetzel, D., Sampedrano, C.C., Aletti, E., Pouchelon, J.L. (2006). Severe pulmonary arterial hypertension due to Angiostrongylosu svasorum in a dog. The Canadian Veterinary Journal 47, 792-795.
PMid:16933559 PMCid:PMC1524835

16. Traversa, D., Di Cesare, A., Meloni, S., Frangipane di Regalbono, A., Milillo, P., Pampurini, F., Venco, L. (2013). Canine angiostrongylosis in Italy: prevalence of Angiostrongylus vasorum in dogs with compatible clinical pictures. Parasitology Research 112, 2473-2480.
http://dx.doi.org/10.1007/s00436-013-3412-5
PMid:23595212 PMCid:PMC3683398

17. Borgarelli, M., Abbott, J., Braz-Ruivo, L., Chiavegato, D., Crosara, S., Lamb, K., Ljungvall, I., Poggi, M., Santilli, R.A., Haggstrom, J. (2015). Prevalence and prognostic importance of pulmonary hypertension in dogs with myxomatous mitral valve disease. Journal of Veterinary Internal Medicine 29, 569–574.
http://dx.doi.org/10.1111/jvim.12564
PMid:25818210

18. Thomas, W.P., Gaber, C.E., Jacobs, G.J., Kaplan, P.M., Lombard, C.W., Moise, N.S., Moses, B.L. (1993). Recommendations for standards in transthoracic two-dimensional echocardiography in the dog and cat. Journal of Veterinary Internal Medicine 7, 247-252.
http://dx.doi.org/10.1111/j.1939-1676.1993.tb01015.x

19. Boon, J.A. (1998). Evaluation of size, function and hemodynamics. In: Boon J.A. (Ed.), Manual of veterinary echocardiography (pp. 151–260). Williams & Wilkins Co, Baltimore.
PMid:9654462

20. Cooper, J.W., Nanda, N.C., Philpot, E.F., Fan, P. (1989). Evaluation of valvular regurgitation by colour Doppler. Journal of the American Society of Echocardiography 2, 56-66.
http://dx.doi.org/10.1016/S0894-7317(89)80030-6

21. Schober, K.E., Baade, H. (2006). Doppler echocardiographic prediction of pulmonary hypertensionin West Highland White Terriers with chronic pulmonary disease. Journal of Veterinary Internal Medicine 20, 912-920.
http://dx.doi.org/10.1111/j.1939-1676.2006.tb01805.x

22. Glaus, T., Schnyder, M., Dennler, M., Tschuor, F., Wenger, M., Sieber-Ruckstuhl, N. (2010). Natural infection with Angiostrongylus vasorum: characterisation of 3 dogs with pulmonary hypertension. Schweizer Archiv für, Tierheilkunde 152, 331-338.
http://dx.doi.org/10.1024/0036-7281/a000076
PMid:20582899

23. Estèves, I., Tessier, D., Dandrieux, J., Polack, B., Carlos, C., Boulanger, V., Muller, C., Pouchelon, J.L., Chetboul, V. (2004). Reversible pulmonary hypertension presenting simultaneously with an atrial septal defect and angiostrongylosis in a dog. Journal of Small Animal Practice 45, 206-209.
http://dx.doi.org/10.1111/j.1748-5827.2004.tb00226.x
PMid:15116890

24. Matos, J. M., Schnyder, M., Bektas, R., Makara, M., Kutter, A., Jenni, S., Deplazes, P., Glaus, T. (2012). Recruitment of arteriovenous pulmonary shunts may attenuate the development of pulmonary hypertension in dogs experimentally infected with Angiostrongylus vasorum. Journal of Veterinary Cardiology 14, 313-322.
http://dx.doi.org/10.1016/j.jvc.2012.01.014
PMid:22575676

25. Kuehn, N.F. (2003). Chronic bronchitis in dogs. In: L. King (Ed.), Textbook of Respiratory Diseases of the Dog and Cat (pp. 379-387). Philadelphia USA: WB Saunders.

26. Paradies, P., Spagnolo, P.P., Amato, M.E., Pulpito, D., Sassanelli, M. (2014). Doppler echocardiographic evidence of pulmonary hypertension in dogs: a retrospective clinical investigation. Veterinary Research Communication 38, 63-71.
http://dx.doi.org/10.1007/s11259-013-9588-4
PMid:24414341

27. Herrtage, M.E., White, R. (2000). Management of tracheal collapse. In: J. Bonagura, RD (Ed) Kirk's Current Veterinary Therapy XIII (pp 796-801). Philadelphia USA: WB Saunders.

28. Hendricks, J.C. (2003). Brachycephalic Airway Syndrome. In: L. King (Ed) Textbook of Respiratory Diseases of the Dog and Cat (pp. 310-318). Philadelphia USA: WB Saunders.

29. Holt, D.E., Brockman, D. (2003). Laryngeal paralysis. In: L. King (Ed) Textbook of Respiratory Diseases of the Dog and Cat (pp. 319-328). Philadelphia USA: WB Saunders.

30. Mason, R.A., Johnson, L.R. (2003). Tracheal collapse. In: L. King (Ed) Textbook of Respiratory Diseases of the Dog and Cat (pp. 346-355). Philadelphia USA: WB Saunders.

24

A REPORT OF A *HEPATOZOON CANIS* INFECTION IN A DOG WITH TRANSMISSIBLE VENEREAL TUMOUR

Namakkal Rajamanickam Senthil, Subramanian Subapriya, Subbaiah Vairamuthu

Centralised Clinical Laboratory
Madras Veterinary College, Chennai - 600007, Tamil Nadu, India

ABSTRACT

In the present study, a case of a *Hepatozoan canis* infection in a dog with a sexually transmissible venereal tumour is reported. Haematological examination revealed marked decrease in haemoglobin, PCV and RBC counts and the blood smear revealed rouleaux formation of RBC, hypochromasia, leptocytes and neutrophilia. Neutrophils were parasitized with both non-nucleated and stained nucleated forms of *H. canis*. Serum biochemistry results showed elevated levels of alkaline phosphatise, whereas blood urea nitrogen, creatinine, total protein, albumin and globulin were in the normal range.

Key words: canine, transmissible venereal tumour, *Hepatozoon canis*

INTRODUCTION

Transmissible venereal tumour (TVT) is a reticuloendothelial tumour in dogs that mainly affects the external genitalia and occasionally the internal genitalia (1). It is sexually transmitted by coitus and other contacts and is also known as infectious sarcoma, venereal granuloma, transmissible lymphosarcoma or sticker tumour. TVT affects the mucosa of the external genitalia and less often, the internal genitalia (2). According to Cohen (3), the exfoliation and transplantation of neoplastic cells during physical contact provide the main mode of transmission onto genital mucosa, and also onto nasal or oral mucosa, during mating or licking of affected genitalia, respectively. Canine hepatozoonosis is caused by *Hepatozoon canis* and transmitted by ingestion of an Ixodid tick, *Rhipicephalus sanguineus* containing mature oocysts (4). *Hepatozoon spp.* are protozoa of the

Corresponding author: Assist. Prof. N.R.Senthil, M.V.Sc.
E-mail address: drnrsenthil@gmail.com
Present address: Centralised Clinical Laboratory
Madras Veterinary College, Chennai- 600007, Tamil Nadu, India

phylum Apicomplexa, some of which parasitize the white blood cells of dogs. At present, two species of *Hepatozoon* have been identified in dogs: *H. canis* which is transmitted by *Rhipicephalus sanguineus*, and *H. americanum* which is transmitted by *Amblyoma maculatum*. Between *H. canis* and *H. americanum* there are differences in morphology, pathogenicity, tissue tropism and clinical signs. In particular, *H. americanum* is much more pathogenic and can be lethal. The dog is infected when it ingests a tick containing sporulated oocysts. The sporozoites are released in the dog's digestive tract, penetrate the intestinal wall and are carried by the blood or lymph to the liver, lymph nodes, kidneys, bone marrow and muscle where schizogony occurs. Numerous merozoites develop, some of them enter neutrophils and monocytes and transform into gametocytes. All *Hepatozoon spp.* share a basic life cycle that includes sexual development and sporogony in a hematophagous invertebrate definitive host, and merogony followed by gamontogony in a vertebrate intermediate host. Definitive hosts for *Hepatozoon spp.* are blood-sucking invertebrates, including ticks, mites, sand flies, tsetse flies, mosquitoes, fleas, lice, reduviid bugs, and leeches (5). To the author's knowledge this is the first report of *H. canis* infection associated with a TVT case in India and hence the case is recorded and discussed.

CASE REPORT

A 14-year-old Spitz female dog with a growth in the caudal vagina protruding from the vulva was presented at the small animal clinics surgery (outpatient unit) of the Teaching Veterinary Hospital at the Madras Veterinary College. On examination the mass was suggestive of TVT by fine needle aspiration cytology (FNAC) sample submitted for cytological examination. Blood samples were collected for haematology in EDTA vials; serum biochemistry and blood smear for Leishman-Giemsa staining were carried out at the centralized clinical laboratory. The whole blood was analysed by auto haematology analyser (BC-2800 Vet) and serum biochemistry in A15 auto analyser. FNAC touch

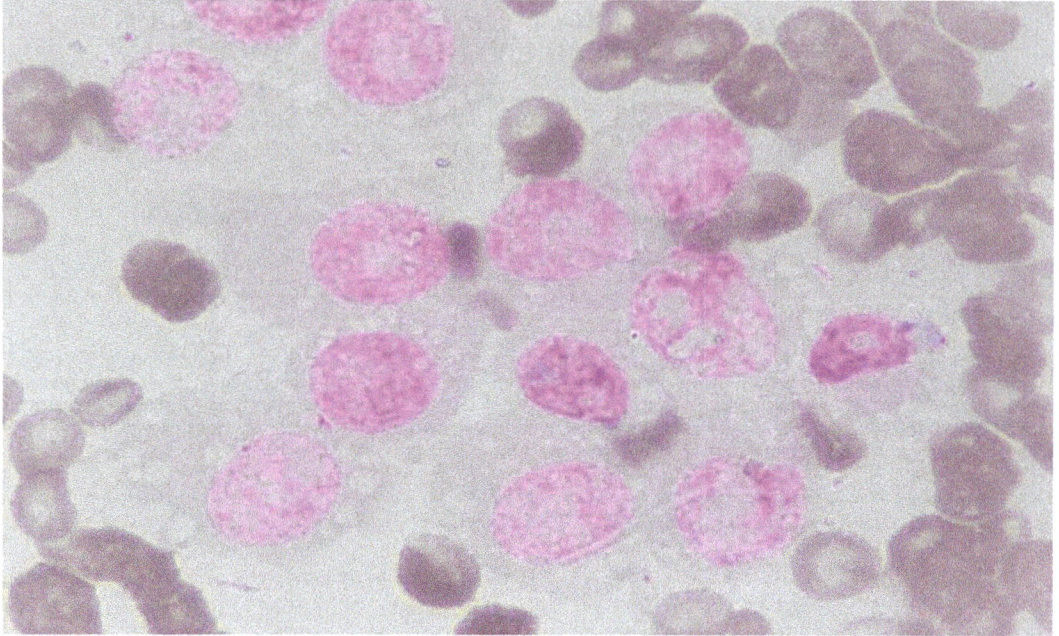

Figure 1. Cytological smear from a vulval mass showing discrete round cells with eccentric round nuclei, uniform granular chromatin pattern and clear, cytoplasmic vacuoles

impression smear was taken from the mass, then stained with Leishman-Giemsa stain for cytological examination.

Cytological smear from the protruding vulval mass showed discrete round cells having eccentric round nuclei with uniform granular chromatin

Table 1. Haemological and sero-biochemical values of *H.canis* infected TVT dog

Haematology	Value	Reference values	Serum Biochemistry parameters	Value	Reference Values
Haemoglobin	3.8 mg/dL	12-18 mg/L	BUN	18.84 mg/dL	10-28 mg/dL
PCV	15.7%	37-55%	Creatinine	1.08 mg/dL	0.5-1.5 mg/dL
RBC	2.72 m /cubic mm	5.5-8.5m/ cmm	Total protein	6.4 g/dL	5.4-7.1 g/dL
WBC	30,700/cubic mm	6000-17000/ cmm	Albumin	1.8 g/dL	2.3-3.8 g/dL
Platelets	5,06,000/cmm	200000-500000/ cmm	Globulin	4.6g/dL	2.3-5.2g/dL
Neutrophils	90%	60-70%	AST	50.0 IU/L	23-66 IU/L
Lymphocytes	8%	20-30%	ALP	476.0 IU/L	20-156 IU/L
Monocytes	2%	0-5%	Total bilirubin	0.40 mg/dL	0.15-.0.50 mg/dL
Blood picture	Rouleaux formation of RBC, Hypochromasia, Leptocytes, Neutrophilia		Direct bilirubin	0.21mg/dL	0.06-0.12mg/dL
Blood Parasite	*Hepatozoan canis*		Calcium	8.81 mg/dL	9-11.3mg/dL

pattern and a single round prominent nucleolus, as shown in Figure 1. The microscopic features of the cytological smear were thus suggestive of TVT. Neoplastic cells ranged from 12-24 μm in diameter and they had moderate amounts of granular and moderately blue staining cytoplasm. Cells revealed clear, distinct, punched out cytoplasmic vacuoles. The vacuoles were similar in size and arranged in linear array along the inner surface of the cell membrane. In addition to the neoplastic cells, normal appearing neutrophils and lymphocytes were seen.

Haematological and serum biochemistry results are showed in Table 1. Haematological examination revealed marked decrease in haemoglobin (3.8g/dl), packed cell volume (PCV) (15.7%) and RBC count (2.7 million cells/mcL), while the blood smear revealed rouleaux formation of RBC, hypochromasia, leptocytes and neutrophilia. Neutrophils were parasitized with both non-nucleated and stained nucleated forms of H. canis, as shown in Figure 2.

Serum biochemistry results showed elevated levels of Alkaline phosphatase (ALP) (476.0 IU/L) whereas BUN, creatinine, total protein, albumin and globulin were in the normal range, as shown in Table 1.

damaged skin and mucosa (6). Stockmann et al. (7) observed tumour formation in the posterior region of the vagina and vestibule-vaginal junction, which was prolapsed out of the vulva of bitches. TVT usually occur in bitches within the age group of 2-8 years (8). In this study an increased level of ALP was observed. According to Kerr (9), increased activities of serum AST, ALT and ALP may be due to liver damage, while increased AST and CK concentrations were thought to be linked to muscle tissue damage. Gavazza et al. (4) and Sarma et al. (10) observed elevation of ALP in H. canis infection. Elevation of ALP seen in this report might be due to progression of schizogony within bone-morrow and hepatocytes, in addition to the spleen.

Kose et al. (11) recorded leucocytosis, haemoconcentration and microcytic hypochromic anaemia in haematological examination of disseminated metastatic TVT. In this report, the complete blood count revealed normocytic and hypochromic anaemia with neutrophillia as observed by Paramjit et al. (12) in a case of hepatozoonosis in a mongrel dog. Ruiz et al. (13) have previously recorded H. canis associated with canine TVT in Argentina. H. canis infection affects spleen, lymph nodes and bone marrow. Clinical signs vary from

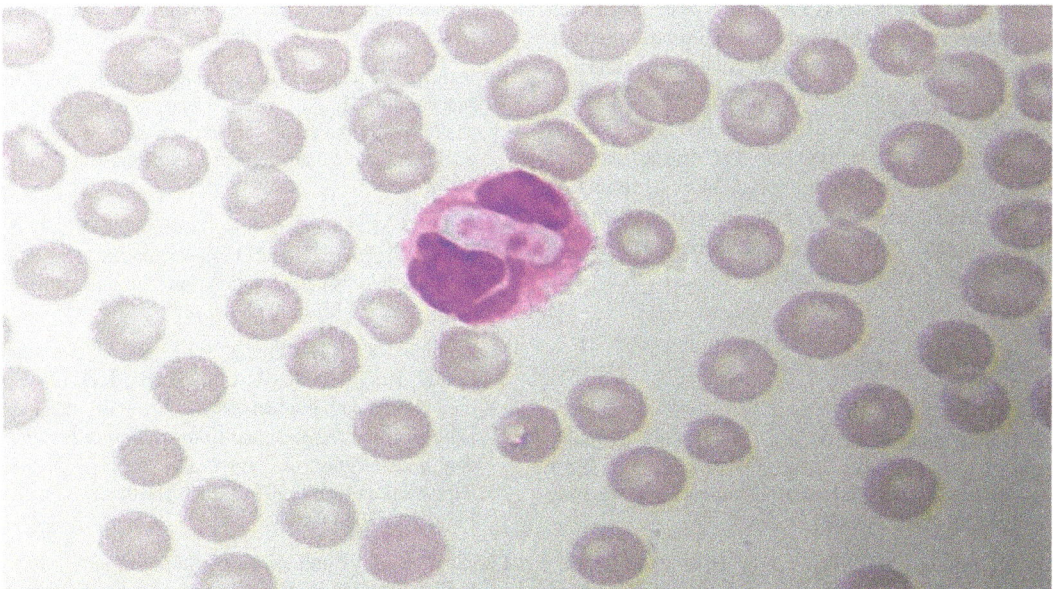

Figure 2. Peripheral blood smear from TVT affected dog showing ellipsoidal shaped *H.canis* gamonts in a neutrophil.

DISCUSSION

The TVT in dogs are transmitted not only by coitus, but also by licking, sniffing, biting, and scrabbling of the tumour affected area or through

asymptomatic, mild or severe, including anaemia and lethargy, depending on the level of parasitemia and the immune status of the subject (4, 14). Hepatozoonosis is often found in association with other infections including blood parasites (15).

The blood picture revealed rouleaux formation of RBCs, hypochromasia, leptocytes, neutrophilia. Rouleaux are stacks of RBCs which form because of the unique discoid shape of the cells. It occurs in inflammatory conditions, connective tissue disorders and in tumours due to the interaction of fibrinogen with sialic acid on the surface of RBCs. This is not an uncommon feature in an anaemic condition. Marino et al. (16) reported that sporadic *Leishmania* amastigotes were found within the canine TVT in three cases, probably transported by infected macrophages often infiltrating the tumour. Moreover, the capacity of tumour cells to internalize amastigotes suggests phagocytic and/or receptor-mediated endocytosis that could be related to the proposed histiocytic phenotype of TVT. A similar pattern of immune-reaction was observed in the present case. In addition to cytological examination of smears for the identification of tumour, the blood smears can necessarily be screened for the presence of parasites like *H. canis* as well.

Chemotherapy has been shown to be the most effective and practical therapy, with vincristine sulfate being the most frequently used drug. Vincristine can be intravenously administered at weekly intervals at a dose of 0.5 to 0.7 mg/m2 of body surface area or 0.025 mg/kg, ranitidine at a dose of 0.2 mg/kg BW, and amoxicillin at a dose of 11mg/kg BW for 5 days (17). In this case, the animal was administered with vincristine sulphate injection at a dose of 0.025 mg/kg BW at weekly intervals and ranitidine injection at a dose of 0.2 mg/kg BW. Oxytetracycline (10 mg/kg BW for 5 days) followed by oral doxycyline (10 mg/kg/day for 21 days) were also administered. Marked reduction in the size of tumors after 5 cycles of treatment was observed and blood smear examination revealed absence of *H. canis* schizonts.

REFERENCES

1. Goldschmidt, M. H., Hendrick, M. J. (2002). Tumours of the skin and soft tissues. In: Meuton, D. J. (Ed.), 4th ed., Tumours in Domestic Animals. (pp. 45-118). Press, Iowa. Iowa State.

2. Chu, R.M., Sun, T.J., Yang, H.Y., Wang, D.G., Liao, K.W., Chuang, T.F., Lin, C.H., Lee, W.C. (2001). Heat shock proteins in canine transmissible venereal tumor. Vet. Immunol Immunopathol. 82, 9-21. http://dx.doi.org/10.1016/S0165-2427(01)00327-0

3. Cohen D. (1985). The canine transmissible venereal tumor: A unique result of tumour progression. Adv Cancer Res. 43, 75-112. http://dx.doi.org/10.1016/s0065-230x(08)60943-4

4. Gavazza, A., Bizzeti, M., Papini, R. (2003). Observations on dogs found naturally infected with *Hepatozoon canis* in Italy. Rev. Méd. Vét. 154, 565-571.

5. Baneth, G., Samish,M., Shkap, V., (2007). Life cycle of *Hepatozoon canis* (apicomplexa: adeleorina: hepatozoidae) in the tick *Rhipicephalus sanguineus* and domestic dog (*Canis familiaris*). J. Parasitol. 93 (2): 283-299. http://dx.doi.org/10.1645/GE-494R.1 PMid:17539411

6. Stettner, N., Brenner, O., Eilam, R., Harmelin, A. (2005). Pegylated liposomal doxorubicin as a chemotherapeutic agent for treatment of canine transmissible venereal tumor in murine models. J. Vet. Med. 67, 1133-1139. http://dx.doi.org/10.1292/jvms.67.1133

7. Stockmann, D., Ferrari, H.F., Andrade, A.L., Lopes, R.A., Cardoso, T.C., Luvizotto, M.C.R. (2011). Canine transmissible venereal tumors: Aspects related to programmed cell death. Braz J. Vet. Pathol. 4, 67-75.

8. Oruc, E., Saglam, Y.S., Cengiz, M., Polat, B. (2011). Cytological diagnosis of breast metastasis of transmissible venereal tumor by fine needle aspiration and the treatment with vincristine sulphate in a dog. Ankara Üniv Vet Fak Derg. 6, 63-69.

9. Kerr, M.G. (2002). Clinical biochemistry and haematology. In: (2nd Ed.), Veterinary Laboratory Medicine (pp.135-147). Blackwell Science Ltd, USA.

10. Sarma, K., Mondal, D.B., Saravanan, M., Kumar, M., Mahendran, K. (2012). Haemato-biochemical changes in Hepatozoon canis infected dog before and after therapeutic management J. Vet. Parasitol. 26 (1): 35-38.

11. Kose, A.M, Cizmeci, S.U, Aydin, I, Dinc, D.A, Maden, M., Kanat, O. (2013). Disseminated metastatic transmissible venereal tumour in a bitch Eurasian J .Vet. Sci. 29, 1, 053-057.

12. Paramjit K., Deshmukh, S., Rajsukhbir, S., Bansal, B.K., Randhawa, C.S., Singla, L.D. (2012). Para-clinico-pathological observations of insidious incidence of canine hepatozoonosis from a mongrel dog: a case report. J .Parasit. Dis. 36(1): 135–138. http://dx.doi.org/10.1007/s12639-011-0092-x PMid:23543040 PMCid:PMC3284626

13. Ruiz, M.F., Zimmermann, R.N., Aguirre, F.O., Forti, M.S. (2013). *Hepatozoon canis* asociado a un tumor venéreo transmisible: singular hallazgo. Vet. Arg. 30, 306.

14. Baneth, G., Weigler, B. (1997). Retrospective case-control study of hepatozoonosis in dogs in Israel. J. Vet. Intern. Med. 11, 365-370. http://dx.doi.org/10.1111/j.1939-1676.1997.tb00482.x PMid:9470163

15. Gondim, L. F. P., Kohayagawa, A., Alencar, N. X., Biondo, A. W., Takahira, R. F., Franco, S. R. V. (1998). Canine hepatozoonosis in Brazil: description of eight naturally occurring cases. Vet. Parasitol. 74, 319-323.
http://dx.doi.org/10.1016/S0304-4017(96)01120-X

16. Marino, G., Gaglio, G., Zanghi, A. (2012). Clinicopathological study of canine transmissible venereal tumour in leishmaniotic dogs. J. Small Anim. Pract. 53, 323–327.
http://dx.doi.org/10.1111/j.1748-5827.2012.01201.x
PMid:22489831

17. Raghunath, M., Sudha Rani Chowdhary, Ch., Vidya Sagar, P., Ravi Kumar, P. (2015). Genital and extra genital TVT in a bitch- a case report. Sch J Agric Vet Sci. 2(1B): 61-62.

25

HEMATOLOGICAL AND BIOCHEMICAL PARAMETERS IN SYMPTOMATIC AND ASYMPTOMATIC LEISHMANIA-SEROPOSITIVE DOGS

Igor Ulchar[1], Irena Celeska[1], Jovana Stefanovska[2], Anastasija Jakimovska[1]

[1]Department of Pathophysiology, Faculty of Veterinary Medicine – Skopje, Ss Cyril and Methodius University, Skopje
[2]Department of Parasitology, Faculty of Veterinary Medicine – Skopje, Ss Cyril and Methodius University, Skopje

ABSTRACT

Leishmaniosis caused by *Leishmania infantum* is vector-born severe enzootic disease in dogs. It includes a wide spectrum of clinical symptoms, but the most characteristic are alterations in the hematopoetic system and renal failure. Also, infected animals could be asymptomatic, so the manifestation of *L. infantum* infection depends on many factors, including host's immunological status. The aim of this survey was to find parameters related with hematopoetic and renal failure (hematology, biochemical parameters – urea, creatinine, serum proteins) in symptomatic and asymptomatic dogs seropositive for canine leishmaniosis. Within the hematological parameters, we found significant differences between symptomatic and asymptomatic dogs in the erythrogram and platelet count, but not in the leukogram. Significant differences between the two groups were found also for urea, creatinine, serum albumin and globulin, but not in serum total protein and A/G ratio. These findings indicate individual variability of the host's response to infection with *L. infantum*.

Key words: leishmaniosis, dog, hematology, biochemistry

INTRODUCTION

Canine leishmaniosis (CanL) is a disease caused by an intracellular protozoan of the genus *Leishmania* that is transmitted to the dog by the bite of some species of the bloodsucking sand flies from the genera *Phlebotomus* in Europe and Asia and *Lutzomyia* in Central and South America (1, 2, 3). The life cycle of *Leishmania* parasite is biphasic with two morphological stages known as promastigotes and amasitgotes. Procyclic promastigotes are attached to the midgut epitehelial cells of *Phlebotomus* or *Lytzomia* female sandflyes, where after replication they differentiate into an infective metacyclic form in the anterior midgut. They are inoculated into the mammalian host by bloodsucking where they transform into amastigotes in macrophages and related cells (4, 5).

The most important species for the dogs is *L. infantum* in the Old World which is synonymous to *L. chagasi* in Central and South America (1). Dogs are considered the main reservoir of *L. infantum* for humans (6). CanL is one of the major zoonoses globally causing severe fatal disease in humans. Clinical manifestation of canine leishmaniosis includes a wide spectrum of clinical symptoms, which in dogs ranges from absence of symptoms to generalized disorders that may result in the host death: fever, anemia, lymphadenopathy, weight loss, emaciation, hepatosplenomegaly, conjunctivitis, renal alterations, keratitis, onychogryphosis and cutaneous lesions (1, 3, 7, 8, 9). Some other organs and systems could also be involved, like heart (10), testis (11), joints (12), liver (13, 14) and brain (7). *L. infantum* is also found in the gastrointestinal system (15, 16), including tongue (17).

Corresponding author: Prof. Igor Ulchar, PhD
E-mail address: iulcar@fvm.ukim.edu.mk
Present address: Faculty of Veterinary Medicine – Skopje
Ss Cyril and Methodius University, Skopje
Lazar Pop-Trajkov 5/7, 1000 Skopje, R. of Macedonia

Leishmania is able to evade the host's non-specific defenses (phagocytosis) to survive and multiply in the macrophage. The progress of the infection depends on the efficiency of the host's immune response. There are two defense effector mechanisms which take part against *Leishmania* parasites: the first one is the release of superoxide (O_2^-) by the neutrophils and macrophages via the NADPH oxidase complex (18), and the second one is the parasiticidal effect of nitric oxide (NO), mediated by interferon (IFN-γ) and tumor necrosis factor (TNF-α) released by macrophages (1, 8, 18, 19, 20, 21, 22). The opposite effect is disease susceptibility manifested with depressed cell mediated immunity with a mixed Th1 and Th2 cytokines response (1, 18). These cytokines are transforming growth factor (TGF-β), IL-10 (18) and iron regulatory protein 2 (IRP2) (22). Affected animals could show decreased antioxidant enzyme activity (23).

The majority of dogs infected with *Leishmania* do not always develop clinical signs (1). Furthermore, seropositivity absence does not prove that a dog is negative for *Leishmania*, because clinically healthy infected dogs could be negative for anti-*Leishmania* antibodies, but positive for *Leishmania* by PCR protocols (24, 25). This fact confirms the importance of asymptomatic dogs with *Leishmania*, because they obviously play a role in the transmission of *Leishmania* parasites. It remains unclear what are the reasons which make one dog resistible or susceptible to the disease. The clinical manifestation of CanL is complex, with many factors involved (age, gender, nutrition, host genetics, coinfections and/or concomitant disease, immunosuppressive conditions, etc.) (1).

As mentioned above, CanL has very variable clinical manifestations, and many different organs could be involved. For this reason, some laboratory tests are necessary for confirming the diagnosis, among them the complete blood count (CBC) and biochemical profile, especially for evaluation of the renal function. The most important and constant hematological change in cases of canine visceral leishmaniosis is non-regenerative anemia (3, 24, 25). Leishmaniosis also causes changes in the white blood cell count (WBC) (3, 24, 25, 26) and thrombocytopenia (1) and even in the disseminated intravascular coagulation (DIC) (27). Another important finding related to CanL is hyperproteinemia, hypoalbuminemia, and decreased albumin/globulin ratio (1, 3, 8, 26). The severe form of CanL is characterized by renal damage with glomerulonephritis due to immune complex deposition, but there are findings which propose

involvement of some other mechanisms too, like migration of T cells into the glomeruli, participation of adhesion molecules, and diminished apoptosis of cells (28). The antibodies involved in the formation of these immune complexes are unknown, although antiactin and antitubulin antibodies are found in dogs with CanL caused by *L. donovani* (29). Renal dysfunction could be the only clinical manifestation of the CanL and immunoinduced glomerulonephritis could progress into chronic renal failure (CRF), which is the principal cause of animal death in CanL (1). So, it is very important for renal disease to be diagnosed early, because it allows better prognosis for the patient and may prolong its life. Despite the high prevalence of renal involvement in the pathogenesis of CanL, azotemia which is typical for renal failure is evident only when the majority of nephrons have become dysfunctional in the final phase of the disease progression.

Majority of the reports are dealing with the seroprevalence of *L. infantum* in dog population (30, 31, 32), while it still remains unclear how the biochemical and hematological status of dogs naturally infected with CanL can be associated with the clinical forms of CanL. The aim of this study was to find some of these parameters: erythrogram, leukogram, biochemical parameters associated with renal function and biochemical parameters associated with plasma protein status in symptomatic and asymptomatic dogs seropositive for CanL.

MATERIAL AND METHODS

This survey was done on a heterogeneous dog population, which included dogs from different breeds and mongrel dogs, with age ranging from 1.5 to 12 years. All investigated dogs were seropositive for CanL, which was confirmed with an indirect fluorescent antibody test (IFAT) (Figure 1). IFAT was performed according to the OIE manual (33). Promastigotes of *L. infatnum* (zymodem MON-1 9MCAN/HR/2003/LLM-1282) isolated from a dog were used for preparation of "in house" antigen. Parasites were fixed with acetone on IFAT slides (according the procedure described in OIE manual) and dog's serums were tested at starting dilution of 1:40, using FITC labeled goat anti-canine IgG (H+L) (Southern Biotech, USA). Based on the previous experiences a titer of 1:80 was considered as positive. Commercial positive and negative control serums (VMRD, cat no. 211-P-LSH and 211-N-LSH) were used for verification of the test results.

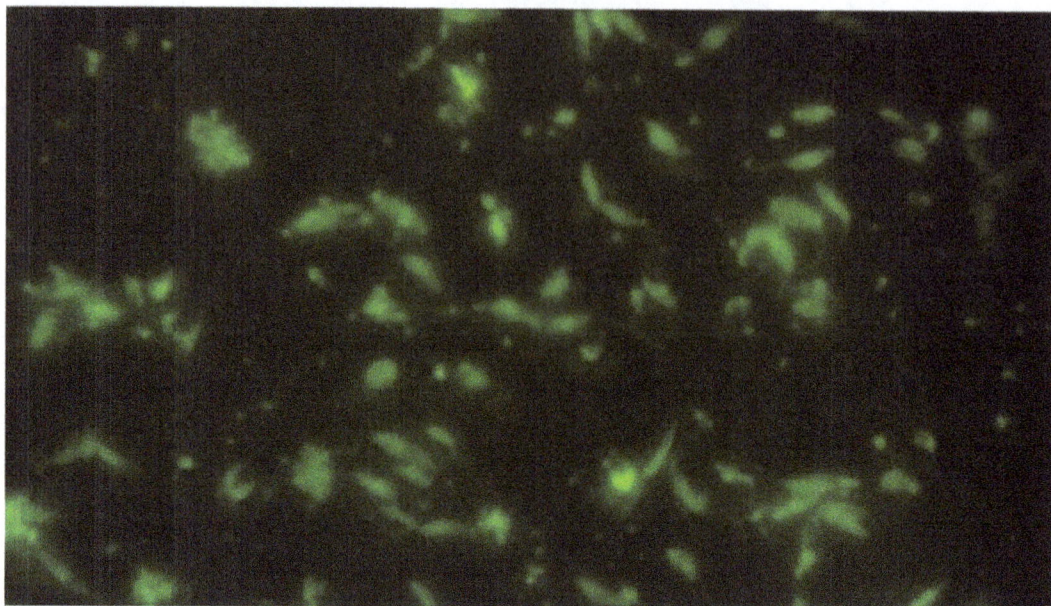

Figure 1. IFAT positive slide (promastigotes with the whole body fluorescence)

There were two groups: one manifesting clinical signs of the disease (symptomatic dogs - SD), and the other group which were dogs infected with *L. infantum*, but without clinical signs of leishmaniasis (asymptomatic dogs - AD). The survey included 42 dogs in total, 21 in the symptomatic and 21 in the asymptomatic group, respectively. Dogs were classified as symptomatic when manifesting at least one of the clinical symptoms classified by Solano-Gallego et al. (2011) (34).

Hemogram analyses included the following parameters: red blood cell count (RBC), hematocrit, hemoglobin concentration, mean corpuscular volume (MCV), mean corpuscular hemoglobin (MCH), mean corpuscular hemoglobin concentration (MCHC), white blood cell count (WBC) and platelet count. Biochemical parameters investigated in this survey where those related with renal function (urea and creatinine), and protein status (total protein – TP, albumin – ALB, globulin – GLO and albumin/globulin ratio – A/G), respectively. IFAT test was done at the Laboratory of Parasitology, and hemogram and biochemical parameters testing were done at the Laboratory of Hematology and Clinical Biochemistry, within the Faculty of Veterinary Medicine in Skopje.

Blood samples for laboratory analysis were collected from V. cephalica antebrachii externa. Samples for hematology testing were taken in VACUETTE® EDTA Tubes (Greiner Bio-One), coated with K_3EDTA and samples for biochemistry testing were taken VACUETTE® Serum Collection Tubes (Greiner Bio-One). Hematological parameters were analyzed on hematology counter SYSMEX 2200 (Germany), according to the standard operative procedure. Biochemical parameters were analyzed on semiautomatic photometer STAT FAX 3300 (Awareness Technology, Inc. USA), Analyses of urea and creatinine were made with standard colorimetric kinetic methods, using commercial kits from Human (Germany), according to the International Federation of Clinical Chemistry and Laboratory Medicine (IFCC) propositions. Analyses of total protein and albumin were made with standard colorimetric biochemical "end-point" methods, also with commercial kits from Human (Germany). Globulin values were estimated using the difference between total protein value and albumin value.

Statistical analysis of gained data included descriptive statistics (mean - M; standard deviation - SD; standard error - SE; minimum and maximum - Min-Max; coefficient of variation - CV) and Student t-test for evaluation of statistical significance of variables' means. Statistical operations were made with STATISTICA for Windows 8.0 (Stat Soft Inc) software.

RESULTS

The values of hematological parameters for both groups of dogs (AD and SD) are shown in Table 1.

Table 1. Hematological parameters: red blood cell count (RBC/10^{12}/L), hematocrit (HCT/%), hemoglobin (HGB/g/dL), MCV (fL), MCH (pg), MCHC (g/dL), white blood cell count (WBC/10^9/L) and platelet count (PLT/10^9/L) in asymptomatic and symptomatic dogs infected with *L. infantum*

	asymptomatic dogs (AD)				symptomatic dogs (SD)			
	M±SD	SE	Min-Max	CV	M±SD	SE	Min-Max	CV
RBC	6.87 ± 0.81*	0.17	5.52-8.32	11.89	4.44 ± 1.72*	0.37	1.73-8.23	38.81
HCT	43.22 ± 6.68*	1.45	29.40-55.40	15.45	29.95 ± 12.29*	2.68	9.20-56.70	41.04
HGB	16.05 ± 2.37*	0.51	11.90-20.80	14.77	10.09 ± 3.75*	0.81	3.90-18.10	37.16
MCV	62.88 ± 6.57	1.43	52.30-74.10	10.44	66.83 ± 6.65	1.45	52.90-75.40	9.95
MCH	23.33 ± 1.76	0.38	19.80-26.60	7.56	22.63 ± 1.17	0.25	21.10-26.00	5.21
MCHC	37.56 ± 5.05	1.10	30.50-44.30	13.45	34.85 ± 3.87	0.84	29.90-42.70	11.12
WBC	13.46 ± 5.25	1.14	5.90-25.20	39.04	11.96 ± 7.91	1.72	3.60-38.20	66.12
PLT	288.80 ± 98.64*	21.52	121.0-598.0	34.15	194.14 ± 151.41*	33.04	3.0-605.0	77.99

* Differences considered as statistically significant for p values < 0.05

As shown in Table 1, statistically significant differences are found for values of RBC, HCT, HGB and PLT, i.e. asymptomatic dogs had these parameters significantly higher than symptomatic dogs.

The values of biochemical parameters for both groups of dogs (AD and SD) are shown in Table 2.

As shown in Table 2, the values of urea, creatinine and globulin are significantly higher, and values of albumin are significantly lower in symptomatic dogs, compared with those in group of asymptomatic dogs.

DISCUSSION

As mentioned above, CanL is a disease with a very variable and complex clinical manifestation, where many different factors are involved. Infection itself does not always cause clinical disease, which is evident in the fact that prevalence of CanL in the endemic regions is lower than 10% (1). Whether the infected animal would remain resistible or a development of clinical disease would occur, depends on many factors, but most important is the immune status of the animal. So, the asymptomatic dogs infected with *L. infantum* are very important as a reservoir of the parasite. Although the clinical symptoms of CanL are very variable, major disorders are related to the hematopoietic system and renal function.

Our findings of RBC value in asymptomatic dogs indicate an equilibrium of erythropoiesis and erythrocyte destruction. The opposite finding was recorded in the group of symptomatic dogs, where the average RBC value was significantly lower (p < 0.05), which indicates occurrence of mild to

Table 2. Biochemical parameters: urea (mmol/L), creatinine (μmol/L), total protein (TP/g/L), albumin (ALB/g/L), globulin (GLO/g/L) and albumin/globulin ratio (A/G) in asymptomatic and symptomatic dogs infected with *L. infantum*

	asymptomatic dogs (AD)				symptomatic dogs (SD)			
	M±SD	SE	Min-Max	CV	M±SD	SE	Min-Max	CV
urea	3.91 ±1.97*	0.43	1.03-9.40	50.44	16.19 ± 22.90*	4.99	0.96-81.20	141.40
creatinine	89.43 ± 26.43*	5.76	8.10-137.00	29.55	228.44 ± 302.34*	65.97	54.00-1341.00	132.34
TP	69.64 ±14.57	3.18	36.40-99.20	20.92	76.07 ± 23.34	5.09	32.00-119.00	30.68
ALB	29.00 ± 6.80*	1.48	18.70-45.90	23.47	22.03 ± 5.70*	1.24	11.40-35.40	25.87
GLO	40.64 ± 15.39*	3.35	7.70-80.50	37.86	54.04 ± 23.05*	5.03	9.00-93.00	42.65
A/G	0.9 ± 0.72	0.16	0.2-3.7	125	0.6 ± 0.53	0.12	0.2-2.5	113.2

* Differences considered as statistically significant for p values < 0.05

severe anemia, which could be a result of decreased erythropoiesis or increased hemolysis. This is also confirmed with high CV (38.81%) in symptomatic dogs, which shows heterogeneity of symptomatic group, where the severity of anemia depends on the individual degree of affection of bone marrow. Values of MCV, MCH and MCHC did not show statistical significant difference between the two groups, which indicates the occurrence of non-regenerative normocytic normochromic anemia, as found by other authors (3, 24, 25). Infection with *L. infantum* causes normocytic normochromic anemia (8), but anemia caused with *L. donovani* complex is normocytic hypochromic (3). The non-regenerative anemia accompanying CanL is commonly explained as a consequence of chronic renal failure (CRF), but there are also findings which suggest that the decrease of erythrocytes in peripheral blood could be result of direct damage of the erythrocytes done by the parasite (3) or result of bone marrow dysfunction (3, 25, 31, 35, 36).

Hematocrit (HCT) as a marker of organism hydratation degree showed statistically significant difference between two groups (p < 0.05). In asymptomatic dogs high value of hematocrit indicated normal water balance regulatory mechanisms, so dehydratation does not occur. In symptomatic dogs HCT was significantly lower, which is confirmed also by other authors (25). HCT decrease could be result of hemodilution, caused by decreased erythropoiesis and/or increased hemolysis, from one side, or it could be due to polydipsia, caused by high blood urea level (urea is substance with high osmolarity). Here the heterogeneity of the group is also seen, with high value of CV (41.04%).

Hemoglobin (HGB) value was also significantly higher in asymptomatic, compared with symptomatic dogs, which is also in accordance with other surveys (25) and this finding shows difference in hemoglobin synthesis capacity in bone marrow. In asymptomatic dogs low CV (14.77%) shows homogeneity of the group. In symptomatic dogs decreased HGB level could be explained with bone marrow dysfunction, due to high parasite load in bone marrow, or by decreased secretion of erythropoietin, caused by chronic renal failure. Here heterogeneity is also obvious, as CV is 37.16%.

White blood cell count (WBC) did not show statistically significant difference between asymptomatic and symptomatic group, although the WBC value of the latter was insignificantly lower. Minimum-maximum range in asymptomatic dogs was very wide, probably as a result of increase of plasmocyte fraction, responsible for occurrence of polyclonal beta and gamma hyperglobulinemia,

which is evident in seropositive dogs with clinical manifestation of CanL (1). Depending on clinical symptoms, in the symptomatic group which was quite heterogenic (CV 66.12%), WBC value ranged from leukopenia, probably because of depletion of white blood cells precursors in bone marrow, to leukocytosis, in accordance with some authors (1). This leukocytosis could be result of concurrent infection with other organism from viral, bacterial (report of concurrent infection with *Streptococcus equisimilis* (37) or parasite origin (*Erlichia canis* as most common (38)). In our study average WBC value in the symptomatic group was insignificantly lower compared with asymptomatic dogs, which differs from findings reported by other authors concerning infection with *L. infantum*, where crucial signs of severe CanL are eosinopenia, lymphopenia and monocytopenia (24, 25, 26), but is similar with those which concerned infection with *L. donovani* complex where total leukocyte count was found normal (3).

Thrombocytopenia is a common hematological finding in dogs affected with CanL (1), as it was also evident in our survey. Possible causes of this disorder are platelet sequestration, platelet consumption during clotting process, decreased or impaired production of megacariocytes and platelets, as well as immuno-mediated process.

Available data about urea and creatinine values in blood during CanL are controversial. In one survey with dogs infected with *L. donovani* complex only urea, but not creatinine was increased, indicating no renal dysfunction and this was evident only in 22.72% of dogs included in the survey (3). In another survey with dogs infected with *L. infantum* the finding was inverse: creatinine, but not urea was increased (26). In our survey blood urea in symptomatic dogs was significantly higher than in the asymptomatic group (p < 0.05), and its average value was very high, beyond the referent maximum. Uremia is considered as an indicator of a late stage of severe CanL, when CRF occurs (1). This CRF is caused by immunoinduced glomerulonephritis. The extremely high CV (141.40%) indicates again heterogeneity of the symptomatic group, where renal failure ranged from mild to severe. In asymptomatic dogs, minimum-maximum range indicates absence of renal dysfunction.

Analogous findings were obtained also for creatinine. Synthesis of creatinine in muscle tissue is relatively constant and in proportion with muscle mass, so significantly higher blood level of creatinine in symptomatic dogs (p<0.05) indicates decreased renal excretion of creatinine. High CV (132.34%) indicates heterogeneity of symptomatic group, and its maximum of 1341.00 µmol/L shows some degree of simultaneous muscle dystrophy, which could contribute to the development of CRF. In the asymptomatic group, the serum level of creatinine and its minimum-maximum range indicate regular protein catabolism and normal glomerular filtration rate (GFR).

Although most of the authors (1, 3, 8, 26) consider hyperproteinemia as important finding in CanL, in our survey the symptomatic dogs had higher serum total protein level compared with the asymptomatic group, but this difference was insignificant. In both groups the minimum-maximum range was within referent values, and CV was low. Also, albumin/globulin ratio (A/G) was found decreased in symptomatic dogs, but this decreasing was statistically insignificant. Both groups had high CV for A/G value (125 for asymptomatic and 113.2 for symptomatic dogs, respectively), which indicates heterogeneity of each group.

However, serum albumin level in symptomatic dogs was significantly lower compared with the symptomatic group ($p < 0.05$), which is in accordance with other authors' findings (1, 3, 8, 26). Normoalbuminemia found in asymptomatic dogs indicates normal protein anabolism and catabolism balance, normal hepatic function and albumin synthesis, and normal renal function, i.e. absence of albumin loss with urine (albuminuria). In symptomatic dogs evident hypoabluminemia is due to renal dysfunction, as well as the consequential albuminuria.

Changes in serum globulin in our survey are analogous to those of serum albumin. Symptomatic dogs showed significant hyperglobulinemia, which is in accordance with findings of other authors (1, 3, 8, 26). This hyperglobulinemia is probably caused by polyclonal beta or gamma hyperglobulinemia. Both groups showed high CV (37.86% in asymptomatic and 42.65 in symptomatic dogs, respectively), which indicates heterogeneity of the immune response of the animal.

As mentioned above, most of the parameters investigated in this survey had high CV in symptomatic dogs, which suggest the heterogeneity of this group. This heterogeneity is also evident in the fact that there were no correlations found between the values of hematological and biochemical parameters.

CONCLUSION

Canine visceral leishmaniosis in the host's organism primarily affects the immune system and depending on the clinical manifestation, thed isease has an impact on thehematological and biochemical status of the animal. The pattern of host's reaction, whether asymptomatic or symptomatic with certain clinical manifestations, depends on the individual immune response. According to our findings, it could be concluded that the clinical manifestation of CanL has an impact on the erythrogram values, i.e. there is a significant difference in the erythrogram between symptomatic and asymptomatic dogs. On the other side, we found that the leukogram could not be a relevant indicator for the disease clinical progression degree in symptomatic and asymptomatic dogs seropositive for *L. infantum*. Biochemical parameters related to the renal function (urea, creatinine) could be used in making prognosis of progressed clinical leishmaniosis. The degree of proteinemia in seropositive asymptomatic and symptomatic dogs could be taken as an indicator of clinical progression of CanL only in cases of significant hyperglobulinemia. There were no correlations found between the values of hematological and biochemical parameters, which indicates individual variability of the host's response to infection with *L. infantum*.

REFERENCES

1. Solano-Gallego, L., Koutinas, A., Miró, G., Cardoso, L., Pennisi, M.G., Ferrer, L., Bourdeau, P., Oliva, G., Baneth, G. (2009). Directions for the diagnosis, clinical staging, treatment and prevention of canine leishmaniosis. Veterinary Parasitology 165, 1–18. http://dx.doi.org/10.1016/j.vetpar.2009.05.022 PMid:19559536

2. Gonçalves, R., Vieira, E.R., Melo, M.N, Gollob, K.J., Mosser, D.M, Tafuri, W.L. (2005). A sensitive flow cytometric methodology for studying the binding of *L. chagasi* to canine peritoneal macrophages. BMC Infectious Diseases, 5, 39. http://dx.doi.org/10.1186/1471-2334-5-39 PMid:15913461 PMCid:PMC1166554

3. Dias, E.L., Batista, Z.S., Guerra, R.M.S.N.C., Calabrese, K.S., Lima, T.B., Abreu-Silva, A.L. (2008). Canine Visceral *Leishmaniosis* (CVL): Seroprevalence, clinical, hematological and biochemical findings of dogs naturally infected in an endemic area of São José de Ribamar Municipality, Maranhão State, Brazil. Ciência animal brasileira, 9(3): 740-745.

4. Bates, P.A. (2007). Transmission of *Leishmania* metacyclic promastigotes by phlebotomine sand flies. Int J Parasitol. 37 (10-3): 1097–1106. http://dx.doi.org/10.1016/j.ijpara.2007.04.003 PMid:17517415 PMCid:PMC2675784

5. Dostálová, A, Volf, P. (2012). *Leishmania* development in sand flies: parasite-vector interactions overview. Parasites & Vectors 5, 276. http://dx.doi.org/10.1186/1756-3305-5-276 PMid:23206339 PMCid:PMC3533922

6. Gramiccia, M., Gradoni, L. (2005). The current status of zoonotic leishmaniases and approaches to disease control. Int J Parasitol. 35, 1169-1180. http://dx.doi.org/10.1016/j.ijpara.2005.07.001 PMid:16162348

7. Sakamoto, K.P., de Melo, G.D., Machado, G.F. (2013). T and B lymphocytes in the brains of dogs with concomitant seropositivity to three pathogenic protozoans: *Leishmania chagasi, Toxoplasma gondii* and *Neospora caninum*. BMC Research Notes 6, 226. http://dx.doi.org/10.1186/1756-0500-6-226 PMid:23758819 PMCid:PMC3701587

8. Sanches, F.P., Tomokane, T.Y, Da Matta, V.L.R., Marcondes, M., Corbett, C.E.P., Laurenti, M.D. (2014). Expression of inducible nitric oxide synthase in macrophages inversely correlates with parasitism of lymphoid tissues in dogs with visceral leishmaniosis. Acta Vet. Scand. 56, 57. http://dx.doi.org/10.1186/s13028-014-0057-z PMid:25195062 PMCid:PMC4172852

9. Verçosa, B.L.A., Lemos, C.M., Mendonça, I.L., Silva, S.M.M.S., de Carvalho, S.M., Goto, H., Costa, F.A.L. (2008). Transmission potential, skin inflammatory response, and parasitism of symptomatic and asymptomatic dogs with visceral leishmaniosis. BMC Veterinary Research 4, 45. http://dx.doi.org/10.1186/1746-6148-4-45 PMid:18990238 PMCid:PMC2613136

10. López-Peña, M., Alemañ, N., Muñoz, F., Fondevila, D., Suárez, M.L., Goicoa, A., Nieto, J.M. (2009). Visceral leishmaniosis with cardiac involvement in a dog: a case report. Acta Vet. Scand., 51, 20. http://dx.doi.org/10.1186/1751-0147-51-20 PMid:19405946 PMCid:PMC2679027

11. Manna, L., Paciello, O., Della Morte, R., Gravino, A.E. (2012). Detection of *Leishmania* parasites in the testis of a dog affected by orchitis: case report. Parasit Vectors 5, 216. http://dx.doi.org/10.1186/1756-3305-5-216 PMid:23021706 PMCid:PMC3481428

12. McConkey, S.E., López, A., Shaw, D., Calder, J. (2002). Leishmanial polyarthritis in a dog. Can Vet J., 43 (8): 607-609. PMid:12170836 PMCid:PMC339396

13. Melo, F.A., Moura, E.P., Ribeiro, R.R, Alves, C.F., Caliari, M.V., Tafuri, W.L., Calabrese, K.S., Tafuri, W.L. (2009). Hepatic extracellular matrix alterations in dogs naturally infected with *Leishmania (Leishmania) chagasi*. Int. J. Exp. Path. 90 (5): 538-548. http://dx.doi.org/10.1111/j.1365-2613.2009.00681.x PMid:19765108 PMCid:PMC2768152

14. Silva, L.C., Castro, R.S, Figueiredo, M.M., Michalick, M.S.M., Tafuri, W.L., Tafuri, W.L. (2013). Canine visceral leishmaniosis as a systemic fibrotic disease. Int. J. Exp. Path. 94 (2): 133-143. http://dx.doi.org/10.1111/iep.12010 PMid:23419132 PMCid:PMC3607142

15. Figueiredo, M.M., Deoti, B., Amorim, I.F., Pinto, A.J.W., Moraes, A., Carvalho, C.S., da Silva, S.M., de Assis, A.C. B., de Faria, A.M.C., Tafuri, W.L. (2014). Expression of regulatory T cells in jejunum, colon, and cervical and mesenteric lymph nodes of dogs naturally infected with *Leishmania infantum*. Infect Immun., 82 (9): 3704-3712. http://dx.doi.org/10.1128/IAI.01862-14 PMid:24935975 PMCid:PMC4187817

16. Pinto, A.J.W., Figueiredo, M.M., Silva, F.L., Martins, T., Michalick, M.S.M., Tafuri, W.L., Tafuri, W.L. (2011). Histopathological and parasitological study of the gastrointestinal tract of dogs naturally infected with *Leishmania infantum*. Acta Vet Scand, 53, 67. http://dx.doi.org/10.1186/1751-0147-53-67 PMid:22166041 PMCid:PMC3269393

17. Viegas, C., Requicha, J., Albuquerque, C., Sargo T., Machado J., Dias I., Pires, M.A., Campino, L., Cardoso, L. (2012). Tongue nodules in canine leishmaniosis – a case report. Parasit Vectors 5, 120. http://dx.doi.org/10.1186/1756-3305-5-120 PMid:22704596 PMCid:PMC3407507

18. Bogdan, C., Röllinghoff, M. (1998). The immune response to *Leishmania*: mechanisms of parasite control and evasion. Int J Parasitol, 28 (1): 121-134. http://dx.doi.org/10.1016/S0020-7519(97)00169-0

19. Loría-Cervera, E.N., Andrade-Narváez, F.J. (2014). Animal Models for the Study of Leishmaniosis Immunology. Rev. Inst. Med. Trop. Sao Paulo, 56 (1): 1-11. http://dx.doi.org/10.1590/S0036-46652014000100001 PMid:24553602 PMCid:PMC4085833

20. Pinelli, E., Killick-Kendrick, R., Wagenaar, J., Bernadina, W., del Real, G., Ruitenberg, J. (1994). Cellular and humoral immune responses in dogs experimentally and naturally infected with *Leishmania infantum*. Infect Immun., 62 (1): 229-235. PMid:8262632 PMCid:PMC186091

21. Pinelli, E., Rutten, V.P.M.G., Bruysters, M., Moore, P.F., Ruitenberg, E.J. (1999). Compensation for decreased expression of B7 molecules on *Leishmania infantum*-infected canine macrophages results in restoration of parasite-specific T-cell proliferation and gamma interferon production. Infect Immun., 67 (1): 237-243. PMid:9864221 PMCid:PMC96302

22. do Nascimento, P.R.P., Martins, D.R.A., Monteiro, G.R.G., Queiroz, P.V., Freire-Neto, F.P., Queiroz, J.W., Lima, Á.L.M., Jeronimo, S.M.B. (2013). Association of pro-inflammatory cytokines and iron regulatory protein 2 (IRP2) with *Leishmania* burden in canine visceral leishmaniosis. PLoS One 8(10): e73873. http://dx.doi.org/10.1371/journal.pone.0073873

23. Souza, C.C., Barreto, T.O., da Silva, S.M., Pinto, A.W. J., Figueiredo, M.M., Rocha, O.G.F., Cangussú, S.D., Tafuri, W.L. (2014). A potential link among antioxidant enzymes, histopathology and trace elements in canine visceral leishmaniosis. Int. J. Exp. Path., 95 (4): 260-270.
http://dx.doi.org/10.1111/iep.12080
PMid:24766461 PMCid:PMC4170968

24. Coura-Vital, W., Marques, M.J., Giunchetti, R.C., Teixeira-Carvalho, A., Moreira, N.D., Vitoriano-Souza, J., Vieira, P.M., Carneiro, C.M., Corrêa-Oliveira, R., Martins-Filho, O.A., Carneiro, M., Reis, A.B. (2011). Humoral and cellular immune responses in dogs with inapparent natural *Leishmania infantum* infection. Vet J. 190 (2), e43-e47.
http://dx.doi.org/10.1016/j.tvjl.2011.04.005
PMid:21596598

25. Nicolato, R.deC., de Abreu, R.T., Roatt, B.M., Aguiar-Soares, R.D.O., Reis, L.E.S., Carvalho, M.G., Carneiro, C.M., Giunchetti, R.C., Bouillet, L.E.M., Lemos, D.S, Coura-Vital, W., Reis, A.B. (2013). Clinical forms of canine visceral leishmaniosis in naturally leishmania infantum-infected dogs and related myelogram and hemogram changes. PLoS One. 8 (12): e82947.
http://dx.doi.org/10.1371/journal.pone.0082947

26. Kargin Kiral, F., Seyrek, K., Pasa, S., Ertabaklar, H., Ünsal, C. (2004). Some haematological, biochemical and electrophoretic findings in dogs with visceral leishmaniosis. Revue Méd. Vét., 155 (4): 226-229.

27. Honse, C.O., Figueiredo, F.B., de Alencar, N.X., Madeira, M.deF., Gremião, I.D.F, Schubach, T.M.P. (2013). Disseminated intravascular coagulation in a dog naturally infected by *Leishmania* (*Leishmania*) *chagas*i from Rio de Janeiro – Brazil. BMC Veterinary Research 9, 43.
http://dx.doi.org/10.1186/1746-6148-9-43
PMid:23497531 PMCid:PMC3599858

28. Costa, F.A.L., Prianti, M.G., Silva, T.C., Silva, S.M.M.S., Guerra, J.L., Goto, H. (2010). T cells,tadhesion molecules and modulation of apoptosis in visceral leishmaniosis glomerulonephritis. BMC Infect Dis., 10, 112.
http://dx.doi.org/10.1186/1471-2334-10-112

29. Pateraki, E., Portocala, R., Labrousse, H., Guesdon, J.-L. (1983). Antiactin and antitubulin antibodies in canine visceral leishmaniosis. Infect Immun. 42 (2): 496-500.
PMid:6642639 PMCid:PMC264456

30. Menn, B., Lorentz, S., Naucke, T.J. (2010). Imported and travelling dogs as carriers of canine vector-borne pathogens in Germany. Parasit Vectors, 3, 34.
http://dx.doi.org/10.1186/1756-3305-3-34
PMid:20377872 PMCid:PMC2857866

31. Momo, C., Jacintho, A.P.P., Moreira, P.R.R., Munari, D.P., Machado, G.F., Vasconcelos, R.deO. (2014). Morphological changes in the bone marrow of the dogs with visceral leishmaniosis. Vet Med Int., 150582.
http://dx.doi.org/10.1155/2014/150582
PMid:24744957 PMCid:PMC3972870

32. Živičnjak, T., Martinković, F., Marinculić, A., Mrljak, V., Kučer, N., Matijatko, V., Mihaljević, Ž., Barić-Rafaj, R. (2005). A seroepidemiologic survey of canine visceral leishmaniosis among apparently healthy dogs in Croatia. Vet Parasitol. 131 (1-2): 35-43.
http://dx.doi.org/10.1016/j.vetpar.2005.04.036
PMid:15946800

33. Office International des Epizooties (OIE) (2008). Manual of standards diagnostic tests and vaccines, Part 2, Section 2.2, Chapter 2.2.11.: Leishmaniosis.

34. Solano-Gallego, L., Miró, G., Koutinas, A., Cardoso, L., Pennisi, M.G., Ferrer, L., Bourdeau, P., Oliva, G., Baneth, G. (2011). LeishVet guidelines for the practical management of canine leishmaniosis. Parasites & Vectors 4, 86.
http://dx.doi.org/10.1186/1756-3305-4-86
PMid:21599936 PMCid:PMC3125381

35. Trópia de Abreu, R., Carvalho, M.dG., Carneiro, C.M., Giunchetti, R.C., Teixeira-Carvalho, A., Martins-Filho, O.A., Coura-Vital, W., Corrêa-Oliveira, R., Reis, A.B. (2011). Influence of clinical status and parasite load on erythropoiesis and leucopoiesis in dogs naturally infected with *Leishmania* (*Leishmania*) *chagasi*. PLoS ONE 6 (5): e18873.
http://dx.doi.org/10.1371/journal.pone.0018873

36. De Tommasi, A.S., Otranto, D., Furlanello, T., Tasca, S., Cantacessi, C., Breitschwerdt, E.B., Stanneck, D., Dantas-Torres, F., Baneth, G., Capelli, G., de Caprariis, D. (2014). Evaluation of blood and bone marrow in selected canine vector-borne diseases. Parasit Vectors. 7, 534.
http://dx.doi.org/10.1186/s13071-014-0534-2
PMid:25441458 PMCid:PMC4261574

37. Ramos-Vara, J.A., Briones, V., Segalés, J., Vilafranca, M., Sordé, A., Miller, M.A. (1994). Concurrent infection with *Streptococcus equisimilis* and *Leishmania* in a dog. J Vet Diagn Invest., 6 (3): 371-375.
http://dx.doi.org/10.1177/104063879400600317

38. Mekuzas, Y., Gradoni, L., Oliva, G., Foglia Manzillo, V., Baneth, G. (2009). *Ehrlichia canis* and *Leishmania infantum* co-infection: a 3-year longitudinal study in naturally exposed dogs. Clin Microbiol Infect., 15 (Suppl. 2): 30-31.
http://dx.doi.org/10.1111/j.1469-0691.2008.02150.x
PMid:19416288

26

ASSESSMENT OF THE EFFECT OF SELECTED COMPONENTS OF EQUINE SEMINAL PLASMA ON SEMEN FREEZABILITY

Miroslava Mráčková, Marta Zavadilová, Markéta Sedlinská

Department of Reproduction, Equine Clinic, Faculty of Veterinary Medicine, University of Veterinary and Pharmaceutical Sciences Brno, Brno, Czech Republic

ABSTRACT

In this study, selected components of seminal plasma in equine semen were evaluated. Levels of enzymes, electrolytes, microelements and some other components were observed. The aim of this study was to find some important differences between the levels of these components and the total sperm motility after freezing and thawing (freezability of the semen). Total of 32 ejaculates from 7 stallions were collected, assessed and prepared in 0,5 ml straws for freezing. After thawing, the sperm motility was analyzed and ejaculates were divided into two groups: "good" freezable and "poor" freezable. The only statistically significant difference between groups of „good" and „poor" freezable ejaculates was in the concentration of vitamin E in the seminal plasma. In the group of „good" freezable ejaculates, the level of vitamin E was significantly lower ($p \leq 0,05$) than in the group of "poor" freezable ejaculates.

Key words: stallion, seminal plasma, semen freezing, vitamin E

INTRODUCTION

Seminal plasma is a very important part of the ejaculate and it is involved in many sperm functions, especially in the metabolism and in events preceding fertilization. But nevertheless, the physiological role of seminal plasma and its components is still not fully understood (1). Also, the effect of seminal plasma on sperm during storage, freezing or cooling is not completely clear.

So far, not many studies about the components of seminal plasma and the freezability of the ejaculate have been conducted. Until now, studies in horses have not shown that it is possible to predict the freezability of semen based on the concentration of some enzymes, microelements (2), total protein or composition of the protein spectrum (3).

Corresponding author: Dr. Miroslava Mráčková, PhD
E-mail address: mrackovam@vfu.cz
Present address: Equine Clinic, University of Veterinary and Pharmaceutical Sciences Brno, Palackého tr. 1/3, 612 42 Brno, Czech Republic

However, questionable or different information is found in certain studies or in studies on other animal species (4).

MATERIAL AND METHODS

Animals and semen collection

In this experiment, 7 licensed stallions were used. The stallions represented various breeds and ranged in age from 4 to 16 years old. During the semen collection, animals were stabled and fed at the Equine Clinic, University of Veterinary and Pharmaceutical Sciences Brno. All of them were in good clinical status and used in breeding with normal fertility. From each stallion 1 to 11 ejaculates were collected, but only 32 ejaculates were used in this study. Four ejaculates were excluded because they did not meet some of the basic quality requirements for semen freezing (2x low percentage of motile sperm, 2x urospermia).

The ejaculates were collected routinely using the Missouri model artificial vagina while stallions were mounted on a dummy with teasing mare standing in front of the phantom.

Evaluation of collected semen

Following collection, each ejaculate was filtered with non-woven semen filter (Minitüb,

Germany) to remove the gel fraction. Overall 36 ejaculates were collected and evaluated. After filtration a macroscopic examination was done: volume, color, odor and viscosity were evaluated. In the microscopic evaluation total sperm motility, concentration and morphology were included. Total sperm motility was assessed by light microscope with phase contrast (enlargement 400x) by one person to eliminate the influence of different observers. Concentration was counted in a Burker chamber and morphology was examined at high power under immersion oil (enlargement 1000x) using Giemsa stain.

Semen processing and freezing

After the macroscopic evaluation of each ejaculate, samples for microscopic evaluation were taken and the ejaculate was centrifuged (1000 G for 10 minutes). Seminal plasma was collected using a sterile syringe and the sediment of the sperm was diluted with French diluent in the concentration of 800 x 10^6 sperm per ml. The diluted semen was transferred to 0,5 ml straws and after 2 hours of equilibration in a fridge (+4°C), it was frozen in liquid nitrogen.

Samples with seminal plasma were kept frozen in a freezer (-18°C) until analysis. After the gathering of all samples, the samples were thawed and examined in the Large Animal Clinical Laboratory at UVPS Brno.

For biochemical analysis, the spectrophotometry analyzer LIASYS (Analyzer Medical System, Italy) was used.

The concentration of microelements was measured by using flame atomic absorption spectrometry 3500 Atomic Absorption Spectrometer (Thermo Electron Corporation).

Evaluation of thawed semen

Frozen-thawed ejaculate was evaluated at least 24 hours after freezing. The straws were thawed in a water bath at 38,5 °C for 30 seconds. Total sperm motility was assessed in a light microscope with phase contrast (enlargement 400x) immediately after thawing, in every case by one person. The total sperm motility after thawing was always the criterion for the evaluation of freezability. Ejaculates were divided into two groups (A, B):

Group A:
Ejaculates with post-thaw sperm motility ≥35% were classified as „good" freezeble (n = 18).
Group B:
Ejaculates with post-thaw sperm motility <35 % were classified as "poor" freezable (n = 14).

Statistical evaluation

Results from group A and B were compared by a nonparametric Wilcoxon signed rank test for unpaired data. In cases where the result from the laboratory was disproportionately high or low, this result was not used in this study. If these extreme results were used, the overall result could be influenced and distorted by them.

RESULTS

Average values of basic parameters of ejaculates in both groups are shown in Table 1. The results of the measured selected parameters, which were monitored in the seminal plasma, are arranged in Table 2. Two parameters which were monitored, but not shown in the table, are cholesterol and vitamin A. In all samples the level of these parameters was zero.

Table 1. Average values of basic parameters of ejaculates in groups A and B (Motility II: motility after thawing)

	Group A (ejaculates with post-thaw motility ≥ 35 %)	Group B (ejaculates with post-thaw motility < 35 %)
	Mean ± SD	Mean ± SD
Volume (without gel fraction) (ml)	68,9±28,36	65,9±46,06
Motility after collection (%)	73,4±5,77	61,4±9,90
Sperm concentration (x10^6/mm^3)	123,6±80,54	129,1±108,74
Morphologically abnormal sperm (%)	28,0±5,88	33,1±13,52
Motility II (%)	41,7±7,07	19,1±12,92
Sperm concentration after thawing (x10^6/mm^3)	889,6±319,90	730,1±361,76
Morphologically abnormal sperm after thawing (%)	32,6±5,88	33,4±13,45

After the statistical analysis of both groups of ejaculates, the only significant difference ($p \leq 0,05$) was in the concentration of vitamin E in the seminal plasma. In the group of ejaculates where motility after thawing was $\geq 35\%$, concentration of vitamin E was significantly lower ($p \leq 0,05$) than in the group of ejaculates with motility $< 35\%$ after thawing.

In this study we tried to find differences in the composition of seminal plasma between „good" and „poor" freezable ejaculates in stallions. The only monitored parameter: vitamin E showed statistically significant differences ($p \leq 0,05$) between the two groups listed above. It is interesting that higher levels of vitamin E were found in the group of „poor"

Table 2. Average values of selected biochemical parameters of ejaculates in groups A and B

Monitored parameter	Group A (ejaculates with post-thaw motility $\geq 35\%$)		Group B (ejaculates with post-thaw motility $< 35\%$)	
	n	Mean±SD	n	Mean±SD
Total protein (g/l)	18	5,9±2,99	14	7,7±4,67
Creatinine (μmol/l)	18	54,3±19,42	13	53,2±21,23
Urea (mmol/l)	18	6,7±0,91	14	6,2±1,26
Alkaline phosphatase (ALP) (μkat/l)	13	65,9±28,96	8	56,4±38,29
Alanine amino-transferase (ALT) (μkat/l)	18	0,2±0,06	14	0,2±0,08
Aspartate-amino-transferase (AST) (μkat/l)	18	0,9±0,81	14	0,9±0,51
Creatinekinase (CK) (μkat/l)	13	2,1±1,56	13	2,2±1,13
Gama-glutamyl-transferase (GMT) (μkat/l)	11	54,6±14,61	6	47,7±18,74
Lactate-dehydrogenase (LDH) (μkat/l)	10	0,5±0,31	9	0,6±0,25
Na^+ (mmol/l)	18	109,6±17,97	14	109,1±20,49
K^+ (mmol/l)	18	21,9±5,77	14	24,5±10,55
Ca (mmol/l)	17	2,3±0,80	12	1,7±1,23
P (mmol/l)	18	0,7±0,44	13	0,8±0,45
Cl (mmol/l)	18	124,7±17,15	14	117,2±17,00
ZnS (μg/l)	18	4,8±2,02	12	4,9±2,29
Cu (μg/l)	17	4,1±2,17	12	5,2±3,11
Mg (μg/l)	18	1,8±0,94	14	1,3±0,63
Se (μg/l)	17	5,7±3,69	13	6,5±3,43
Vitamin E (mmol/l)	18	0,015±0,0269[*]	14	0,068±0,0720[*]

[*] $p \leq 0,05$

DISCUSSION

The results of some studies show that seminal plasma negatively affects sperm during short term and also long term storage (5-7). Some other studies denote that in humans (8), and also in stallions (9-11) the presence or adding specific amounts of seminal plasma before storage seems to improve sperm motility during cooled storage and also after thawing. However, the effect of seminal plasma differs significantly between individual stallions (12, 13).

freezable ejaculates (mean 68 μmol/l), while in the group of „good" freezable ejaculates the mean value of vitamin E was only 15 μmol/l. During semen cryopreservation in humans, the adding of vitamin E to extender in a dose 200 μmol has positive effects on sperm motility in samples from fertile and also subfertile men. When vitamin E in a dose 100 μmol was added, no positive effect on sperm motility was observed (14). Similar observations were made in boars (15), but adding vitamin E to the extender had no effect on sperm motility. When levels of vitamin E were measured in the fresh ejaculate of men (16), no correlation between vitamin E (α-tocopherol) and sperm motility was found. It is a question if the difference between concentrations of vitamin E in our two groups of ejaculates is not just an accidental finding because of the very low concentration of this vitamin in stallion seminal plasma or if sperm motility after freezing and thawing is really influenced by vitamin E. This vitamin is well known as an antioxidant. It is possible that lower use of vitamin E in the antioxidant processes in „poor" freezable ejaculates is the reason for its higher level in this group of ejaculates. However, more samples and further studies are necessary for confirmation or refutation of the results of our study.

The antioxidant role of vitamin E and selenium is very closely related. In the study of Mahmoud et al. (17) it was demonstrated that supplementation of selenium and vitamin E in parenteral form in rams has a positive effect on the quality and quantity of semen. Similar observations were made in stallions (18). The authors proved that oral supplementation with selenium, vitamin E and zinc in stallions leads to the improvement of some quality parameters in ejaculate, especially the improvement of sperm motility. However, the results of another study did not show any improvement of sperm motility in fresh ejaculate and in ejaculate after 24 hours of storage at 5°C when stallions and pony stallions were supplemented with a combination of vitamin E, vitamin C, L-carnitine and folic acid (19). Over the last few years there has been a lot of work on antioxidants, fat acid or commercially available feed additive dietary supplementation, but the results are not very conclusive (20-22). Unfortunately, in none of the studies the levels of supplemented substances were not monitored in seminal plasma.

In this study not only vitamin E was determined, but also selenium. No statistically significant difference was found in the concentration of selenium. From the observations of Bertelsmann et al. (23) it is obvious that in stallions the level of selenium in the blood does not corresponded with the level of selenium in seminal plasma, but the concentration of selenium positively correlated with sperm motility in fresh ejaculate.

In this study, no correlation between the monitored elements was found. The monitored elements were Zn, Cu, Mg, Ca and P. This concurs with the work of Barrier-Battut et al. (2). In humans, a strong correlation between zinc concentration in seminal plasma and sperm motility exists (24, 25), but correlations with other elements has not been confirmed (26). From this view, a measurement of seminal plasma zinc concentration in fertile and subfertile stallions would be interesting.

Concentrations of Na, K and Cl did not significantly differ between both observed groups. The role of these ions during sperm cooling and freezing, as well as the influence on sperm motility before and after storage is still not very clear. There are some studies about these ions in seminal plasma, but the results differ. Also, connection or correlation with semen quality or freezability is still not clear enough (1, 27-30).

The total protein was higher in the group of „poor" freezable ejaculates, but the difference was not statistically significant. It is known that protein concentration is lower in pre-spermatic fraction of ejaculate and the highest protein concentration is in the first phase of spermatic fraction in stallions (31). The total protein seems not to be a very important parameter in stallion ejaculate, but further research of single proteins in seminal plasma could give us some valuable information (1).

Also enzyme concentrations which were monitored in this study are not useful for ejaculate freezability predictions. It has been seen that gama-glutamyl-transferase (GMT) has an important role in sperm protection against oxidative stress, so it was expected that this enzyme could be a good marker for semen freezability (32, 33). Pesch et al. (29) and Kareskoski and Katila (1) found a correlation between GMT concentrations in seminal plasma and sperm motility. In our study, the concentration of this enzyme was higher in the group of „good" freezable ejaculates, but without statistical significance.

A very strong positive correlation between the concentration of lactate-dehydrogenase (LDH) and sperm motility was found (29), but in our study LDH concentrations were almost the same in both groups of ejaculates. Another difference between the „good" and „poor" freezable group was in the concentration of alkaline phosphatase (ALP) but without statistical significance.

Concentrations of ALP were slightly higher in the group of „good" freezable ejaculates. In stallions, as well as in dogs, ALP is an indicator of ejaculation (34, 35). In the study by Kareskoski et al. (30) there was a clear difference between ALP concentrations in seminal plasma in fertile and subfertile stallions. The same result was found in dogs, where there was also a correlation between the concentration of ALP and ejaculate freezability (36). Average values of other monitored enzymes: aspartate-amino-transferase (AST), creatine kinase (CK) and alanine amino-transferase (ALT) was the same in both groups or the difference was minimal.

Creatinine and urea are well known markers for the detection of urine in ejaculate. In both groups, levels of creatinine and urea were almost the same. In all of the samples, the border for urospermia was not exceeded.

Evaluation of the effect of seminal plasma components on sperm and the freezability of ejaculate is complicated. Only little information is available about some of the components, while concerning other components information is not complete, clear or uniform. So, in this part of the research there is still a lot of work and verification to be done.

ACKNOWLEDGEMENT

This project was supported by grant no. IGA 59/2013/ FVL.

REFERENCES

1. Kareskoski, M., Katila, T. (2008). Components of stallion seminal plasma and the effect of seminal plasma on sperm longevity. Anim Reprod Sci, 107, 249-256.
http://dx.doi.org/10.1016/j.anireprosci.2008.04.013
PMid:18556156

2. Barrier-Battut, I., Delajarraud, H., Legrand, E., Bruyas, J-F., Fieni, F., Tainturier, D., Thorin, C., Pouliquen, H. (2002). Calcium, magnesium, cooper, and zinc in seminal plasma of fertile stallions, and their relationship with semen freezability. Theriogenology 58, 229-232.
http://dx.doi.org/10.1016/S0093-691X(02)00744-6

3. Brinsko, S,P, Blanchard, T.L., Varner, D.D., Schumacher, J., Love, C.C., Hinrichs, K., Hartmen, D. (2011). Manual of equine reproduction. 3rd ed. (pp. 19-192). Mosby, Missouri

4. Trein, C.R., Zikler, H., Bustamante-Filho, I.C., Malschitzky, E., Jobim, M.I.M., Sieme, H., Mattos, R.C. (2008). Equine seminal plasma proteins related with semen freezability. Anim Reprod Sci, 107, 252-253.
http://dx.doi.org/10.1016/j.anireprosci.2008.05.129

5. Jasko, D.L., Moran, D.L., Farlin, M.E., Squires, E.L. (1991). Effect of seminal plasma dilution or removal on spermatozoa motion characteristics of cooled semen. Theriogenology 35, 1059-1067.
http://dx.doi.org/10.1016/0093-691X(91)90354-G

6. Braun, J., Sakai, M., Hochi, S., Oguri, N. (1994). Preservation of ejaculated and epididymal stallion spermatozoa by cooling and freezing. Theriogenology 41, 809-818.
http://dx.doi.org/10.1016/0093-691X(94)90497-7

7. Alghamdi, A.S., Troedsson, M.H., Xue, J.L., Crabo, B.G. (2002). Effect of seminal plasma concentration and various extenders on post-thaw motility and glass wool - Sephadex filtration of cryopreserved stallion semen. Am J Vet Res 63, 880-885.
http://dx.doi.org/10.2460/ajvr.2002.63.880
PMid:12061536

8. Ben, W.X., Fu, M.T., Mao, L.K.,Ming, Z.W., Xiong, W.W. (1997). Effects of various concentration of native seminal plasma in cryoprotectant on viability on human sperm. Arch Androl 39, 211-216.
http://dx.doi.org/10.3109/01485019708987918
PMid:9352032

9. Aurich, J.E., Kuhne, A., Hoope, H., Aurich, C. (1996). Seminal plasma effects membrane integrity and motility of equine spermatoza after cryopreservation. Theriogenology 46, 791-797.
http://dx.doi.org/10.1016/S0093-691X(96)00237-3

10. Katila, T., Anderson, M., Reilas, T., Koskinen, E. (2002). Post-thaw motility and viability of fractionated and frozen stallion ejaculates. Theriogenology 58, 241-244.
http://dx.doi.org/10.1016/S0093-691X(02)00783-5

11. Morrell, J.M., Pihl, J., Dalin, A.M., Johannisson, A. (2012). Restoration of seminal plasma to stallion spermatozoa selected by colloid centrifugation increase progressive motility but is determinal to chromatin integrity. Theriogenology 78, 345-352.
http://dx.doi.org/10.1016/j.theriogenology.2012.02.009
PMid:22494676

12. Aurich, J.E., Kuhne, A., Hoope, H., Aurich, C. (1998). Effect of seminal plasma on stallion semen quality after cryopreservation. J Reprod Fertil Abstr Ser. 15: 34.

13. Ackay, E., Reilas, T., Andersson, M., Katila, T. (2006). Effect of seminal plasma fractions on sperm survival after cooled storage. J Vet Med A, 53, 481-485.
http://dx.doi.org/10.1111/j.1439-0442.2006.00882.x
PMid:17054486

14. Taylor, K., Roberts, P., Sanders, K., Burton, P. (2009). Effect of antioxidant supplementation of cryopreservation medium on post-thaw integrity of human spermatozoa. RBM online 18: 184-189.

15. Pech-Sansores, A.G.C., Centurion-Castro, F.G., Rodriguez-Buenfil, J.C., Segura-Correa, J.C., Ake-Lopez, J.R. (2011). Effect of the addition of seminal plasma, vitamin E and incubation time on post-thawed sperm viability in boar semen. Tropical and Subtropical Agroecosystems 14, 965-971.

16. Therond, P., Auger, J., Legrand, A., Jouannet, P. (1996). α-tocopherol in human spermatozoa and seminal plasma: relationship with mitility, antioxidant enzymes and leukocytes. Molecular Human Reproduction 10, 739-744.
http://dx.doi.org/10.1093/molehr/2.10.739

17. Mahmoud, G.B., Abdel-Raheem, S.M., Hussein, H.A. (2013). Effect of combination of vitamin E and selenium injections on reproductive performance and blood parameters of Ossimi rams. Small Ruminant Res 113, 103-108.
http://dx.doi.org/10.1016/j.smallrumres.2012.12.006

18. Contri, A., De Amicis, I., Molinari, A., Faustini, M., Gramenzi, A., Robbe, D., Carluccio, A. (2011). Effect of dietary antioxidant supplementation on fresh semen quality in stallion. Theriogenology 75, 1319-1326. http://dx.doi.org/10.1016/j.theriogenology.2010.12.003 PMid:21295825

19. Deichsel, K., Palm, F., Koblischke, P., Budik, S., Aurich, C. (2008). Effect of a dietary antioxidant supplementation on semen quality in pony stallions. Theriogenology 69, 940-945. http://dx.doi.org/10.1016/j.theriogenology.2008.01.007 PMid:18358523

20. Franco, J.S.V., Chaveiro, A., Góis, A., da Silva, F.M. (2013). Effects of α-tocopherol and ascorbic acid on equine semen quality after cryopreservation. J Eq Vet Sci, 33, 787-793. http://dx.doi.org/10.1016/j.jevs.2012.12.012

21. Schmid-Lausigk, Y., Aurich, C. (2014). Influences of a diet supplemented with linseed oil and antioxidants on quality of equine semen after cooling and cryopreservation during winter. Theriogenology 81, 966-973. http://dx.doi.org/10.1016/j.theriogenology.2014.01.021 PMid:24576708

22. Blomfield, J., Tucker, L., McLeay, L., Morris, L.H.A. (2014). Evaluation of antioxidant dietary supplementation on semen quality parameters in New Zealand Standard bred stallions. J Eq Vet Sci, 34, 89. http://dx.doi.org/10.1016/j.jevs.2013.10.061

23. Bertelsmann, H., Keppler, S., Holtershinken, M., Bollwein, H., Behne, D., Alber, D., Bukalis, G., Kyriakopoulos, A., Sieme, H. (2010). Selenium in blood, semen, seminal plasma and spermatozoa of stallions and its relationship to sperm quality. Reprod Fertil Dev, 22, 886-891. http://dx.doi.org/10.1071/RD10032 PMid:20450841

24. Fuse, H., Kazama, T., Ohta, S., Fujiuchi, Y. (1999). Relationship between zinc concentrations in seminal plasma and variuos sperm parameters. International Urology and Nephrology 31, 401-408. http://dx.doi.org/10.1023/A:1007190506587

25. Colagar, A.H., Marzony, E.T., Chaichi, M.J. (2009). Zinc levels in seminal plasma are associated with sperm quality in fertile and infertile men. Nutrition Research 29, 82-88. http://dx.doi.org/10.1016/j.nutres.2008.11.007

26. Wong, W.Y., Filk, G., Groenen, P.M., Swinkels, D.W., Thomas, C.M., Copius-Peereboom, J.H., Merkus, H.M., Steegers-Theunissen, R.P. (2001). The impact of calcium, magnesium, zinc, and cooper in blood and seminal plasma on semen parameters in men. Reprod Toxicol, 15, 131-136. http://dx.doi.org/10.1016/S0890-6238(01)00113-7

27. Amann, R.P., Pickett, B.W. (1987). Principles of cryopreservation and a review of cryopreservation of stallion spermatozoa. J Eq Vet Sci, 7, 145-173. http://dx.doi.org/10.1016/S0737-0806(87)80025-4

28. Kareskoski, M., Reilas, T., Andersson, M., Katila, T. (2006). Motility and plasma membrane integrity of spermatozoa in fractionated stallion ejaculates after storage. Reprod Dom Anim, 41, 33-38. http://dx.doi.org/10.1111/j.1439-0531.2006.00647.x PMid:16420325

29. Pesch, S., Bergmann, M., Bostedt, H. (2006). Determination of some enzymes and macro- and microelements in stallion seminal plasma and their correlations to semen quality. Theriogenology 66, 307-313. http://dx.doi.org/10.1016/j.theriogenology.2005.11.015 PMid:16413936

30. Kareskoski, M., Reilas, T., Sankari, S., Andersson, M., Guvenc, K., Katila, T. (2010). Alkaline and acid phosphatase, β-glucuronidase and electrolyte levels in fractionated stallion ejaculates. Reprod Dom Anim, 45, 396-374. http://dx.doi.org/10.1111/j.1439-0531.2009.01579.x PMid:20074319

31. Koskinen, E., Karlsson, M., Reilas, T., Sankari, S., Esala, A-L., Katila, T. (2002). Catalase activity and total protein in fractionated stallion seminal plasma. Theriogenology 58, 337-340. http://dx.doi.org/10.1016/S0093-691X(02)00767-7

32. Kohdaira, T., Kinoshita, Y., Konno, M., Oshima, H. (1986). Distribution of G-glutamyl-transpeptidase in male reproductive system of rats and its age-related changes. Andrologia 18, 610-617. http://dx.doi.org/10.1111/j.1439-0272.1986.tb01839.x PMid:2880528

33. Hinton, B.T., Lan, Z.J., Rudolph, D.B., Labus, J.C., Lye, R.J. (1998). Testicular regulation of epididymal gene expression. J Reprod Fertil, Suppl. 53, 47-58.

34. Kutzler, M.A., Solter, P.F., Hoffmann, W.E., Volkmann, D.H. (2003). Characterization and localization of alkaline phosphatase in canine seminal plasma and gonadal tissues. Theriogenology 60, 299-306. http://dx.doi.org/10.1016/S0093-691X(02)01366-3

35. Turner, R.M.O., McDonnell, S. (2003). Alkaline phosphatase in stallion semen: chracterization and clinical applications. Theriogenology 60, 1-10. http://dx.doi.org/10.1016/S0093-691X(02)00956-1

36. Kosiniak-Kamysz, K., Bittmar, A., Podstawski, Z. (2007). Alkalina phosphatase activity as a marker of dog semen freezability. Zootehniesi Biotehnologii 40, 131-135.

27

THE PREVALENCE OF *PASTEURELLA MULTOCIDA* FROM FARM PIGS IN SERBIA

Oliver Radanovic, Jadranka Zutic, Dobrila Jakic-Dimic,
Branislav Kureljusic, Bozidar Savic

Institute of Veterinary Medicine of Serbia, Vojvode Toze 14, 11000 Belgrade, Serbia

ABSTRACT

The investigations covered a total of 234 lungs from necropsied pigs with different pneumonic lesions, from 6 farrow-to-finish pig farms during 2013 and 2014. The samples were inoculated on selective culture media and aerobically incubated at 37°C and in carbon dioxide condition. The isolated bacterial colonies were further characterised morphologically and biochemically. The identification was confirmed using the BBL Crystal, E/N, G/P ID Kit (Becton Dickinson). For determination of the type of *Pasteurella multocida*, the PCR method was used. The findings showed that bacteria were isolated from 202 (86%) out of 234 examined lung samples. The pure isolates of *Pasteurella multocida* were obtained from 71 (35 %) samples. Out of the remaining 29 (14%) examined lung samples, 9, 8, 7 and 5 examined lung samples were shown as mixed cultures of *Pasteurella multocida* and *Streptococcus* spp., *Arcanobacterium pyogenes*, *Actinobacillus pleuropneumoniae* and *Haemophilus parasuis*, respectively. The PCR method confirmed that all 15 investigated strains of *P. multocida* belong to type A.

Key words: *Pasteurella multocida*, lung, pig

INTRODUCTION

Some of the most important problems in modern pig farming are closely related to respiratory diseases. Respiratory diseases in pigs are spread worldwide, striking substantial financial damage on livestock production systems (1, 2). One of the features of modern pig farming is spatial agglomeration with large numbers of individuals in limited spaces. This benefits respiratory pathogens which subsequently keep a high virulence level *in vivo* (3).

Among a number of factors that can cause these type of diseases, viruses and bacteria have the most important role (4). Out of many non-specific factors that can contribute to the emergence and the development of respiratory diseases, some of the most significant are overcrowded housing, bad

hygiene, high humidity, high concentration of toxic gases, sudden temperature changes, disregarding veterinary-sanitary and biosafety measures etc.

These conditions serve in favor of persisting infectious agents in aerosol on one hand, and creating "ambient stress" on the other, which leads to immunosuppression (2). Thus, a majority of authors agree that the prevalence of respiratory diseases increases if the concentration of biological agents in their environment rises, or if the immune system in the lung tissue weakens caused by some other cause. Lung infections are usually caused by a number of factors affecting the organism at the same time, rather than individually. Most common combination of factors includes a mixed virus and bacterial infection. Pathogenic bacteria which can cause respiratory infections are *Pasteurella multocida* (*P. multocida*), *Actinobacillus pleuropneumoniae* (*A. pleuropneumoniae*), *Bordetella bronchiseptica*, *Streptococcus* spp. *Haemophilus parasuis* (*H. parasuis*), *Actinobacillus suis* (*A. suis*), *Arcanobacterium pyogenes* (*A. pyogenes*) and *Salmonella enterica subsp. enterica* serovar *Choleraesuis* (4, 5, 6). Some authors agree that some of aforementioned pathogens (such as *P. multocida*) can be considered the primary respiratory pathogen, because of their ability to cause lesions in the lung tissue on their own (7).

Corresponding author: Dr. Oliver Radanović, PhD
E-mail address: radanovic.oliver@gmail.com
Present address: Institute of Veterinary Medicine of Serbia
Department of Microbiology, Vojvode Toze 14,
11000 Belgrade, Serbia

The goal of this study was to determine the incidence and identify the bacteria causing pneumonia in pigs, with an accent on the incidence of *P. multocida*.

MATERIAL AND METHODS

The pneumonic pig lungs were examined in this study. The samples originated from 6 commercial farrow-to-finish pig farms. The pigs were bred in confined production systems and the technology recommended for this type of livestock breeding

Kit (Becton Dickinson, USA). For the isolation of *A. pleuropneumoniae* and *H. parasuis*, additional blood agar plates with a *Staphylococcus aureus* streak as a source of the NAD, were incubated in jar with reduced oxygen and enhanced carbon dioxide content. Colonies suspicious to *A. pleuropneumoniae* and *H. parasuis* were subcultured on chocolate agar with PolyVitex (bioMerieux, France) and identified with Gram-stains, haemolysis activity on sheep blood agar, positive CAMP test, requirement NAD and urease production. For typing of *P. multocida* isolates, the PCR method was used according to Jaglic et al. (8).

Table 1. Incidence of certain bacteria strains isolated from 202 samples from the pig lungs

Bacterial species	No. isolates	% isolates
Pasteurella multocida	71	35.14
Haemophilus parasuis	29	14.35
Actinobacillus pleuropneumoniae	25	12.37
Streptococcus spp.	23	11.38
Arcanobacterium pyogenes	15	7.42
Mixed infection including Pasteurella multocida	29	14.35
Multiple species of bacteria	10	4.95
Total	202	99.96

was used. The farms where this study was conducted did not use immunization as a form of prevention against bacteria which cause pneumonia in pigs. PRRS and porcine circovirus 2 (PCV2) were both detected in those farms. The lungs sampled from the necropsied pigs were deposited in sterile PVC bags and transported to the Institute of Veterinary Medicine of Serbia for further examination.

Samples were inoculated on agar with 5 % sheep blood, Columbia and MacConkey agar (HiMedia), and incubated aerobically at a temperature of 37°C for 24-48 h. Bacterial isolates were identified using standard bacteriological methods. The identification was confirmed using the BBL Crystal E/N, G/P, ID

RESULTS

Out of total of 234 pig lungs sampled for bacterial presence, 202 (86%) were found positive. *P. multocida* had the highest occurrence rate found in the lung samples with 71 (35%), followed by 29 samples (14%) for *H. parasuis*, 25 samples (12%) for *A. pleuropneumoniae*, 23 samples (11%) for *Streptococcus* spp. and 15 samples (7%) for *A. pyogenes*. From 10 (5%) lung samples, multiple different non specific microorganisms were isolated. Results are presented in Table 1.

Furthermore, mixed cultures of bacteria were established in 29 (14%) samples, where in addition

Table 2. Combination mixed culture of bacteria isolates from pig lungs

Combination of bacterial species	No. samples	% of different combination
Pasteurella multocida + *Streptococcus* spp.	9	31.03
Pasteurella multocida + *A. pyogenes*	8	27.58
Pasteurella multocida + *A. pleuropneumoniae*	7	24.13
Pasteurella multocida + *H. parasuis*	5	17.24
Total	29	99.98

to *P. multocida*, *Streptococcus* spp. was isolated from 9 (31%) samples, A. pyogenes 8 (27%), *A. pleuropneumoniae* 7 (24%) and *H. parasuis* 5 (17%). Results are presented in Table 2.The PCR method confirm that all 15 investigated selected strains of *P. multocida* belong to type A.

DISCUSSION

A high percentage of *P. multocida* isolates shows that currently this microorganism is one of the most important pathogens among pneumonia causing bacteria in pigs in the farms from which the samples were collected in this study.

The importance of *P. multocida* as a main pathogen causing pneumonia in pigs was confirmed by Dutra et al. (9). Holko et al. (10) cited that *P. multocida* caused pneumonia in 44% of pigs tested. A lower percentage of 33% isolation of *P. multocida* from lung pigs was found in Serbia (11). The PCR method confirms that all 15 investigated strains of *P. multocida* belong to type A, which is in agreement with the reports of Stepniewska (12).

Radanovic et al. (13) found that mixed infections were determined in 6% of lung tissue samples, while other authors report an incidence of mixed bacterial infections to be 8.29% (14). It is important to note that the incidence of infections caused by mixed bacteria cultures increased on 14% in the pig farms in Serbia.

Mixed infections of lung tissue are also reported by researchers, who, among other bacterial causative agents, also report a prevalence of viruses which cause pneumonia in pigs, especially a coinfection with the PRRS virus. Choi et al. (15) report a prevalence of coinfection with PRRS and *P. multocida* to be 10.4%, PRRS and *M. hyopneumoniae* of 7% and PRRS and *A. pneumoniae* to be 6.2%. Also, the mixed infections have been described in several studies (16, 17, 18, 19). In these studie,s the more common mixed infections were *P. multocida* with viruses or bacterial agents.

All of the farms from which the samples were collected reported the presence of either PRRS or PCV2, or both viruses. In previous research in Serbia, the positive samples of PRRSV were found in all examined regions, in 14 of 20 (70%) examined farms (20). Also, PCV2 is a ubiquitous virus of pigs, and all of 12 examined farms have experienced PMWS over the time. One or both viruses tend to produce both local (lung tissue) or systemic immunosuppression, which is believed to help develop lethal bacterial pneumonia (21). The result of immunosuppression is lower defensive activity towards different microbial agents, especially to

bacterial antigens, which leads to the conclusion that the control of these viral infections is of great importance concerning the respiratory disease control.

These results and other similar findings, must be well explained regarding the global trend in the recent years. It has been determined that, after the infection with PRRS and PCV2, bacterial isolates often differ both between the animals in the same group, and between different production groups in the same farm. The explanation for this occurrence can be found in the individual differences between animals, their different ability to react to antigens and the diverse immune status of rears as the result of the immunosuppressive activity of the aforementioned viruses.

CONCLUSION

Bacteriological examination of pig lungs with pneumonic lesions showed the presence of bacterial pathogens in 86%, which points to the significance of bacterial causative agents in the ethiopathogenesis of pig pneumonia in this studied farms.

The high prevalence of *P. multocida* (35%) and the prevalence of *P. multocida* in mixed infections (14%) was also found. Such a high percentage of the isolation of   *P. multocida* indicated its important role in the occurrence of respiratory infections of swine on our farms with intensive production systems. Compared to the previous period, the incidence of mixed bacterial infections was higher.

REFERENCES

1. Bochev, I. (2007). Porcine respiratory disease complex (PRDC): A review. I. Etiology, epidemiology, clinical forms and pathoanatomical features. Bulg. J. Vet. Med. 10, 131-146.

2. Savić, B., Radanović, O., Žutić, M., Pavlović, I., Jakić-Dimić, D. (2011). Prevalenca bakterijskih uzročnika pneumonija svinja. IX Simpozijum Veterinara "Zdravstvena zaštita, selekcija i reprodukcija svinja". Zbornik radova. 77-82. Srebreno Jezero.

3. Woeste, K. Grosse, E. (2007). Transmission of agents of the porcine respiratory disease complex (PRDC) between swine herds; a review. Part 2-Pathogen transmission via semen air and living/nonliving vectors. Deutsche. Tierarzt. Wochenschrift. 114, 364-373.
PMid:17970334

4. Baker, R.B. (2005). Diseases of the respiratory system. Proceedings of the North Carolina healthy hogs seminar. Clinton. 1-19. PMCid:PMC4147871

5. Halbur, P.G. (1997). Porcine respiratory disease complex, Proceedings of the North Carolina healthy hogs seminar. 1-15.

6. Lee, A. (2013). Mycoplasmal pneumonia in pigs, 1-3. http://www.dpi.nsw.gov.au

7. Tigga, M., Ghosh, R.C., Malik, P., Choudhary, B.K., Tigga, P., Nagar, D.K. (2014). Isolation, characterization, antibiogram and pathology of Pasteurella multocida isolated from pigs, Vet. World 7, 363-368. http://dx.doi.org/10.14202/vetworld.2014.363-368

8. Jaglic, Z., Kucerova, Z., Nedbalcova, K., Pavlik, I., Alexa, P., Bartos, M. (2005). Characterisation and comparison of Pasteurella multocida isolated from different species in the Czech Republic: capsular PCR typing, ribotyping and dermonecrotoxin production. Vet. Med. – Czech. 50 (8): 345–354

9. Dutra, V., Chitarra, C., Paula, D.A. (2013). Detection of Pasteurella multocida by qPCR Associated with Ppneumonic lung in pigs slaughtered in M Grosso Brazil. Int. J. Sc. 2,25-31.

10. Holko, I., Urbanova, J., Holkova, T., Kmet, V. (2004). Diagnostics of main bacterial agents of porcine respiratory diseases complex (PRDC) using PCR detection of Mycoplasma hyopneumoniae. Vet. Med. – Czech. 49, 35–41.

11. Radanović, O., Savić, B., Kureljušić, B., Ivetić, V., Žutić, M. (2010). Učestalost izolacije Pasteurella multocida iz pluća prasadi iz kategorije odgoja.Proceedings of the XII Symposium of Epidemiological days with international participation. Oplenac-Topola. 99-102.

12. Stepniewska, K., Markowska-Daniel, I. (2013). Phenotypic and genotypic characterization of Pasteurella multocida strains isolated from pigs in Poland. Bull Vet Inst Pulawy 57, 29-34.

13. Radanović, O., Žutić, M., Ivetić, V., Savić, B., Stanojević, S. (2008). Significance of Pasteurella multocida in respiratory disease complex of swine. Proceedings of the X Symposium of Epidemiological days with international participation. Tara. 253-255.

14. Žutić, M., Ivetić, V., Radanović, O., Žutić, J., Jakić-Dimić, D., Savić, B., Pavlović, I., Stanojević, S. (2009). Investigations of representation of certain bacteria strains in lungs of pigs with pneumonia. Vet. Glasnik 63, 3-15. http://dx.doi.org/10.2298/VETGL0902003Z

15. Choi, Y.K., Goya, S.M., Joo, H.S. (2003). Retrospective analysis of etiological agents associated with respiratory diseases in pigs. Can. Vet. J. 44, 735-737. PMid:14524628 PMCid:PMC340270

16. Hansen, M.S., Pors, S.E., Jensen, H.E., Bille-Hansen V., Bisgard, M., Flachs, E.M., Nielsen O.L. (2010). An investigation of the pathology and pathogens associated with porcine respiratory disease complex. in Denmark. J. Comp. in Denmark. J. Comp. Pathology. 143,120-131. http://dx.doi.org/10.1016/j.jcpa.2010.01.012 PMid:20181357

17. Opriessnig, T., Gimenez-Lirola, L.G., Halbur, P.G. (2011). Polymicrobial respiratory disease in pigs. Anim. Health. Res. Rev. 12,133-48. http://dx.doi.org/10.1017/S1466252311000120 PMid:22152290

18. Weissenbacher-Lang, C., Kureljušić, B., Nedorost, N., Stixenberger, D., Binanti, D., Viehmann, M., Weissenböck, H. (2014). Association between Pneumocystis carinii and bacterial lung pathogens in pigs with pneumonia. Proc. 23rd IPVS Congress,Cancún, Mexico, 08.06.–11.06.2014. p. 53.

19. Pors, S.E., Hensen, M.S., Christensen, H., Jensen, H.E., Petersen, A., Bisgard, M. (2011). Genetic diversity and associated pathology of Pasteurella multocida isolated from porcine pneumonia. Vet. Microbiol. 150, 354-361 http://dx.doi.org/10.1016/j.vetmic.2011.02.050

20. Petrović, T., Miličević, V., Radulović-Prodanov, J., Maksimović-Zorić, J., Lupulović, D., Došen, R., Lazić, S. (2011). Molecular detection and genetic analysis of Serbian PRRSV isolates. Euro PRRS Symposium. Proceedings pp. 50-56. 12-14 October Novi Sad.

21. Truszczyński, M., Pejsak, Z. (2010). Immunosuppression as the cause of swine diseases of multifactorial etiology. Meycyna Wet. 66, 370-373.

28

THE ART AND SCIENCE OF CONSULTATIONS IN BOVINE MEDICINE: USE OF MODIFIED CALGARY – CAMBRIDGE GUIDES

Kiro R. Petrovski, Michelle Mc Arthur

School of Animal and Veterinary Sciences, the University of Adelaide, SA, Australia

ABSTRACT

This article describes few steps of the application of the modified Calgary-Cambridge Guides (CCG) to consultations in bovine medicine. A review of pertinent clinical communication skills literature in human medicine was integrated with the burgeoning research within veterinary medicine. In particular, there are more recent studies examining companion animal veterinarian's communication skills and outcomes which can be extrapolated to practitioners. This was integrated into a teaching example of a reproductive case consultation. The first article deals with the 1) Preparation, 2) Initiating the Session and 3) Gathering Information sections. The aim of the modified CCG is to provide a set of skills to facilitate a relationship-centred approach to consultations in bovine medicine, both at the individual animal and population level. They were initially developed for human medicine and expanded recently for use in veterinary medicine. The CCG enable the practitioner to facilitate interacting with that particular client at the time of the consultation. It is likely that the majority of practitioners do use many of the skills recommended by the modified CCG. These skills are often gained through experience. However, they may not use the skills intentionally and with purpose for a specific communication goal or outcome. Practitioners can improve their communication skills using the set of skills as recommended by the modified CCG. They allow the practitioner to gain insight into the client's understanding of the problem, including underlying aetiology, epidemiology and pathophysiology. The guides also provide opportunity to understand client's expectations regarding the outcome, motivation and willingness to change and adherence.

Key words: modified Calgary-Cambridge guides, practitioner, client, consultation

INTRODUCTION

Successful bovine consultation relies on good communication skills and a healthy client-practitioner relationship. The objective is to create conducive conditions aiming to establish an effective relationship. Key facets of an effective relationship include appreciating the other's perspective which inherently involves taking time to understand the other party's story as well as shared decision making and ultimately a collaborative approach. Specific effective and efficient communication skills to help achieve the above include both verbal and nonverbal components. Multiple benefits may be realised from collaborative relationship-centred communication

Corresponding author: Dr. Kiro R. Petrovski, PhD
E-mail address: kiro.petrovski@adelaide.edu.au
Present address: The University of Adelaide
School of Animal and Veterinary Sciences
JS Davies building G13, Roseworthy Campus, Roseworthy, Australia

styles and inherent skills. These benefits include anticipated increased adherence to recommendations (1), and improved client and veterinarian satisfaction (2, 3). However, ineffective communication, as determined from the client's perspective, is one of the leading causes of complaints at the Veterinary Surgeons Board of South Australia. While clients are typically more informed in recent times, mostly due to freely available data on the internet, the practitioner works with a professional, whose job it is to know intimately the health and husbandry of his/her stock. As such, the practitioner –client-patient relationship, like those in other production animal settings, is typically a unique and specialised communication domain.

Practitioners are required on farms for individual patient and/or herd problem consultations and both require in effect a case management approach. Despite the recent changes in the cattle industry, particularly dairy, including larger herd size, less contact of labour per patient and decreased importance of treatment of individual animals, case management is still required. This is true for smaller farms, but also for large dairy enterprise-type farms, provided the intervention is economically justified and/or addresses animal welfare issues. Given the cost associated with economically justified consultation, involving the judicious use of ancillary techniques and laboratory testing, it is even more important that a complete and thorough history is gathered with the client. A very early empirical study suggested that significant reduction in diagnostic tests in human medicine and thereby costs could be achieved with thorough information gathering and clinical examination (4). Additionally, the practitioner will need to develop proficiency in clinical examination as well as the appropriate choice of diagnostic techniques. To achieve a successful outcome, the practitioner must be inquisitive, critically reflective, and observant. This will prevent overlooking any abnormality in either the animal/s, or the environment.

In dealing with clinical cases practitioners usually use the tailored traditional case management skills that involve the following steps:

a. Collection of data or clinical findings
  i. Client concern
  ii. Gathering history
  iii.Clinical examination
  iv. Ancillary examination techniques
  v. Collection and assaying appropriate samples

b. Analysis of data or evaluation of clinical findings
  i. Generation of a list of problems
  ii. Generation of a list of differential diagnoses (for each problem; diagnostic hypotheses)
  iii. Rule in or out differential diagnosis
  iv.Establishing final diagnosis

c. Development of a management plan
  i. Determining a prognosis
  ii. Treatment plan
  iii.Establishing a programme to prevent recurrent and new cases

The Calgary-Cambridge Guides (5) are a widely accepted model for teaching communication skills in human (6) and veterinary medicine (7). The Calgary Cambridge Guides integrate the content of a clinical case with effective communication skills (5). The modified Calgary Cambridge Guides (MCCG) were developed by Radford et al. (8) to suit the veterinary clinical setting. It can be easily adopted in all areas of clinical veterinary practice. The MCCG are used to break-down the management of the clinical case (consultation) into seven key components: 1. Preparation, 2. Initiating the Session, 3. Gathering Information, 4. Physical examination,

5. Explanation and Planning, 6. Closing the Consultation, 7. Providing Structure, and 8. Building the Relationship (5). The aim of this article which is designed to integrate clinical content with history gathering skills; thus, introducing the first three components of the model. Despite their equal importance, the skills associated with 'Explanation and Planning', 'Closing the Consultation', 'Building the Relationship' and 'Structuring the Consultation' which run after or in parallel to the discussed skills will not be the focus of this article.

Specifically, to help illustrate skills delineated in the MCCG, this article will focus on a fertility case of an individual cow ('Margery'). The specific information relating to this case is italicised. Some issues are not italicised as they are more general than specific and may be used in every day practice. The terminology used in this article has been adjusted to the typical language used in previous literature regarding the MCCG model. A consultation in this article encompasses the management of a clinical case, intervention, visit or a session. A client in this article refers to farm owner, manager, stockman, and/or attendant. A patient is the animal attended by the practitioner. The list of skills follows the originally developed by Kurtz et al. (5) for human practitioners with slight modifications to veterinary profession. The list of skills will be included as an appendix to the series or articles in the second part.

PREPARATION

Preparation for a bovine consultation involves the practitioner familiarising themselves with the past history of the client and, when applicable, the patient (Skill 0a) as well as anticipation of potential difficulties or conflicts regarding the client or the patient itself (Skill 0b).

Establishing context

Skill 0a (Familiarises with past history relating to client and animals(s)):
The modern veterinary practice will likely have a good filing system and appropriate computer software for management of clinical cases. Such systems should result in the rapid and easy retrieval of information. It is a good idea to familiarise with the previous history and clinical record of the farm, and if applicable of the patient to be examined.

E.g. *The client (Mr Jack Bentley) is a regular client of your clinic, but you have never before been on his property or have met him. From the clinic records you have found that Mr Bentley has a mixed breed farm (Jersey, Holstein Friesian and their crosses) of 120 cows that are well looked after, milking through 15 a-side herring bone milking parlour, mainly pastoral system with some supplemental feed when feed shortage occurs and some concentrate in the parlour. Each cow has her own name and identification number. Clinical records indicate that there are no obvious problems on the farm. Margery has not been seen previously for health problems at all.*

Skill 0b (Anticipates potential conflict of difficulties, relating to the client, the animal and to systems and infrastructures):

The filing system should also allow for adding special notes on the requirements of the client (e.g. client requires more time on explanations, client very knowledgeable of the subject) or the patient itself (e.g. may charge). It is important to approach the bovine consultation without pre-conceived ideas of their complexity or alternatively their simplicity.

Creating a professional, safe and effective environment

The creation of a professional, safe and effective environment should be tailored to the appropriate needs during the consultation (Skill 0c).

Skill 0c (Ensures facilities/environment are professional and appropriate to anticipated needs):

Independent of the previous relationship with the client, the practitioner should arrive on the farm presentable, in appropriate clothing and in a tidy vehicle. Professionalism of this type leaves a good impression. Furthermore, disinfecting working shoes upon arrival and departure is a biosecurity requirement. A spray bottle filled with ready-to-use disinfectant is enough for this purpose. Finally, equipment should be clean and presentable (e.g. packed in a sterilisation pack, individually covered, and/or no residuals such as manure or saliva from the previous consultation).

For conducting a safe and complete clinical examination of the patient, appropriate facilities are required. It is the practitioner's duty to ensure that the working environment is safe and fit for purpose (e.g. operating crush, proper yards and raceway available). Old, damaged facilities may endanger the practitioner, the client or the patient.

E.g. *the client has no crush for restraining Margery. The alternative is to use the dairy shed but the milking facilities are currently in use. This may require Margery to be examined on another occasion or in a portable crush brought in by the practitioner.*

Observation

Skill 0d (Continuous observation of the animal, the client and the environment):

The observation of the patient, the client and the environment should continue throughout the visit. The cattle patient cannot describe its symptoms. Hence, the observations of abnormalities (signs) made by the client are essential in forming a full picture about the case. The client should be observed for their competency in working with cattle, their attitude to handling cattle, honesty and the interest in the business as whole. E.g. *an inexperienced client may be the reason for Margery not being seen in heat.*

Furthermore, observation of the environment may provide clues for detecting risk factors that may have contributed to the incidence of the disorder. Unfortunately, the effects of the environment are often overlooked, and may not have received the consideration they deserve. The environment should be observed for the general state of the farm, location of the farm, topography, pasture, housing, walking surfaces, access to potentially dangerous goods and availability of feedstuffs and water, coupled with the cow comfort.

E.g. *not having enough feedstuffs on the farm may indicate that malnutrition may be the reason for Margery not cycling (e.g. negative energy balance) or the slippery walking surfaces may prevent normal oestrous behaviour and heats may be missed.*

Finally, practitioners should learn to ask only questions to which answers are not obvious. In some situations asking specific questions may be embarrassing (e.g. having been presented with a calving problem the sex of the patient should not be enquired). In these situations, the practitioners should take the obvious information as part of the history, without asking the questions.

INITIATING THE SESSION

Initiating the session encompasses the time from meeting the client, and sometimes the patient, until the reason for the visit is discussed.

Establishing Initial Rapport

An effective partnership is difficult to develop without first establishing initial rapport. Initial rapport is a first impression of the genuine and potential compatibility of a person and their capacity to work together. It characterised by establishing common ground through mutually objective topics. These topics might include the patient of interest or the weather in order to establish connection with the client and ability to connect mentally and emotionally with the other party; thus promoting trust and mutual respect (9).

Skills 1 (Greets the client; obtains/confirms client's name and the name/identity of the animal) & 2 (Introduces self, role and nature of the consultation; obtains consent):

The initial few minutes of the consultation, particularly when meeting for the first time, will likely shape the relationship between the practitioner and the client, as well as the nature of future interactions. An introduction of the practitioner to the client (if they have not met previously) usually begins the consultation as well as the usual greetings of the day and the reason for the visit. Sometimes, it may be a good idea to indulge in a little general conversation before discussing the case. Conversation about the weather, a recent sporting event, and the recent introduction of an industry policy are the easiest and often most comfortable themes to discuss.

E.g. *'Good morning Mr Bentley (or Jack) ... My name is Dr John...'* (shakes hands if the client is comfortable with this). *''How are you this morning? ...it has been cold the last few days, hasn't it? ...* or *'I hope the price increase of the milk/meat last week is going to help the business ...'*

This will likely help relax the atmosphere and the client does not feel like they are being interrogated and ***Skill 3 (Demonstrates interest, concern and respect for the client and the animal)*** demonstrates respect and interest in the client, the farm and the patient of interest.

By examining the body language of the client, the practitioner may be able to determine a suitable time to start the conversation about the case *(Skill 3a. Attends to client's and animal's physical comfort).* It is important to note that in an urgent clinical case (e.g. severe bleeding), it is still important to follow these guides. However, the practitioner after Skills 1 & 2, will immediately deal with the case and while doing so inherently addresses the other aspects of developing initial rapport by meeting the client's needs.

Identifying the reason for the consultation

Following the development of initial rapport, it is important to ascertain the reason for the consultation. This is traditionally known as the client's concern/complaint.

Skill 4 (Identifies the client's problem or the issues that the client wishes to address):

The reason for the consultation is the concern expressed by the client. It must be clearly established and verified with open-ended questions. Open-ended questions allow the client to provide as much information as they feel necessary and to explore their own concerns freely. e.g. 'What is the problem today?' or 'What can we do for you today?' or 'How can I help today?'

e.g. *'How can I help with Margery today?'* or *'You mentioned over the phone that you have a cow with a problem. What is the problem that you have called for?'* or *'You mentioned over the phone to the receptionist that Margery has a problem with not cycling. Can you clarify that for me?'*

The list of common complaints includes drooling from the mouth, swelling, lethargy, lameness, mastitis, distension of the abdomen, trouble breathing, diarrhoea, abnormal skin, abnormal milk, and dehydration. It is beyond the scope of this article to address all these in a single example. In our example the following reason for the consultation has been obtained:

'Margery has calved three months ago. I have not seen her in heat at all after calving. She is a high producer though.'

Therefore, the primary reason for the consultation in our case is that Margery is a non-cycling cow.

Skill 5 (Listens attentively to the client's opening statement, without interrupting or directing the client's response):

It is important that the practitioner listens attentively to the client's observations and response to questions, and actively determines as well as acknowledges the client's perspective. The skills associated with attentive listening are well described in Boudreau et al. (10). Amongst other features, attentive listening is an active and perceptual process and involves noticing non-verbal cues, verbal language and can assist in gathering diagnostic data. Attentive listening can be a difficult skill to consistently achieve and may be more difficult to learn than the clinical interview itself (10). Furthermore, a study of human medicine residents reported that patients are interrupted after an average of 12 seconds (11) and in a companion animal veterinarian study, clients were interrupted after just 11 seconds (12) thus suggesting attentive listening is indeed a challenging skill. An attentive listener should understand that the fact *'Margery is a high producer'* mentioned at the start of the consultation means something to the client. This should stimulate further questioning, of an open-ended type, regarding the normal post-partum anoestrus interval of low versus high producing cows on the farm or the value of Margery for the client. If this questioning is omitted the client may feel disappointed that this was not completely understood.

Skill 6 (Checks and screens for further problems):

Finally, the client may have a range of concerns he/she wishes to raise. Dysart et al. (12) reported that open-ended questions designed to check for additional concerns resulted in veterinary clients expressing a fuller range of concerns. It is believed in human medicine literature that patients have multiple concerns and the first concern expressed is not always the most important (13). It is important to ascertain this at the outset, in order to efficiently structure the consultation and address all needs. Additionally, Dysart et al. (12) reported clients were four times more likely to voice late arising concerns when an initial solicitation for additional concerns was omitted. Furthermore, a study of physicians and their patients found that the way a solicitation of concerns is worded affects the likelihood that a patient will disclose their full range of concerns (14). The authors reported that the question "Is there something else you want to address today" resulted in a reduction of patient unmet concerns rather than 'Is there anything else you to want to address in the visit today' or a variant 'Do you have any questions?' A more effective solicitation would be. 'So you've noticed a drop in milk production … Is there something else?'

E.g. *'So you have noticed that Margery is not coming in heat. Did you have something else you wanted to raise with me today?'*

The loop of asking for any additional concerns from the client can be repeated until he/she says that everything seems to be addressed (e.g. 'I think that's all').

Skill 7 (Negotiates agenda taking both the client's and practitioner's needs into account):

When there are multiple problems in the same patient, the practitioner should negotiate the order of addressing problems using a logical explanation for the agenda. Effective solicitation of needs is likely to allow for effective time allocation in the consultation and does not lead to longer consultations (14, 15) as well as reducing late arising concerns (15). During negotiation of the order of addressing concerns, the practitioner should take into account multiple factors including the needs of the client, ensuring efficiency with the agenda, acknowledging the physical or time constraints of the practitioner or the facility, as well as biosecurity requirements.

E.g. *'So, we'll look at the infected hoof first and then we'll talk about the milk yield … is that okay?'* It is most likely that the client will wish to prioritise the chief clinical concern, rather than other aspects the practitioner deems equally important. There are two agendas in every consultation; the practitioner and the clients. An aspect of the art of communication is being able to meet both needs in a relatively short time frame.

E.g. *'We will discuss Margery's problem in detail and then we will talk about the farm and the herd. Does this sound reasonable?'* or *'So, we will look at problem with the fertility first and then we will check the leg. I think this is better to prevent contamination to the reproductive organs with bugs from the foot….pause…is that okay?'*

GATHERING INFORMATION

Gathering information includes four important steps in case management namely 1) gathering a history, 2) clinical examination, 3) ancillary examination techniques and 4) collecting and assaying appropriate samples. Addressing all four steps in gathering information is not within the scope of this article; gathering a history is the focus. For the other three steps in gathering information (clinical examination, ancillary examination techniques and collection and assaying appropriate samples) readers are referred to numerous textbooks and reviews on clinical examination of cattle examples.

Gathering a history

Gathering a precise, complete and relevant history is a key step to an accurate diagnosis and in fact contributes 60-80% of the data for diagnosis in human medicine (16). The clinical content of gathering history, particularly for a non-experienced practitioner, may be aided by examination checklists allowing for consistency in obtaining initial information. In general, there are two types of histories; the complete and the focussed history (16). A complete history is usually gathered for a first consultation and includes the client's problem list, the clinical (patient and disorder) data, the client's perspective and background information including general history (Table 1). A more focussed interview is often used for follow-up appointments and is the same as the complete history, but includes only selective discussion of pertinent background information. It is important to ensure that during each consultation, regardless of time between visits, those changes to management practice are routinely sought.

Table 1. Elements of gathering history

Element	Some important components
Patient data	Species, breed, identification, sex, age, colour, production status, stage in lactation
Presenting problem	• Major signs observed (SOCRATES: Site, Onset, Character, Radiation, Alleviation, Time, Exacerbation, Severity) • Context of what were the circumstances when signs were observed (epidemiological parameters, place, nutrition, past or concurrent problems / treatments, activity, recent travel) • Associated signs (e.g. fever, diarrhoea, discharge).
Review of body regions and/or organ systems	Rarely done in practice: e.g. gastro-intestinal, respiratory, cardio-vascular, genito-urinary, integumentary, nervous, musculo-skeletal, lymphatic, and sensory
Client's perspective	• Effect of the disorder on client's lifestyle • Effects of the disorder on farm management • Pride in the society
	Reasons why the problem has occurred Management ideas about the problem

The accuracy of information provided by clients may be variable due to a number of factors, many of which are inherent to the professional nature of the farming client. It is important to remember that the client is an expert in his/her own right. The client has expertise in the farm and its management, characteristics of their stock and their own capacity for management. An aspect of this expertise may be elucidated through careful and accurate observations which clients make when describing clinical concerns. History obtained from such a client may be of great assistance in establishing the diagnosis. Other clients may be less observant or not experienced enough to detect the abnormalities. Therefore, history obtained from such a client may have some level of inaccuracy and relies upon the expertise of the practitioner in deciphering this. Some inaccuracy may reflect how closely cattle are being monitored (*i.e.* beef *vs.* dairy cattle, dry *vs.* milking cows). On very rare occasions, the answers to the questions may be deliberately untrue in an attempt to cover incompetency, fraudulent action or negligence. The accuracy of the answers has to be carefully assessed during the examination process. Consequently, it is vital that a collaborative relationship is established to enable both parties to work together in collecting an accurate history.

Exploration of client's problems

Skill 8 (Encourages client to tell the story of the animal's problem/s from when it first started to the present in their own words):

The practitioner should encourage the client to tell the story in the client's own words and guide the client towards the necessary detail, clarity and completeness for diagnostic accuracy (17). Often, a client will come with a pre-prepared narrative of the concerns and it requires patience on the part of the veterinarian to listen to the full account. The payoff is considerable. Hearing the client's full narrative gives the practitioner insight into how the client is understanding and interpreting events and at what level. Additionally, the client may provide detail that the practitioner may have overlooked (17).

E.g. *'Can you walk me through what you have seen with Margery from calving to now?'* or *'You told me that Margery has not cycled since calving. Can you tell me how her calving was?"*

Skill 9 (Uses open and closed questions, appropriately moving from open to closed):

A 'cone' or 'funnel' approach to question asking is suggested as most efficacious in the clinical interview. Questioning about the history should progress from open-ended (e.g. How's her appetite?' or *'Can you tell me how was Margery's calving?'*) to more narrow open-ended questions *'Can you describe the force that you used to pulled her calf?'* to closed-ended questions (e.g. 'How many times was she sick' or *'How often per do day you check if Margery is in heat?'*). Open-ended questions permit the client to tell his/her story in their own words, from their own perspective, and to give the client space to ensure his/hers agenda is met. The effective use of open-ended questions in veterinary medicine is believed to increase client adherence and satisfaction as well as prevent premature hypothesis generation (18). Interestingly, open-ended questions were used in 10/65 (15%) of companion animal veterinary consultations, thus veterinarians relied on a series of closed-ended questions to gather a complete history from their client (19). Closed-ended questions serve an important purpose in clarifying details, ensuring completeness of the history and ultimately ensuring the practitioner's agenda is covered. It is of interest to note the difference between open- and closed-ended questions as outlined in Table 2; in so much as every closed-ended question can easily become an open-ended question.

Table 2. Examples of open- and closed - ended questions for gathering information

Open-ended questions	Closed-ended questions
Tell me about Margery's walking.	How long has Margery been walking awkwardly?
Describe to me what you have seen.	Did you notice if she was able to walk in a straight line?
What has Margery been offered in the feed bunk?	Does Margery have easy access to the feed bunk?
How is Margery acting in the presence of humans?	Does Margery run away from you?
How do you feel about this outcome?	Are you happy with this outcome?

It is imperative that the questioning is non-judgmental (e.g. *'Are you sure you have not missed her being in heat?'*) and without the use of leading questions (e.g. *'Margery's calving was OK, wasn't it?'*). Anecdotally, it is often suggested that closed-ended questions can save time. However, used in isolation they often produce misleading or inaccurate answers and may require a return to the same issue later in the consultation; thus suggesting a false economy. In fact, open-ended questions are part of a cluster of skills inherent to relationship-centred styles of communication which are associated with increased patient satisfaction and similar, if not reduced, consultation length (20).Enquiry type and tact are particularly important for the chronology of the disorder, as many clients may feel responsible for not taking action when the first abnormalities were observed and, therefore, may try to cover their oversight or neglect.

Skill 10 (Listens attentively, allowing the client to complete statements without interruptions and leaving time for the client to think before answering):

To be effective at gathering information, practitioners must learn to get the right balance between listening and questioning. This is an important aspect of the practitioner's 'bedside manner' and is essential if the appropriate information is to be gathered. The client should be allowed to finish their statement without interruption. Another related problem occurs when there is too much unstructured questioning which can come across as an interrogation. Once interrupted with sub-questions or paraphrasing of the first expressed problem, the client may not feel confident introducing new issues (21).

Skill 11 (Facilitates the client responses verbally and non-verbally):

It is important to encourage the client to complete their response. There are several ways to achieve this goal including encouragement and silence (16). The first, encouragement, is in the form of verbal utterances "Yes... (pause)... go on", "Uh huh" or nonverbally by head nodding and other facial and nonverbal indicators expressing interest. Second, silence or a momentary pause often gives enough space for the client to finish their thought. Interestingly, when teachers were trained to pause for three seconds at key times following question asking, students were more inclined to ask questions, spoke for longer duration and even those quieter students contributed. Similar effect has been reported in human medicine and is expected to be valid for clients presenting cattle problems.

Skill 12 (Picks up verbal and non-verbal cues from the client, checks out and acknowledges as appropriate):

Clients will use nonverbal methods to communicate the message a staggering 80% of the time and actual verbal utterances account for the remaining 20% or sometimes less (22). Accordingly, the practitioner will need to attend to both the verbal message and nonverbal cues expressed by the client. Noticing the cue is the first step, responding and acknowledging it, the second. This can be achieved by stating, where the practitioner notices a look of discomfort in the form of facial expressions or hand movements "Am I right in thinking you have been unhappy with the treatment provided in the past?" or noticing the cue, can be as simple as repeating the cue expressed by the client, for example "Wished you had called earlier...?" "Financially stressed...?" Interestingly, acknowledging the patient's cues has been found to shorten consultations (22), quite possibly due to patients not needing to raise the same issues repeatedly in an attempt to be understood or worse, giving up.

"You seem to be concerned about the results I have given you. Would you like to discuss this now or do you want to have a think first and we can discuss this at the next visit?"

Skill 13 (Clarifies statements that are vague or need amplification):

Clients may provide responses which are vague and will require prompts for clarity, detail or completeness from the practitioner. Additionally, the way each person perceives an experience is likely different from another. For example a client responds, in the case of Margery, with *"a lot of discharge from the vagina"* the definition of "a lot" and for that matter "discharge" may be different from that of the practitioner. Consequently clarifying questions such as *"Could you please describe what you mean by a lot of vaginal discharge?"* are invaluable for accuracy.

Skill 14 (Periodically summarises to verify own understanding of what the client has said):

It is advisable that the practitioner overtly repeats the verbal information provided by the client. Repetition demonstrates understanding of the information obtained from the client, allows the client time to confirm or change the meaning and ensures accuracy (16). Specifically, two skills are of interest; paraphrasing and summarising. A paraphrase involves using the practitioner's own words to clarify or encourage the client to continue e.g. *"So you've had a difficult time lately with Margery..."*. A summary can represent an internal summary or a summary designed to be used at various times throughout the gathering information phase (16). It should include both the client's perspective as well as the clinical information obtained. (e.g. *"You have noticed that Margery had some discharge from the vagina for about a week that began approximately two weeks after calving and you thought it might have been related to her decreased appetite... (pause) ... is there something else?* While summaries are a vital aspect of information gathering, when repeatedly inaccurate, clients may experience the physician as being inattentive and not understanding their concerns (23).

Skill 15 (Uses concise, easily understood language, avoiding or adequately explaining jargon):

The use of non-technical terms during the gathering history phase helps to ensure the client understands questions being asked of them. For example, the client will easily understand in heat, but may be unfamiliar with the term oestrus. Interestingly, an North American report written in 2005 reported the majority of adults read at an 8th grade level but most health information is written at a year 10 reading level (24). Moreover, a study of medical residents found that they significantly overestimated the health literacy of their patients and erroneously made judgements of their patients' capacity for understanding based on their completed year of high school (25). Taken together, these results strongly advocate the use of client-friendly language.

Additional skills for understanding client's perspective

The client's perspective incorporates the beliefs, ideas, concerns, role of the individual patient/herd on the farm, expectations and how the problem affects client's life as well as the management of the enterprise. An appreciation and incorporation of the client's perspective is fundamental to the development of a collaborative approach. Numerous positive outcomes have been realised with human medicine clinicians employing a relationship-centred style of communication including patient satisfaction (26), loyalty and commitment to the individual practitioner, as well as enhanced adherence to treatment and recommendations (27). Similar benefits are expected for veterinarians.

Skills 16a (Determines and acknowledges client's ideas and concerns regarding each problem):

The client may request a bovine consultation with a preconceived notion or diagnosis of the presenting problem. The client's formulation may or may not be accurate. However, in formulating this diagnosis, for example *"Margery having inactive ovaries"*, the client may have ideas about how to treat the inactivity, what the effect will be and concerns related to its management. It is important that the practitioner determines these ideas and concerns early in the consultation and importantly, acknowledges them with questions such as:

"What do you think is the cause?", "Have you got any ideas about what is happening here?" and/ or *"Is there something that particularly concerns you?"*

The client responds: *'Margery is not cycling. She is certainly looking the same as Mooie who had inactive ovaries.'* At this point the practitioner is well aware of the client's formulation and is better equipped to manage the client's expectations of diagnosis and treatment based on this formulation. Without this information, discussion of the diagnosis and treatment plan may be met with resistance as the client may be confused or shocked by the information provided by the practitioner. This can negatively affect adherence and the ongoing collaborative relationship.

Skill 16b (Determines and acknowledges client's expectations):

The client will have expectations about the care provided by the practitioner, the outcomes and perhaps the process for the consultation. It is useful to determine these expectations with questions such as "It seems you have thought a lot about this. What were you thinking is the best course of action?" or "What were you hoping for today?"

E.g. *"OK, Jack. Seems you have thought a lot about Margery's problem and researched this issue on the internet. She does share some similar symptoms to Mooie. However, Margery has active ovaries and probably is cycling regularly but has not been detected. It is very likely she is a high producer to have so-called 'silent heats'. We can leave it to run its course hoping you will detect her at the next cycle or we can use hormonal treatment to use fixed time artificial insemination. What would be the preferred option for Margery today?"*

Skill 16c (Determines and acknowledges how each problem affects the client):

Finally, it is essential that the practitioner determines how each noted problem impacts the management of the enterprise and life of the client. For example, *"I get the sense that you want to change your heat detection, and you have concerns about your production and lifestyle. Please, let me know how this affects you."* A question of this type provides an excellent entry point to understanding the client's perspective and helps to plan treatment within the capacity of the client with minimal changes to the management of the cattle enterprise. Ultimately, understanding this information should enhance adherence to treatment and the recommended course of action as it is specifically tailored to the needs of that particular client.

In our example of Margery being one of the cows characterised with a 'silent heat' the client is interested in how to recognise these cows. With the second explanation, the client is interested immediately how to recognise these cows. The practitioner could explain that the use of more 'in heat' observations per day or oestrus detection aids may assist is a logical continuation of the discussion.

Skill 17 (Encourages expression of the client's feelings and thoughts):

In determining the client's perspective, it is important for the practitioner to allow the client to express the thoughts and feelings with regard to the information provided and decisions made. These issues will also need to be addressed as required.

"Jack, I think you have read a lot about non-cycling cows. Do you agree with what we have discussed? Tell me what you think about it."

CONCLUSIONS

Appropriate communication skills are essential to successful companion and production animal veterinary practice, including practitioners. The MCCG as exemplified above, provides a useful framework for integrating clinical communication skills with clinical content; a must for effective consultations. The MCCG are relevant to all veterinary practitioners from production to equine to companion animal veterinarians. Communication both verbal and non-verbal is a cornerstone skill in building a relationship with the client and directly influences the outcome of the consultation, treatment and adherence to recommendations (18, 28).

ACKNOWLEDGMENTS

KRP was responsible for the idea, preliminary write up and clinical aspects of the article. MMM was responsible for the theoretical basis and contributed to the writing and editing of the manuscript.

REFERENCES

1. Kanji, N., J. B. Coe, Adams, C. L., Shaw J. R. (2012). Effect of veterinarian-client-patient interactions on client adherence to dentistry and surgery recommendations in companion-animal practice. J Am Vet Med Assoc. 240(4): 427-436. http://dx.doi.org/10.2460/javma.240.4.427 PMid:22309015

2. Coe, J.B., Adams, C.L. Bonnett, B.N. (2008). A focus group study of veterinarians' and pet owners' perceptions of veterinarian-client communication in companion animal practice. Journal of the American Veterinary Medical Association 233(7): 1072-1080. http://dx.doi.org/10.2460/javma.233.7.1072 PMid:18828715

3. Shaw, J.R., Adams, C. L., Bonnett, B.N., Larson, S., Roter, D.L (2012). Veterinarian satisfaction with companion animal visits. Journal of the American Veterinary Medical Association 240(7): 832-41. http://dx.doi.org/10.2460/javma.240.7.832 PMid:22443436

4. Sandler, G. (1979). Costs of unnecessary tests. British Medical Journal. 7(2): p. 21-4. http://dx.doi.org/10.1136/bmj.2.6181.21

5. Kurtz, S., Silverman, J., Benson, J., Draper, J. (2003). Marrying content and process in clinical method teaching: Enhancing the Calgary-Cambridge guides. Academic Medicine. 78 (8): 802-809. http://dx.doi.org/10.1097/00001888-200308000-00011 PMid:12915371

6. Gillard, S., Benson, J., Silverman, J. (2009). Teaching and assessment of explanation and planning in medical schools in the United Kingdom: cross sectional questionnaire survey. Med Teach. 31 (4): 328-331. http://dx.doi.org/10.1080/01421590801953018 PMid:19142799

7. Adams, C.L., Kurtz, S.M. (2006). Building on existing models from human medical education to develop a communication curriculum in veterinary medicine. J Vet Med Educ. 33 (1): 28-37.
http://dx.doi.org/10.3138/jvme.33.1.28
PMid:16767635

8. Radford, A., Stockley, P., Silverman, J., Taylor, I., Turner, R., Gray, C. (2006). Development, teaching, and evaluation of a consultation structure model for use in veterinary education. J Vet Med Educ. 33(1): 38-44.
http://dx.doi.org/10.3138/jvme.33.1.38
PMid:16767636

9. Moulton, L. (2007). The naked consultation: A practical guide to primary consultation skills. Abingdon, UK: Radcliffe.

10. Boudreau, J.D., Cassell, E. Fuks, A. (2009). Preparing medical students to become attentive listeners. Med Teach. 31 (1): 22-29.
http://dx.doi.org/10.1080/01421590802350776
PMid:19140065

11. Rhoades, D.R., McFarland, K.F. Finch, W.H., Johnson, A.O. (2001). Speaking and interruptions during primary care office visits. Fam Med. 33 (7): 528-532.
PMid:11456245

12. Dysart, L.M., Coe, J.B., Adams, C.L. (2011). Analysis of solicitation of client concerns in companion animal practice. Journal of the American Veterinary Medical Association. 238 (12): 1609-1615.
http://dx.doi.org/10.2460/javma.238.12.1609
PMid:21671816

13. Beckman, H., Frankel, R. (1984). The effect of physician behaviour on the collection of data. Annals of Internal Medicine. 9 (9): 517-521.

14. Heritage, J., Robinson, J.D., Elliott, M.N., Beckett, M., Wilkes, M. (2007). Reducing patients' unmet concerns in primary care: the difference one word can make. Journal of General Internal Medicine. 22 (10): 1429-33.
http://dx.doi.org/10.1007/s11606-007-0279-0
PMid:17674111 PMCid:PMC2305862

15. Brock, D.M., Mauksch, L. B., Witteborn, S., Hummel, J., Nagasawa, P., Robins, L.S. (2011). Effectiveness of intensive physician training in upfront agenda setting. Journal of General Internal Medicine. 26 (11): 1317-1323.
http://dx.doi.org/10.1007/s11606-011-1773-y
PMid:21735348 PMCid:PMC3208461

16. Silverman, J.D., Kurtz, S., Draper, J. (2005). Skills for communicating with patients. 2nd ed. Oxford: Radcliffe Publishing.

17. Lipkin, M., Putnam, S.M., Lazare, A. eds (1995). The Medical Interview: Clinical Care Education and Research. Springer-Verlag: New York.
http://dx.doi.org/10.1007/978-1-4612-2488-4

18. Shaw, J. (2006). Four core communication skills of highly effective practitioners. Veterinary Clinics of North America-Small Animal Practice. 36 (2): 385-396.
http://dx.doi.org/10.1016/j.cvsm.2005.10.009
PMid:16442449

19. McArthur, M. Fitzgerald, J. (2013). Companion animal veterinarians' use of clinical communication skills. Aust Vet J. 91 (9): 374-380.
http://dx.doi.org/10.1111/avj.12083
PMid:23980830

20. Abdel-Tawab, N. Roter, D. (2002). The relevance of client-centred communication to family planning settings in developing countries: lessons from the Egyptian experience. Social Science and Medicine. 54, 1357-1368.
http://dx.doi.org/10.1016/S0277-9536(01)00101-0

21. Gask, L., Usherwood, T. (2002). ABC of psychological medicine. The consultation. BMJ. 324 (7353): 1567-1569.
http://dx.doi.org/10.1136/bmj.324.7353.1567
PMid:12089097 PMCid:PMC1123505

22. Levinson, W., Gorawara-Bhat, R., Lamb, J. (2000). A study of patient clues and physician responses in primary care and surgical settings. Journal of the American Medical Association 284, 1021-1027.
http://dx.doi.org/10.1001/jama.284.8.1021
PMid:10944650

23. Quilligan, S., Silverman, J. (2012). The skill of summary in clinician-patient communication: a case study. Patient Educ Couns. 86 (3): 354-359.
http://dx.doi.org/10.1016/j.pec.2011.07.009
PMid:21821377

24. Safeer, R.S., Keenan, J. (2005). Health literacy: the gap between physicians and patients. Am Fam Physician. 72 (3): 463-468.
PMid:16100861

25. Bass, P.F., Wilson, J. F., Griffith, C. H., Barnett, D. R. (2002). Residents' ability to identify patients with poor literacy skills. Acad Med. 77 (10): 1039-1041.
http://dx.doi.org/10.1097/00001888-200210000-00021
PMid:12377684

26. McMillan, S.S., Kendall, E., Sav, A., King, M. A., Whitty, J. A., Kelly, F., Wheeler, A. J. (2013). Patient-centered approaches to health care: a systematic review of randomized controlled trials. Med Care Res Rev. 70 (6): 567-596.
http://dx.doi.org/10.1177/1077558713496318
PMid:23894060

27. Robinson, J.H., et al. (2008). Patient-centered care and adherence: definitions and applications to improve outcomes. J Am Acad Nurse Pract. 20 (12): 600-607. http://dx.doi.org/10.1111/j.1745-7599.2008.00360.x PMid:19120591

28. Kleen, J.L., Atkinson, O., Noordhuizen, J. (2011). Communication in production animal medicine: modelling a complex interaction with the example of dairy herd health medicine. Irish Veterinary Journal. 64. http://dx.doi.org/10.1186/2046-0481-64-8 PMid:21777495 PMCid:PMC3156738

29

PCR ASSAY WITH HOST SPECIFIC INTERNAL CONTROL FOR *STAPHYLOCOCCUS AUREUS* FROM BOVINE MILK SAMPLES

Zafer Cantekin[1], Yasar Ergun[2], Hasan Solmaz[3], Gamze Özge Özmen[1], Melek Demir[1], Radhwane Saidi[4]

[1]*Mustafa Kemal University, Faculty of Veterinary Medicine, Department of Microbiology, Tayfur Sokmen Campus 31000 Hatay, Turkey*
[2]*Mustafa Kemal University, Faculty of Veterinary Medicine, Department of Obstetrics and Gynecology, Tayfur Sokmen Campus 31000 Hatay, Turkey*
[3]*Yüzüncü Yıl University, Faculty of Pharmacy, Department of Pharmaceutical Microbiology, Campus, 65100 Van, Turkey*
[4]*Department of Agronomy, Telidji Amar University, P. O. Box 37G, 03000 Laghouat, LBRA, Algeria*

ABSTRACT

Staphylococcus aureus is considered as one of the most important and common pathogens of bovine mastitis. Polymerase Chain Reaction is frequently proposed in the diagnosis of *S. aureus* directly from milk samples instead of classical culture. However, false-negative results may occur in the polymerase chain reaction analysis performed directly from clinical material. For the purpose of disclosing the false negative results, the use of internal amplification controls can be beneficial. Therefore, in this study a new polymerase chain reaction technique with host specific internal amplification control was developed by optimizing *S. aureus*-specific primers in combination with bovine specific primers. The effectiveness of the developed technique in this study was attempted in milk samples from bovine subclinical mastitis. This technique has the potential to detect *S. aureus* from bovine milk samples or dairy products.

Key words: bovine milk, internal control, polymerase chain reaction, *Staphylococcus aureus*

INTRODUCTION

Staphylococcus aureus, one of the most prevalent pathogens of clinical and subclinical bovine mastitis, can spread rapidly throughout the herd if management precautions are not taken (1, 2). *S. aureus* is one of the most important and common pathogens of bovine mastitis. It causes significant economic losses in the dairy industry (3). *S. aureus* damages milk-producing tissue and significantly decreases milk yield. In the early stages of infection, damage may be reversible, but when diagnosis is delayed, tissue damage is excessive and irreversible (4). Therefore, a rapid and reliable method of identifying the bacteria responsible for mastitis is important for disease management in the herd (5). Moreover, *S. aureus* infections are considered a serious problem that may affect public health because they can be transmitted by milk and milk products (6).

While different methods have been used to detect these agents, bacterial culture is considered the gold standard method for identifying mastitis-causing microorganisms. However, conventional culture is slow, requiring 24–48 h, and needs labour intensive study for definitive identification (7, 8). Therefore, it is of commercial interest to accelerate this procedure by investigating alternative rapid DNA-based methods. PCR methods for detecting *S. aureus* in milk samples to identify cow mastitis have been proposed (9, 10, 11). However, PCR analyses from direct clinical material can result in false negative results caused by inhibitors in

Corresponding author: Dr. Zafer Cantekin, PhD
E-mail address: zcantekin@hotmail.com
Present address: Mustafa Kemal University, Faculty of Veterinary Medicine, Department of Microbiology, Tayfur Sokmen Campus 31000 Hatay, Turkey

the clinical specimens (12, 13). Therefore the use of internal amplification controls with different strategies is recommended to determine false negative results of PCR analyses from direct clinical material or food samples (14, 15).

The aim of the present study was to develop PCR analyses with internal amplification control to detect *S. aureus*. A specific primer set for *S. aureus* was used and combined with bovine-specific primers.

and Sau 1645) specific for *S. aureus*, and 5 pmol primers (12SM-FW and 12SBT-REV2) specific for bovine gene.

Amplification was carried out after an initial denaturation at 95°C for 3 min. The PCR protocol was: 60 s of template denaturation at 94°C, 60 s of different primer annealing temperatures at 54°C, and 90 s of primer extension at 72°C (total of 35 cycles), with a final extension at 72°C for 5 min. The amplified PCR products were electrophoresed

Table 1. Properties of primers used in the study

Primer names	Target Gene	GC Contents (%)	Melting Temperature	Sequences of primers	Length of amplicons	References
Sau 327	23S rRNA	45	63 °C	5'-GGACGACATTAGACGAATCA-3'	1318 bp	10
Sau 1645		45	63 °C	5'-CGGGCACCTATTTTCTATCT-3'		
12SM-FW	12S rRNA gene sequences	39	65 °C	5'-CTAGAGGAGCCTGTTCTATAATCGATAA-3'	346 bp	17
12SBT-REV2		37	65 °C	5'-AAATAGGGTTAGATGCACTGAATCCAT-3'		

MATERIAL AND METHODS

Samples and Primers

Total of 50 milk samples from subclinical bovine mastitis were obtained from cattle farms in the Hatay region (The clinical samples were taken with permission with MKÜ Local Ethics committee; Meeting Date 17.06.2010: Meeting No: 2010/02: Decision No: 30) and nucleic acids were extracted from milk samples using the phenol–chloroform method. Extracted DNA was stored at -20°C (16).

Primers for *S. aureus* (Sau 327 and Sau 1645) and Bovine specific (12SM-FW and 12SBT-REV2) were used in this study. Simplex PCR protocols and procedures were carried out according to the recommendations in the literature for those primers. The properties of the primers used in this study are shown in Table 1.

Optimisation of internally controlled PCR mix

All procedures and protocols for multiplex PCR assays were optimized according to Henegariu et al., (18). The amplification mixture for multiplex PCR was carried out in a final volume of 25 µL. The mixture consisted of 200 ng of extracted DNA template, different amounts of 1.5U of *Taq*DNA polymerase (Vivantis Technologies), 2 µL of 10x PCR buffer (10X ViBuffer A without MgCl$_2$), 3 mM MgCl$_2$, 200 µM each of dNTPs (Vivantis Technologies), 20 pmol of primer pair (Sau 327

in 1.5% agarose gel and stained with ethidium bromide (0.5 mg/mL), and the DNA bands were visualised under UV light.

RESULTS

Simplex PCR reaction results

In the PCR analyses of milk samples, 3 of 50 samples were found to be *S. aureus* by simplex PCR and the specific amplification products (1318 bp). They are shown in Figure 1. *S. aureus*–specific bands were amplified very effectively with simplex PCR.

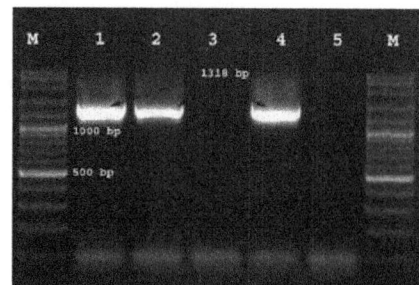

Figure 1. Results of simplex PCR from milk samples with *S. aureus* specific primers. M: 100bp plus marker. Lanes 1, 2, and 4: *S. aureus*-specific bands with Sau 327 and Sau 1645 primers (1318 bp). Lane 5: Distilled Water (Negative Control)

Multiplex PCR reaction results

In the PCR analysis results, specific bands for bovine gene as an internal control and specific bands for *S. aureus* were amplified effectively in the same PCR mixture; the amplification products are shown in Figure 2.

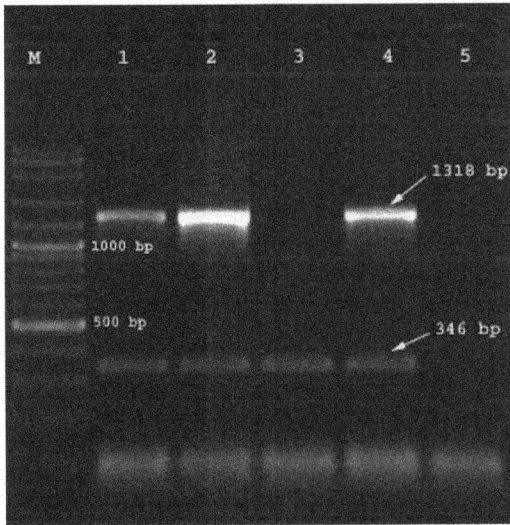

Figure 2. Results of multiplex PCR from milk samples. M: 100bp plus marker. 1–4: bovine-specific bands with 12SM-FW and 12SBT-REV2 primers (346 bp); 1, 2, and 4: *S. aureus*–specific bands with Sau 327 and Sau 1645 primers (1318 bp); 5: Distilled Water (Negative Control)

DISCUSSION

Staphylococcus aureus is considered an important and common pathogen causing bovine mastitis that can also be dangerous to human health. There are some studies including PCR detection of *S. aureus* from bovine milk samples (9, 10, 11). However, in the PCR analyses from clinical material false negative results can be encountered due to inhibitory substances. In order to avoid these false negative results, using internal control was recommended (12, 13). Particularly, using of host specific internal control can be useful to determine false negative results due to mistakes in sampling, DNA extraction or preparing PCR mixtures and thermal cycler failures (14, 15, 19). Therefore, a PCR technique with host specific internal control was developed in this study by combining *S. aureus* specific primers and cow specific primers.

In this study a preliminary type, a specific primer set for *S. aureus*, was combined with specific bovine gene primers to develop an easy and rapid multiplex PCR system with high specificity. Using this optimised combination, a PCR analysis

with an internal control specific for bovine genes was developed to detect *S. aureus*. The primer sets successfully amplified the target genes in the multiplex PCR without nonspecific or additional bands. There was no difficulty in discriminating between each band for the target strain (1318 bp) and the internal control (346 bp). Despite the low numbers of positive samples used in this study, the authors are confident that the developed technique will be reproducible in larger experiments.

At the end of the optimisation experiments, the best amplification results were obtained by decreasing 10x PCR buffer (2 µL) and host-specific primers 12SM-FW and 12SBT-REV2 (internal control, 5 pmol) and increasing to 20 pmol primers (Sau 327 and Sau 1645) specific for *S. aureus*. While low and high concentrations of $MgCl_2$ negatively affected the multiplex PCR, the best results were obtained with 3 mM of $MgCl_2$ concentration. The other important parameter was the annealing temperature: the best results were obtained at 54°C. The effects of these parameters were found to be in agreement with the recommendations of Henegariu et al. (18) and Phuektes et al. (20).

Despite the small number of samples analysed, the results of this preliminary study showed that this method can be used as a reliable and effective method for the diagnosis of *S. aureus* in the individual bovine milk or bulk milk samples. This technique should be tried for *S. aureus* detection from bovine milk products

In conclusion, conventional PCR has already become widespread and is less expensive than other molecular techniques. The developed technique in this study might have the potential to detect *S. aureus* from bovine clinical samples. This method can be used for detecting *S. aureus* in the bovine milk or milk products. The technique can also be extended to detect other contagious mastitis pathogens, such as *Streptococcus agalactiae* and *Trueperella pyogenes*.

REFERENCES

1. Sommerhäuser, J., Kloppert, B., Wolter, W., Zschöck, M., Sobiraj, A., Failing, K. (2003). The epidemiology of Staphylococcus aureus infections from subclinical mastitis in dairy cows during a control programme. Vet Microbiol., 96, 91- 102. http://dx.doi.org/10.1016/S0378-1135(03)00204-9

2. Le Marechal, C., Thiery, R., Leloir, Y. (2011). Mastitis impact on technologic properties of milk and quality of milk products- review. Dairy Sci Technol., 91, 247-282. http://dx.doi.org/10.1007/s13594-011-0009-6

3. Halasa, T., Nielen, M., De Roos, A.P., Van Hoorne, R., De Jong, G., Lam, T.J., Van Werven, T., Hogeveen, H. (2009). Production loss due to new subclinical mastitis in Dutch dairy cows estimated with a test-day model. J Dairy Sci., 92, 599-606.
http://dx.doi.org/10.3168/jds.2008-1564

4. Belschner, A.P., Hallberg, J.W., Nickerson, S.C., Owens, W.E. (1996). Staphylococcus aureus mastitis therapy revisited. Proceedings of the National Mastitis Council Annual Meeting, (pp. 116-122), Madison, Wisconsin

5. Taponen, S., Simojoki, H., Haveri, M., Larsen, H.D., Pyorala, S. (2006). Clinical characteristics and persistence of bovine mastitis caused by different species of coagulase-negative staphylococci identified with API or AFLP. Vet Microbiol., 115, 199-207.
http://dx.doi.org/10.1016/j.vetmic.2006.02.001
PMid:16527434

6. Le Loir, Y., Baron, F., Gautier, M. (2003). Staphylococcus aureus and food poisoning. Genet Mol Res., 2, 63-76.

7. NMC (1999). Laboratory and field handbook on bovine mastitis. National Mastitis Council, p.139, Madison, Wisconsin

8. Koivula, M., Mäntysaari, E.A., Pitkälä, A., Pyörälä, S. (2007). Distribution of bacteria and seasonal and regional effects in a new database for mastitis pathogens in Finland. Acta Agric Scand. A. 57, 89-96.
http://dx.doi.org/10.1080/09064700701488941

9. Khan, M.A., Kim, C.H., Kakoma, I., Morin, E., Hansen, R.D., Hurley, W.L., Tripathy, D.N., Baek, B.K. (1998). Detection of Staphylococcus aureus in milk by use of polymerase chain reaction analysis. Am J Vet Res., 59, 807-813.

10. Riffon, R., Sayasith, K., Khalil, H., Dubreuil, P., Drolet, M., Lagace, A. (2001). Development of a rapid and sensitive test for identification of major pathogens in bovine mastitis by PCR. J Clin Microbiol., 39, 2584-2589.
http://dx.doi.org/10.1128/JCM.39.7.2584-2589.2001
PMid:11427573; PMCid:PMC88189

11. Ahmadi, M., Rohani, S.M.R., Ayremlou N. (2010). Detection of Staphylococcus aureus in milk by PCR. Comp Clin Pathol., 19, 91-94.
http://dx.doi.org/10.1007/s00580-009-0901-0

12. Wilson, I.G., Cooper, J.E., Gilmour, A. (1994). Some factors inhibiting amplification of the Staphylococcus aureus enterotoxin c1 gene (sec+) by PCR. Int J Food Microbiol., 22, 55-62.
http://dx.doi.org/10.1016/0168-1605(94)90007-8

13. Kim, C.H., Khan, M.A., Morin, E., Hurley, W.L., Tripathy, D.N., Kehrli, M., Jr Olouch, A.O., Kakomal, I. (2001). Optimization of the PCR for detection of Staphylococcus aureus nuc gene in bovine milk. J Dairy Sci., 84, 74-83.
http://dx.doi.org/10.3168/jds.S0022-0302(01)74454-2

14. Hoorfar, J., Malorny, B., Abdulmawjood, A., Cook, N., Wagner, M., Fach, P. (2004). Practical considerations in design of internal amplification controls for diagnostic PCR assays. J Clin Microbiol., 42, 5, 1863-1868.
http://dx.doi.org/10.1128/JCM.42.5.1863-1868.2004

15. He, X., Shi, X. (2010). Internal amplification control and its applications in PCR detection of foodborne pathogens. Wei Sheng Wu Xue Bao 50, 2, 141-147.

16. Sambrook, J., Russell, W. (2001). Molecular cloning: a laboratory manual (3rd ed.), A8.9-A8.10. (pp.2049-2050), Cold Spring Harbor Press, New York

17. Lopez-Calleja A.I., Fajardo I.G, Rodriguez, V., Hernandez, M.A., Garcia, P.E., Martin, R. (2005). PCR detection of cows' milk in water buffalo milk and mozzarella cheese. Int Dairy J., 15, 1122-1129.
http://dx.doi.org/10.1016/j.idairyj.2004.12.003

18. Henegariu, O.N., Heerema, A., Dlouhy, S.R., Vance, G.H., Vogt, P.H. (1997). Multiplex PCR-critical parameters and step-by-step protocol. Biotechniques 23, 504-511.

19. Helps, C., Reeves, N., Egan, K., Howard, P., Harbour, D. (2003). Detection of Chlamydophila felis and feline herpes virus by multiplex real-time PCR analysis. J Clin Microbiol., 6, 2734-2736.
http://dx.doi.org/10.1128/JCM.41.6.2734-2736.2003

20. Phuektes, P., Mansell, P.D., Browning, G.F. (2001). Multiplex polymerase chain reaction assay for simultaneous detection of Staphylococcus aureus and streptococcal causes of bovine mastitis. J Dairy Sci., 84, 1140-1148.
http://dx.doi.org/10.3168/jds.S0022-0302(01)74574-2

PERMISSIONS

LIST OF CONTRIBUTORS

Barna S. Tomislav and Milovanović M. Aleksandar
Department of Reproduction, Scientifi c Veterinary Institute "Novi Sad", Rumenački put 20, 21000 Novi Sad, Republic of Serbia

Lazarević I. Miodrag and Gvozdić M. Dragan
Faculty of Veterinary Medicine, University of Belgrade, Bulevar Oslobođenja 18, 11000 Belgrade, Republic of Serbia

Rossen Georgiev Stefanov and Desislava Vasileva Abadjieva
Institute of Biology and Immunology of Reproduction-BAS, bul. Tsarigradsko Shose 73, p.c. 1113, Sofia, Bulgaria

Georgi Anev
Agricultural Institute, BG – Turgovishte, Bulgaria

Miroslav Radeski, Aleksandar Janevski and Vlatko Ilieski
Animal Welfare Center, Faculty of Veterinary Medicine Lazar Pop Trajkov 5-7, 1000 Skopje, Macedonia

Riccardo Benedetti
Department of Environmental Science, University of Camerino, Via Gentile III da Varano 62032 Camerino (MC), Italy

Mirko Barabucci and Alessandra Pigliapoco
Veterinary Clinic "Pigliapoco, Leoni, Barabucci", C.da Valle 6, 62100 Macerata (MC), Italy

Simona Cannas and Clara Palestrini
Department of Veterinary Science and Public Health, University of Milan Via Celoria 10, 20133, Milan, Italy

Kiril Krstevski, Dine Mitrov, Slavcho Mrenoshki, Iskra Cvetkovikj, Aleksandar

Janevski, Aleksandar Dodovski and Igor Djadjovski
Veterinary Institute, Faculty of Veterinary Medicine, Ss. Cyril and Methodius University in Skopje, Republic of Macedonia

Ivancho Naletoski
Animal Production and Health Section, Joint FAO/IAEA Division, International Atomic Energy Agency, Vienna, Austria

Kirovski Danijela
Department of Physiology and Biochemistry, Faculty of Veterinary Medicine, University of Belgrade, 11000 Belgrade, Serbia

Sladojević Željko
Veterinary Station „Veterina system Sladojević", 78400 Gradiška Bosna and Herzegovina, Republic of Srpska

Šamanc Horea
Department of Farm Animal Disease, Faculty of Veterinary Medicine, University of Belgrade, 11000 Belgrade, Serbia

Lainšček Raspor Petra and Kirbiš Andrej
Institute for Food Hygiene and Bromatology, University of Ljubljana, Veterinary Faculty, Ljubljana, Slovenia

Toplak Ivan
Institute for Microbiology, University of Ljubljana, Veterinary Faculty, Ljubljana, Slovenia

Igor Dzadzovski and Aleksandar Janevski
Farm Animal Health Department, Faculty of Veterinary Medicine Skopje, Ss. Cyril and Methodius University, Skopje

Irena Celeska and Igor Ulchar
Department of Pathophysiology, Faculty of Veterinary Medicine Skopje, Ss. Cyril and Methodius University, Skopje

Danijela Kirovski
Department of Physiology and Biochemistry,
Faculty of Veterinary Medicine,
University of Belgrade

Chrcheva-Nikolovska Radmila, Sekulovski Pavle, Jankuloski Dean and Angelovski Ljupco
Faculty of Veterinary Medicine, Ss Cyril and Methodius University, Lazar PopTrajkov 5-7, 1000 Skopje, Republic of Macedonia

Daniela Belichovska
Faculty of Ecological Resources Management, MIT University in Skopje

Zehra Hajrulai-Musliu and Risto Uzunov
Food Institute, Faculty of Veterinary Medicine
Ss. Cyril and Methodius University in Skopje

Katerina Belichovska
Institute for Animal Biotechnology, Faculty of Agricultural Sciences and Food
Ss. Cyril and Methodius University in Skopje

Mila Arapcheska
Faculty of Biotechnical Sciences, St. Kliment Ohridski University in Bitola

Cvetkovikj Aleksandar and Radeski Miroslav
1Veterinary Institute, Faculty of Veterinary Medicine, University Ss. Cyril and Methodius in Skopje

Blazhekovikj-Dimovska Dijana
Fishery Department, Faculty of Biotechnical sciences, University St. Kliment Ohridski in Bitola

Kostov Vasil
Fishery Department, Institute of Animal Science, University Ss. Cyril and Methodius in Skopje

Mirko Prodanov
Food Institute, Faculty of Veterinary Medicine
Skopje University "Ss. Cyril and Methodius" in Skopje

Miroslav Radeski
Veterinary Institute, Faculty of Veterinary Medicine Skopje, University "Ss. Cyril and Methodius" in Skopje

Vlatko Ilieski
Institute for Reproduction and Biomedicine, Faculty of Veterinary Medicine
Skopje, University "Ss. Cyril and Methodius" in Skopje

Ivica Gjurovski, Branko Angelovski, Toni Dovenski, Dine Mitrov and Trpe Ristoski
Faculty of Veterinary Medicine, "Ss Cyril and Methodius" University in Skopje
Lazar Pop Trajkov 5-7, 1000 Skopje, Republic of Macedonia

Zapryanova Dimitrinka
Department of Pharmacology, Animal Physiology and Physiological Chemistry, Faculty of Veterinary Medicine, Trakia University, 6000, Stara Zagora, Bulgaria

Dodovski Aleksandar and Krstevski Kiril
Veterinary Institute, Faculty of Veterinary Medicine, University "Ss. Cyril and Methodius" Skopje, Macedonia

Naletoski Ivancho
Joint FAO/IAEA Division of Nuclear Techniques in Food and Agriculture, Vienna, Austria

Ralica Kyuchukova, Aleksandra Daskalova, Deyan Stratev and Alexander Pavlov
Department of Hygiene and Technology of Foods, Faculty of Veterinary Medicine, Trakia University, Bulgaria

Anelia Milanova and Lubomir Lashev
Department of Pharmacology, Physiology of Animals and Physiological Chemistry, Faculty of Veterinary Medicine, Trakia University, Bulgaria

Saganuwan Alhaji Saganuwan and Patrick Azubuike Onyeyili
Department of Veterinary Physiology, Pharmacology and Biochemistry College of Veterinary Medicine, University of Agriculture, Makurdi, Benue State, Nigeria

Elena Atanaskova Petrov and Goran Nikolovski
Department of Internal Medicine of Small Animals, Faculty of Veterinary Medicine, Ss. Cyril and Methodius University in Skopje, Macedonia

Toni Dovenski
Department of Reproduction, Faculty of Veterinary Medicine, Ss. Cyril and Methodius University, Skopje, Macedonia

Gordana Petrushevska
Department of Pathology, Medical Faculty,Ss. Cyril and Methodius University in Skopje, Macedonia

Ivica Gjurovski and Trpe Ristoski
Department of Pathology, Faculty of Veterinary Medicine, Ss. Cyril and Methodius University in Skopje, Macedonia

Pandorce Trenkoska
Veterinary Clinic D-r Naletoski, Str. 1244/3, Skopje, Macedonia

Plamen Trojacanec and Ksenija Ilievska
Department of Surgery, Faculty of Veterinary Medicine, Ss. Cyril and Methodius University in Skopje, Macedonia

Vania Marutsova and Rumen Binev
Department of Internal Diseases, Faculty of Veterinary Medicine, Trakia University, Students' Campus, 6000 Stara Zagora, Bulgaria

Plamen Marutsov
Department of Veterinary Microbiology, Infectious and Parasitic Diseases, Faculty of Veterinary Medicine, Trakia University, Students' Campus, 6000 Stara Zagora, Bulgaria

Tanja Švara, Mitja Gombač and Milan Pogačnik
Institute of Pathology, Forensic and Administrative Veterinary Medicine

Irena Zdovc
Institute of Microbiology and Parasitology, Veterinary Faculty University of Ljubljana, Gerbičeva 60, 1000 Ljubljana, Slovenia

Zsolt Becskei
University of Belgrade, Faculty of Veterinary Medicine, Department for Animal Breeding and Genetics, Belgrade, Serbia

Tamara Ilić and Sanda Dimitrijević
University of Belgrade, Faculty of Veterinary Medicine, Department of Parasitology, Belgrade, Serbia

Nataša Pavlićević and Ferenc Kiskároly
Veterinary Specialist Institute Subotica, Subotica, Serbia

Tamaš Petrović
Scientific Veterinary Institute Novi Sad, Novi Sad, Serbia

Adeolu Adedapo, Omotayo Babarinsa and Ademola Oyagbemi
Department of Veterinary Physiology, Biochemistry and Pharmacology, University of Ibadan, Ibadan, Nigeria

Aduragbenro Adedapo
Department of Pharmacology and Therapeutics, University of Ibadan, Ibadan, Nigeria

Temidayo Omobowale
Department of Veterinary Medicine, University of Ibadan, Ibadan, Nigeria

Chiara Locatelli, Daniela Montrasio, Ilaria Spalla, Giulia Riscazzi,
Matteo Gobbetti, Alice Savarese, Stefano Romussi and Paola G. Brambilla
Department of Veterinary Sciences and Public Health (DIVET), Università degli Studi di Milano, Via Celoria 10, 20133 Milan, Italy

Namakkal Rajamanickam Senthil, Subramanian Subapriya and Subbaiah Vairamuthu
Centralised Clinical Laboratory Madras Veterinary College, Chennai - 600007, Tamil Nadu, India

Igor Ulchar, Irena Celeska and Anastasija Jakimovska
Department of Pathophysiology, Faculty of Veterinary Medicine – Skopje,
Ss Cyril and Methodius University, Skopje

Jovana Stefanovska
Department of Parasitology, Faculty of Veterinary Medicine – Skopje, Ss Cyril and Methodius University, Skopje

Miroslava Mráčková, Marta Zavadilová and Markéta Sedlinská
Department of Reproduction, Equine Clinic, Faculty of Veterinary Medicine, University of Veterinary and Pharmaceutical Sciences Brno, Brno, Czech Republic

Oliver Radanovic, Jadranka Zutic, Dobrila Jakic-Dimic, Branislav Kureljusic and Bozidar Savic
Institute of Veterinary Medicine of Serbia, Vojvode Toze 14, 11000 Belgrade, Serbia

Kiro R. Petrovski and Michelle Mc Arthur
School of Animal and Veterinary Sciences, the University of Adelaide, SA, Australia

Zafer Cantekin, Gamze Özge Özmen and Melek Demir
Mustafa Kemal University, Faculty of Veterinary Medicine, Department of Microbiology, Tayfur Sokmen Campus 31000 Hatay, Turkey

Yasar Ergun
Mustafa Kemal University, Faculty of Veterinary Medicine, Department of Obstetrics and Gynecology, Tayfur Sokmen Campus 31000 Hatay, Turkey

Hasan Solmaz
Yüzüncü Yıl University, Faculty of Pharmacy, Department of Pharmaceutical Microbiology, Campus, 65100 Van, Turkey

Radhwane Saidi
Department of Agronomy, Telidji Amar University, P. O. Box 37G,
03000 Laghouat, LBRA, Algeria

Index

A

Abrus Precatorius, 106-115
Acute Infl Ammation, 88-91
Adipose Tissue, 2, 46, 48, 50, 59-60, 64, 125
Air Quality, 77-78, 80-81
Animal Based Measures, 15
Artificial Insemination, 10, 13

B

Backyard Poultry, 93-94
Biliary Clearance, 37, 40-41
Bovine Consultation, 176-178, 183
Breeding Ostriches, 59, 64
Bromosulfophthalein, 37-38, 40
Bromosulfophthalein (BSP) Clearance, 37
Brucellosis, 27-28, 32, 34-36

C

Calgary-cambridge Guides, 176-177, 184
Canine Leishmaniosis (CANL), 158
Canonical Case Study, 106
Cardiotoxicity, 138, 142
Cardiotoxicity Study, 138
Chios Sheep, 46-47, 49
Ciprofl Oxacin, 100-101, 103
Circovirosis, 82-83, 85
Clinical Ketosis, 37, 121-123, 125
Clinical Samples, 27-28, 31-33, 99, 189
Common Carp, 100, 103-104
Complex Morphology, 116
Compulsive Disorders, 24-26
Corn Silk, 138-139, 141-144
Crested Porcupine, 129-131

D

Dairy Cattle Welfare, 15-16, 20-21
Dairy Cows, 1-2, 6-9, 15-16, 22-23, 37, 40-41, 50, 121-122, 125-128, 189-190
Diabetic Rats, 52-57, 143

Diet Supplement, 52
Different Extenders, 10-11, 13-14

E

Enrofloxacin, 100-105

F

Fatty Acids, 46, 48, 57-65, 122, 125
Fertility, 2, 7-8, 10, 13, 126-127, 166, 177, 180
Fi N Damage, 66-68, 70-75
Fi Sh Welfare, 66, 75
Fluoroquinolones, 100, 103-104

G

Gas Chromatograph with a Flame-ionization De-tector (GC-FID), 59
Gastrointestinal Disease, 24, 26

H

Hematological Parameters, 121-122, 128, 158, 160-161
Hepatitis E Virus, 42, 44-45
Hepatozoon Canis, 153, 156
Histopathology, 82-83, 86, 116-119, 138, 140-141, 165
Hyperglycemia, 48, 52, 54
Hypodermosis, 133-137

I

Immunohistochemical Detection, 116-117
Immunohistochemistry, 82-87
Internal Control, 187, 189
Internal Myiasis, 133

K

Ketotic Holstein Cows, 37

L

Lactating Cows, 121-122, 125
Larval Stage, 133
Laying Hens, 77, 81
Leaf Extract, 106, 108-110, 112, 114, 143
Liver of Pigs, 42

M

Mammary Tumor, 116-117
Metabolic Profile, 46
Metalloenzyme, 88
Molecular Assays, 27
Molecular Characterization, 34, 93
Monogastric, 106-107, 111
Motility, 10-14, 166-171

N

Newcastle Disease (ND), 93
Non-ruminant Animals, 46
Nucleotide Sequencing, 93-95, 99

O

Oestridae, 133, 136
Oxidative Stress, 13, 52-53, 57-58, 144, 169

P

Pasteurella Multocida, 172-173, 175
Pigeon Paramyxovirus Type 1 (PPMV-1), 93-94
Pleuritis, 129, 131
Polymerase Chain Reaction, 35, 94, 187, 190
Porcine Circovirus Type 2, 82, 86
Post-weaning Multisystemic Wasting Syndrome, 82
Poultry Housing Systems, 77
Progesterone Eia Test, 1-2, 6-7
Pyloric Leiomyoma, 24-25

Q

Quill Injury, 129, 131

R

Rainbow Trout, 66-68, 72-75, 100, 102, 104
Real Time Pcr, 27-33
Reproduction, 1-2, 6-8, 10, 13-14, 21, 77, 116, 122, 126, 166, 170
Respiratory Disease, 82, 145-146, 148-150, 174-175
Ruminants, 28, 46, 50, 121, 125-126

S

Screening, 15, 17, 20-21, 105, 113, 144
Selected Indicators, 15-16, 19
Semen Freezing, 166
Seminal Plasma, 10, 13, 166-171
Septicaemia, 129
Shelter Dog, 24
Slaughterhouse, 42-45
Sperm Extenders, 10
Staphylococcus Aureus, 106, 131, 173, 187, 189-190
Storage Periods, 10

T

Transmissible Venereal Tumour, 153, 156-157
Tricuspid Regurgitation, 145-149

U

Undercooked Pork Meat, 42

W

Welfare Indicator, 66-67

www.ingramcontent.com/pod-product-compliance
Lightning Source LLC
Chambersburg PA
CBHW062002190326
41458CB00009B/2948